GU01080792

Biological Rhythms in Clinical Practice

Biological Rhythms in Clinical Practice

Edited by

J Arendt
Department of Biochemistry,
University of Surrey,
Guildford

D S Minors
Department of Physiological Sciences,
University of Manchester,
Manchester, UK

J M Waterhouse
Department of Physiological Sciences,
University of Manchester,
Manchester, UK

WRIGHT
London Boston Singapore Sydney Toronto Wellington

Wright
is an imprint of Butterworth Scientific

 PART OF REED INTERNATIONAL P.L.C.

First published 1989

© **Butterworth & Co. (Publishers) Ltd, 1989**

British Library Cataloguing in Publication Data

Biological rhythms in clinical practice.

1. Biological rhythms
I. Arendt, J. II. Minors, D. S. III. Waterhouse,
John M. (John Malcolm), *1932–*
612'.022

ISBN 0–7236–0961–6

Library of Congress Cataloging-in-Publication Data

Biological rhythms in clinical practice / edited by
    J. Arendt, D.S. Minors, J.M. Waterhouse.
        p. cm.
    Includes bibliographies and index.
    ISBN 0–7236–0961–6
    1. Clinical chronobiology. I. Arendt, J. II. Minors,
D.S. III. Waterhouse, J. M. (James M.)
    [DNLM: 1. Biological Clocks. 2. Circadian Rhythm.
QT 167 B61525]
    RB148.B56   1989
    612'.022—dc20
    DNLM/DLC
    for Library of Congress   89–15897
                                                         CIP

Photoset by Scribe Design, Gillingham, Kent
Printed and bound by Hartnolls Ltd, Bodmin, Cornwall

Preface

Periodicity is inherent in human behaviour, physiology and pathology. Although universal experience tells us that this is so, the concept of time-related variations in medicine has been greatly neglected. The last few years have, however, seen an explosion of interest in the study of biological rhythms and the application of this knowledge to medical problems. The importance of time factors in the diagnosis and treatment of disease and in the understanding of the disease process is now recognized.

The manipulation of some rhythmic processes to optimize response to treatment or simply to improve well-being in large populations such as shift-workers, once a remote possibility, now appears feasible in the near future.

With these important developments and the recent establishment of chronobiology as a science in its own right we felt that a volume on medical chronobiology would be both timely and useful.

We have attempted to cover all those areas of chronobiology of practical interest to the clinician and of interest to those studying medicine, physiology, pharmacology and biochemistry. An exception is the subject of sleep, an area where we felt that sufficient material already exists.

If we have succeeded in our objectives it is entirely due to the unstinting efforts of our contributors, all international experts in their field. They have provided in-depth, up to the minute coverage of their subjects. We were fortunate, indeed, to gather together such a group of people. We hereby express to them our most grateful thanks.

J. Arendt
D. S. Minors
J. M. Waterhouse

Contributors

G. Wynne Aherne
Department of Biochemistry, University of Surrey, Guildford, Surrey, UK

J. Arendt
Department of Biochemistry, University of Surrey, Guildford, Surrey, UK

Peter J. Barnes
Department of Thoracic Medicine, National Heart and Lung Institute, London, UK

Chantal Canon
Fondation Adolphe de Rothschild, 75940 Paris, France

Stuart Checkley
Institute of Psychiatry, Maudsley Hospital, Denmark Hill, London, UK

W.J.M. Hrushesky
Department of Medicine and Microbiology/Immunobiology, Albany Medical College of Union University, Albany, NY, USA

M. G. Koopman
Department of Nephrology, Academic Medical Centre, Amsterdam, The Netherlands

Peter Leathwood
Nestec Ltd, Nestlé Research Centre, Vers-chez-les-Blanc, 1000 Lausanne 26, Switzerland

Björn Lemmer
Johann Wolfgang Goethe-Universität, Zentrum der Pharmakologie, Frankfurt am Main, FRG

Francis Lévi
Fondation Adolphe de Rothschild, Paris, France

D.S. Minors
Department of Physiological Sciences, University of Manchester, Manchester, UK

Alain Reinberg
Fondation Adolphe de Rothschild, Paris, France

R.v. Roemeling
Division of Medical Oncology, Albany Medical College of Union University, Albany, NY, USA

M.H. Smolensky
University of Texas School of Public Health, Health Sciences Center, Houston, TX, USA

R.B. Sothern
Department of Medicine, University of Minnesota, Minneapolis, MN, USA

Eve Van Cauter
Department of Medicine, The University of Chicago, Chicago, IL, USA and Institute of Interdisciplinary Research, Université Libre de Bruxelles, Belgium

J. M. Waterhouse
Department of Physiological Sciences, University of Manchester, Manchester, UK

Contents

Part 1

Biological rhythms in principle

Chapter 1

Basic concepts and implications

J. Arendt, D.S. Minors and J. M. Waterhouse

The subject of our book is rhythms – the regular repetition of some process – that will be of interest to the clinician. For the most part, we have restricted ourselves by concentrating on circadian rhythms, those with a cycle length (period) of about 24 h. However, we do make some forays into other fields such as circannual (seasonal) rhythms (Chapter 7) and ultradian (short period) rhythms when the pulsatile release of hormones is measured (Chapter 3).

What are circadian rhythms?

A study of circadian rhythms requires as frequent and regular sampling over the 24 h as possible (see Chapter 14). In return, this imposes certain restrictions upon the sampling methods that are acceptable, an issue to which we will return.

However, having agreed that means exist for the frequent and unobtrusive sampling of a physiological or biochemical variable, it is then necessary to establish what kind of rhythmicity exists under normal circumstances. Such measurements indicate that most physiological and biochemical variables are not constant over the 24 h but rather show a rhythmic change. In most cases, lowest values are found nocturnally, though most hormones are an exception to this, with highest values being found then (Chapters 3 and 10).

Intuitively this might be expected on the grounds that we are mobile, eat, drink and live in a socially active and alerting environment in the daytime, in contrast to our inactivity and fasting and the quiet environment at night. If this argument were correct then the rhythms would not be observed in individuals living in an environment from which all rhythmic factors had been removed. Such an environment has been achieved experimentally in a protocol described as a Constant Routine. In this, volunteers are required to stay awake continuously for 24 h in an environment of constant light, temperature, noise, etc.; they are also required to eat an identical snack each hour so that total intake over the 24 h is normal. In such conditions body rhythms persist, even if with slightly diminished amplitude. It is argued that the rhythmicity that persists in these circumstances must originate from inside the body – it is called the endogenous component – and is attributed to some form of body clock. In the following sections we will give a brief outline of the mechanisms controlling circadian rhythms and the properties of the internal clock; the interested reader is referred to several reviews and books [1–4].

The endogenous component and zeitgebers (time-givers)

The properties of the internal clock have been investigated by placing individuals in time-free environments such as the Arctic during the summer, in underground caves and in specially constructed isolation units. In such circumstances the individual's times of retiring, rising and eating will no longer be dictated by the external world but rather by the internal clock. These experiments have established that the rhythms continue, generally with remarkably little day-to-day variation, but with a period closer to 25 than 24 h. For this reason such rhythms are described as circadian, from the latin *circa* – about and *dies* – a day.

In our normal environment such circadian rhythms are synchronized to a period of 24 h by external rhythmic changes known as zeitgebers. The nature of these zeitgebers depends upon the living organisms under consideration. For example, in many animals and plants it is the alternation of light and dark that adjusts the internal clock each day, and in predatory animals it is the rhythmic availability or absence of food. For humans living in society and able to make use of artificial lighting and preserved food, the situation is evidently rather different. The structure imposed upon them by society as a whole is likely to play a major role. There are only certain times of the day when it is acceptable or socially convenient to sleep, go shopping, make a noise, expect eating facilities etc. Even if we could be independent with regard to lighting and food, we still have to go to bed at the 'normal' time in order to have enough sleep before getting up for work, etc. the next day. Nevertheless, access to bright light, for example sunlight, has powerful synchronizing effects on some human rhythms (see Chapter 10).

The exogenous component

The external environment not only adjusts the internal clock but also exerts a direct effect upon the rhythms measured under normal circumstances. Thus the rhythm of deep body temperature in individuals living in the normal rhythmic environment demonstrates a higher daytime value than when the individuals are studied again under Constant Routine conditions; by contrast, when a subject is allowed to sleep, values are lower than during the comparable hours of a Constant Routine. These direct effects of the external environment and our sleep/waking cycle are termed exogenous (in contrast to the endogenous clock) and the normal overt circadian rhythms are considered to result from the sum of endogenous and exogenous components, the relative sizes of which are a characteristic of each variable. Moreover these two components are normally in phase with each other, for example, both raising body temperature during the daytime and lowering it in the night.

Advantages and disadvantages of a circadian system

The advantage of possessing a circadian clock is that it enables the individual to adjust better to a rhythmic world. Thus, a circadian system enables the body to prepare for waking – by increasing blood pressure, plasma adrenaline and body temperature towards the end of the sleep period – and to prepare for sleep – by enabling us to 'tone down' in the evening.

At first, such a system would appear to be in opposition to one of the central tenets of physiology – homoeostasis. In fact, this is not true. Homoeostatic mechanisms are still of the greatest importance; they are means by which the body can respond to all the multifarious changes that are part of being a living organism in a hostile environment. However, superimposed upon such a system is the ability to predict rhythmic changes in the environment. This ability seems to be brought about by circadian changes in the set-point of the homoeostatic mechanisms. Moore-Ede [5] has drawn attention to these differences by distinguishing reactive homoeostasis (the conventional type) from predictive homoeostasis (that causing the endogenous component of a circadian rhythm).

There are, however, disadvantages inherent in endogenous 'clocks'. These arise essentially since cultural and technological evolution have outstripped biological evolution. For example, both rapid time-zone change, following a long-distance flight, and night work lead to conflict between the new external time cues and the internal clock whose various endogenous rhythms adapt relatively slowly to the enforced phase shift. Presumably adaptation could be instantaneous if our rhythmic physiology depended entirely upon exogenous control.

Recent work has been directed towards facilitating this adaptive process (Chapters 10, 11 and 13).

Implications of circadian rhythms to medicine

Accepting that circadian rhythms are a normal part of health, we should not only make use of this fact in the diagnosis and treatment of disease but also expect that disorders of the circadian timing system itself might play a role in some diseases or occupational health problems.

Abnormalities of the circadian system

Individuals who by choice – social 'loners' – or by misfortune – the blind and in some cases the aged – are exposed less than normal to zeitgebers are likely to show irregularity of circadian rhythms. Indeed, in extreme cases, free-running rhythms with a period of 25 h might be expected (see Chapter 10).

In some cases, the ability of normal zeitgebers to adjust the circadian system to an exact 24 h will be less than normal. In these circumstances, regular sleeping habits are lost – particularly after changes in the sleep/waking cycle, say after a weekend – and insomnia develops.

Finally, as described in Chapter 9, there is some evidence that the relative timing of different rhythms can be upset in some forms of depression.

The use of chronobiology in diagnosis

As has been stressed by Halberg [6], the knowledge that variables show circadian rhythmicity in health implies that normal values must be expressed not only with any correction necessary for age, weight and sex of the patient but also with respect to the *time* of diagnosis. (See Part 2 for the application of this concept to the major physiological systems: a discussion of the self-monitoring of different variables – 'autorhythmometry' – at various times of day is to be found, in Chapter 13.) Such a concept is particularly important when the amplitude of a circadian rhythm is marked, as with many hormones, for example (Chapter 3).

Important endocrine challenge tests, both of suppression and stimulation of certain hormones, give very different responses at different times of day. In addition to the normal daily variation, it is important to bear in mind that shift workers and time-zone travellers may well be in an abnormal phase of their normal rhythm at the time of diagnosis.

It is well known that circadian rhythms alter in some disease states; some, for example airway resistance (Chapter 5), increase in amplitude; some become more irregular in their timing; some, in the case of renal rhythms in oedematous conditions, even become inverted (Chapter 6); and some become ultradian at the expense of their normal circadian rhythmicity.

In other circumstances, markers of a particular disease state (arthritic pain; allergy, Chapter 7; and plasma-borne tumour markers, Chapter 12, for example) show rhythmicity. In addition, a knowledge of circadian rhythms can help us understand the aetiology of disease. This is clear when the cases of the nocturnal exacerbation of the dyspnoea of asthma (Chapter 5) and the circadian peak in the frequency of onset of cardiac infarction (Chapter 4) are considered.

The element of time in treatment

To some extent, the timing of treatment follows from a knowledge that symptoms show circadian rhythmicity; treatment is needed most when symptoms are worst. This is an obvious point, but the position is not so straightforward if the drug takes some time to reach its site of action, for example the synovial fluid, or if there are certain 'critical' times of the day when control is particularly important (reducing the early morning rise in blood pressure in hypertensives; Chapter 4).

There is also the recent evidence that indicates that the uptake, metabolism and elimination of a drug, together with its therapeutic and toxic effects can all show circadian changes. An introduction to chronopharmacology is to be found in Chapter 2 and recent developments using chronopharmacological concepts are to be found in Chapter 12. There are two major areas where these chronopharmacological considerations are important. First, with chronic medication the correct timing of a drug might reduce the amount that is required to be effective; this might have economic benefits as well as reduce the chance of long-term side effects. Second, particularly in cancer chemotherapy (Chapter 12), the limitations to treatment are generally the toxic effects upon the patient; a suitable timing here can increase the amount of drug or number of treatments that can be given, so improving patient outcome.

Measuring circadian rhythms

The assessment of circadian rhythms has benefitted greatly from recent developments that have permitted more frequent measurements to be made. Some of the requirements for this are:

1. The method involves the automatic recording and storage of data while the subject or patient is living a normal lifestyle.
2. The measurement is non-invasive.
3. If a sample of plasma is required then the smaller its volume, the better.
4. Non-invasive alternatives to plasma sampling are found.

The electronic and biochemical advances of recent years have enabled such desirable changes to take place. For example:

1. It is now routine to record and store large amounts of temperature, electroencephalographic and performance data – obtained under 'field' conditions – on either magnetic tape or microchips.
2. Blood pressure can be reliably measured by automatic inflation of a sphygmomanometric cuff; cardiac output can be measured by the use of ultrasound together with the principle of the Doppler shift.
3. The volume of blood or plasma required for analysis of ions has decreased with the development of microanalytical flame photometers, etc. The field of endocrinological rhythms received a considerable boost with the development of radioimmunoassay techniques; as a result, specific assays of a large number of hormones can now be performed upon small volumes of plasma. Accordingly, multiple-sampling techniques become more acceptable.
4. Alternative fluids to blood have been used; the most common are urine and saliva. Often the concentration of substance that is being investigated is very low in such transcellular fluids; again, the development of high-sensitivity methods of analysis has enabled this not to be a limiting factor.

During the course of this book many more examples of the advantages to be gained from such developments will be found. Chronobiology is a new field and yet begins to make exciting contributions to clinical studies and practice; this promise should develop, so that *time* takes its rightful place in the processes of diagnosis and treatment.

References

1. Wever R. *The Circadian System of Man*, Springer-Verlag, new York (1979)
2. Minors, D.S. and Waterhouse, J.M. *Circadian Rhythms and the Human*, John Wright, Bristol (1981)
3. Moore-Ede, M.C., Sulzman, F.M. and Fuller, C.A. *The Clocks that Time Us*. Harvard, Cambridge, MA (1982)
4. Aschoff, J. Circadian timing. *Ann. N.Y. Acad. Sci.*, **423**, 442–468 (1984)
5. Moore-Ede, M.C. Physiology of the circadian timing system: predictive versus reactive homeostasis. *Amer. J. Physiol.*, **250**, R737–R752 (1986)
6. Halberg, F., Halberg, J., Halberg, F. and Halberg, E. Reading, 'riting, 'rithmetic – and rhythms: a new 'relevant' 'R' in the educative process. *Persp. Biol. Med.*, **17**, 128–141 (1973)

Chapter 2

An introduction to chronopharmacology

G. Wynne Aherne

Introduction

Throughout the ages, chemicals and biological compounds have been used to treat illnesses and diseases with varying degrees of success. The use of drugs is not without considerable cost, both in financial and clinical terms. Besides the vast financial burden of providing effective drug treatments, iatrogenic disease, caused by the misuse of therapeutic agents, is a common occurrence.

Most drugs exert their effects by interfering in some way with normal physiological and biochemical processes. Therefore, no matter how safe a drug is considered to be there is a risk that toxic side effects will occur. These may be severe, for example in the case of antineoplastic agents. Toxic effects can be dose dependent and predictable. Others are unpredictable, occur in individual patients and are not necessarily dose dependent.

Where appropriate it has been common practice to adjust the dose of a drug given to individual patients using a pharmacological end point. This practice continues to be acceptable for drugs such as anticoagulants, digoxin, antihypertensives, insulin and glucose where easily measured end points are apparent. In anticancer therapy, dosage is often reduced or delayed in the face of life-threatening toxicity in the form of severe myelosuppression and renal or hepatic impairment.

In some cases it is not appropriate to titrate drug dosage against effect. This is the case for phenytoin and other antiepileptic agents where seizures occur with variable frequency. However, it is now recognized that a measure of drug concentration or distribution within the body is more closely related to effectiveness and toxicity than the dose itself.

Pharmacology is concerned with the effectiveness of drugs in man and can be divided into pharmacodynamics (what the drug does to the body) and pharmacokinetics (what the body does to the drug). Whilst pharmacodynamic studies have been carried out for many years, it is only relatively recently that pharmacokinetic studies were made possible with the advent of specific sensitive analytical techniques for the measurement of drugs in biological fluids. It is now evident that for many classes of drugs there is a closer correlation of therapeutic effect and/or toxicity with plasma concentration (or some other pharmacokinetic parameter) than with the dose of drug itself. Indeed, for a small but clinically important number of drugs, therapeutic drug monitoring has been successfully used to ensure that the plasma concentration of a drug in an individual subject lies within a particular therapeutic window.

Whilst it is now recognized that an individual's response to a drug can be markedly affected by idiosyncratic variations in absorption, metabolism and elimination, other factors, e.g. type and timing of meals, diet, posture and concomitant drug therapy, are also known to alter pharmacokinetics and hence drug effect. Until the last few years, little work has been carried out on the effect of time of drug administration on therapeutic outcome. This is in spite of the fact that biological rhythms have been recorded and investigated for many years. This chapter aims to define the principles of chronopharmacology and to show how increased therapeutic success may be possible by taking into account the time of day of drug administration.

Chronopharmacology

Historical aspects

The term chronopharmacology – the study of time-dependent variations in pharmacology – was first coined in the 1960s although chronopharmacological examples had been described many years earlier. For example, Agren and coworkers [1] showed that mice, used to assay insulin for therapeutic use, were more susceptible to insulin-induced convulsions if the hormone was given in the morning rather than the evening. In 1960, Halberg [2] showed that a dose of endotoxin killed 95% of mice when it was given in the early afternoon but only 10% if given at midnight. This study illustrates the quite remarkable effects that the time of day can have on the pharmacology of administered compounds. Many other examples of chronopharmacological effects are now available in the literature indicating a rapid recent growth of interest in the subject. In 1982, the circadian variations in drug disposition of over 20 drugs were reviewed [3]. Since this time the publication of the proceedings of several international symposia and congresses and the rapid increase in the number of published papers reflect the growing interest in, and impact of, chronopharmacology.

Definitions

Several aspects of chronopharmacology have been studied in both experimental and clinical settings: (a) the pharmacology of a drug as a function of administration time and how these effects can be modulated; (b) the effect of drugs on endogenous biological rhythms; (c) modification of the timing of dose schedules to improve the therapeutic index of the compound.

Three terms have been defined (Figure 2.1) which describe interdependent aspects of chronopharmacology [4]: the *chronopharmacokinetics* of a drug, the *chronesthesy* of the target organs or cells and the *chronergy* or overall effects.

Chronopharmacokinetics refer to the rhythmic variations in the mathematical parameters that describe the absorption, distribution and elimination of an administered compound. There are now numerous examples in the scientific literature of chronopharmacokinetic differences observed in both animals and man. Figures 2.2 and 2.3 illustrate the type and magnitude of the time-dependent variations observed. A threefold variation in disappearance half-life occurred in groups of six rats dosed at four time points with 1 mg/kg (i.v.) cytosine arabinoside, an effective anticancer drug. Maximum half-life (54 ± 3 min) occurred at 06:00 h

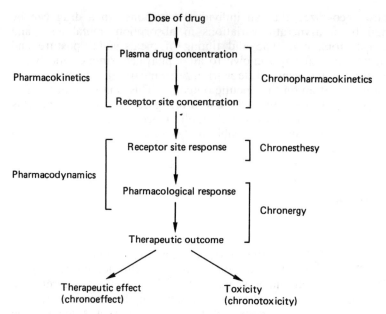

Figure 2.1 Pharmacology and chronopharmacology

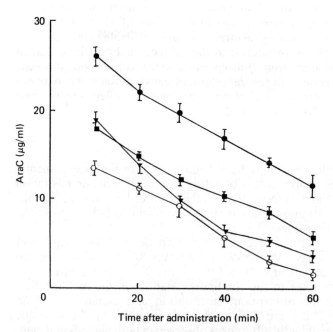

Figure 2.2 The chronopharmacokinetics of cytosine arabinoside. Serum cytosine arabinoside (AraC) was measured in rats ($n=6$) following intravenous injection of AraC (1 mg/kg) given at 06:00 (●), 12:00 (■), 18:00 (▼) and 24:00 h (○) (L:D 12:12, lights on 06:30 h). $t_{\frac{1}{2}} = 54 \pm 3, 33 \pm 1, 37 \pm 2, 16 \pm 1$ min and AUC (area under curve) = $17 \pm 2, 8 \pm 1, 11 \pm 1, 9 \pm 1$ μg/ml per h at these times respectively. Results are given ± S.E.M.

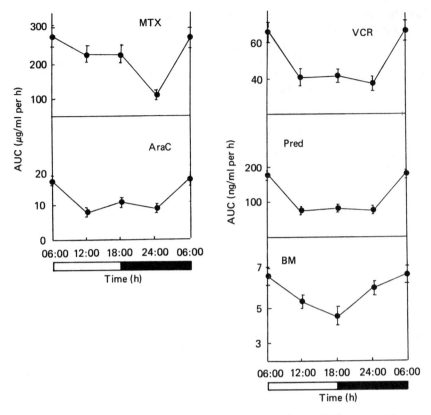

Figure 2.3 Circadian variations in AUC of some anticancer drugs. AUC measured in groups of rats (*n*=6) for five drugs used in cancer chemotherapy. Drugs were administered intravenously at 06:00, 12:00, 18:00 and 24:00 h (L:D 12:12) at the following doses: bleomycin (BM), 0.5 mg/kg; vincristine (VCR), 0.1 mg/kg; cytosine arabinoside (AraC), 1 mg/kg; methotrexate (MTX), 2 mg/kg; prednisolone (Pred), 1 mg/kg.

and minimum half-life at 24:00 h (16 ± 1 min) with corresponding variations in the area under the curve (AUC), 9 ± 1 μg/ml per h and 17 ± 2 μg/ml per h respectively. Similar variations in pharmacokinetics have been observed for other anticancer agents (Figure 2.3). Interestingly, in the rat, all these drugs showed maximum plasma exposure dosing at 06:00 h. For statistically significant chronopharmacokinetic effects to be seen, at least four time points throughout a 24-h period should be studied under standardized conditions. As with all pharmacokinetic studies, sufficient sampling time points for proper evaluation of parameters, e.g. half-life ($t_{1/2}$), AUC, time to peak concentration, etc. should be used. Studies that use only two administration time points can be criticized because they are unlikely to indicate the true rhythm and may be misleading if no difference in pharmacology between the two times is observed (see Chapter 14).

Chronesthesy is defined as the rhythmic changes in biological susceptibility and may include changes in the quantity or quality of receptors, cell permeability or metabolic processes within the cell, e.g. DNA synthesis. Such changes as these mean that at some times of the day a biological system may be completely unresponsive to a dose of drug or given drug concentration that at other times may be highly effective.

Rhythmic changes in the pharmacodynamics of a compound have been defined as chronergy and are manifested by changes in the desired therapeutic response as well as changes in the severity of side effects or toxicity of the drug. Chronergy is determined by both the chronesthesy and chronopharmacokinetics of the administered compound.

Relationship between changes in pharmacokinetics and therapeutic outcome

For some drugs, e.g. cisplatin [5], it has been possible to relate rhythmic changes in pharmacokinetics directly to rhythmic changes in therapeutic response and/or

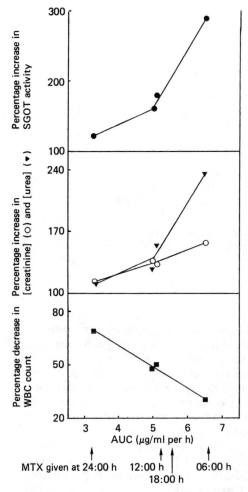

Figure 2.4 The relationship between circadian variations in pharmacokinetics and toxicity of methotrexate. The percentage change in peripheral white blood cells (WBC), urea and creatinine concentration and SGOT activity following a 200 mg/kg i.v. dose at 06:00, 12:00, 18:00 and 24:00 h to groups of six rats related to AUC μg/ml per h of a 2 mg/kg i.v. dose of drug. SGOT, serum glutamic oxaloacetic transaminase; MTX, methotrexate. The rats were kept in 12:12 L:D; lights on at 06.30 h

toxicity in man. It is difficult to carry out properly controlled experiments in human subjects since differences caused by endogenous rhythms due to genuine biological clocks are difficult to distinguish from the response of the body to a wide variety of environmental factors. Such environmental factors can be much more carefully controlled in animal experiments. In this laboratory it has been possible to relate directly changes in the pharmacokinetics of the antifolate drug, methotrexate, with changes in toxicity measured by the fall in peripheral white cell count (WBC) as well as by measures of liver (serum glutamic oxaloacetic transaminase (SGOT)) and kidney toxicity (serum creatinine and urea).

Groups of rats ($n=6$) were dosed at four different time points with methotrexate (200 mg/kg i.v.). A well-marked time-related variation in the severity of toxicity was observed (Figure 2.4). Maximum toxicity occurred after administration at 06:00 h. (The animals were housed on a lighting schedule of 06:30–18:30 h light, 18:30–06:30 h dark.) Minimum toxicity was observed when the drug was given at midnight. The severity of the observed toxic reactions bore a direct relationship to the pharmacokinetic parameters of methotrexate (2 mg/kg i.v.) [6].

The results depicted in Figure 2.4 also suggest that a rhythm in some parameters of toxicity may only become apparent above a certain dose (or drug concentration) indicating that chronopharmacology experiments may need to be repeated at different dose levels. Also, for some drugs, chronic rather than acute dosing may be required before a chronopharmacological difference is observed.

In our laboratory, the chronopharmacology of another anticancer drug, 6-mercaptopurine, has been studied. In this case it was not possible to demonstrate a direct relationship between changes in pharmacokinetics and effect. Groups of rats ($n=6$) were dosed at four different time points with 6-mercaptopurine (37.1 mg/kg i.p.). The AUC over 2.5 h was significantly lower following administration at 18:00 h than following drug administration at 06:00, 12:00 or 24:00 h (Figure 2.5). However, at none of the dosing times was it possible to measure or detect

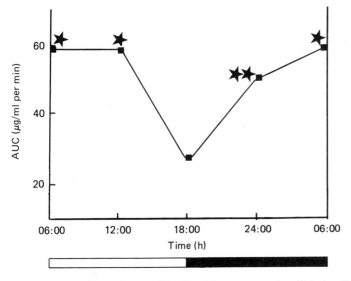

Figure 2.5 The chronopharmacokinetics of 6-mercaptopurine. Rats ($n=6$) were dosed at 06:00, 12:00, 18:00 and 24:00 h with 37.1 mg/kg i.p. (12:12 L:D, lights on at 06:00 h) and plasma drug concentrations were measured over 2.5 h. $^*P<0.02$, $^{**}P<0.05$ compared to 18:00 h time point (paired Student's t test)

any toxicity as measured by myelosuppression or changes in hepatic or renal function. Whether this is due to the use of a dose of 6-mercaptopurine that was too low remains to be determined, but the mode of action of 6-mercaptopurine requires that intracellular active drug metabolites are formed. The amount of these metabolites formed after one single dose of drug may not be sufficient for toxicity to become apparent. Chronopharmacokinetic effects, however, may be important determinants for successful 6-mercaptopurine therapy. In one clinical study [7], in children with acute lymphoblastic leukaemia, night-time administration of 6-mercaptopurine resulted in greater drug exposure than morning administration. These results may partly explain the results of a retrospective study [8] in which children with acute lymphoblastic leukaemia who had had their maintenance dose of 6-mercaptopurine and methotrexate in the evening had a lower risk of disease relapse than children receiving their medication in the morning.

For some drugs, the peak of therapeutic response (chronergy) need not coincide with the peak of blood/plasma concentrations. This has been shown for ethanol [9] and theophylline [10]. We illustrated this experimentally during a study of the chronopharmacology of morphine in mice. Mice were injected with morphine i.p. (10 mg/kg), at four time points (06:00, 12:00, 18:00 and 24:00 h), and 30 min later the analgesic response was measured by the foot-licking response using a hot plate set at 55°C. Immediately afterwards the animals were sacrificed and blood was obtained for plasma morphine determination by radioimmunoassay. Greatest morphine plasma concentrations at 35 min post dose were measured in samples obtained following drug administration at 06:00 h. However, greatest analgesic effect at 30 min (latency of response measured in seconds) was obtained in animals dosed at 12:00 h. Thus circadian variations in both the pharmacokinetics and pharmacology of morphine were demonstrated although the peak responses of each did not occur following the same time of administration. The important pharmacokinetic determinant for morphine, a centrally acting drug, is presumably the drug concentration at the opiate receptors. Further experimentation may show that the maximum drug concentrations in the central nervous system at 30 min occurred at 12:00 h, the time of maximum analgesia.

Factors that determine circadian variations in pharmacology

Significant circadian variations in the pharmacokinetics and pharmacodynamics of several classes of drug have now been documented and it is clear that elimination and metabolic processes are not equally effective over 24 h. It should not be assumed therefore that a particular dose of drug will be equally effective throughout the day. The magnitude of the circadian differences in drug handling will not be the same for all drugs (or each dose of drug) and is determined by the amplitude of the circadian variation of the main mode of elimination, e.g. liver metabolism, renal excretion etc., for that drug.

Several factors and processes involved in pharmacology (Figure 2.6) are susceptible to temporal variations and the variation observed in the overall outcome of drug therapy will depend on how these factors interact with each other throughout the day. The concentration of drug in plasma is determined by factors such as drug absorption, metabolism and excretion, and transport of drug into cells. Similarly, pharmacodynamic aspects of a drug will also be determined by circadian rhythms within an organ or cell.

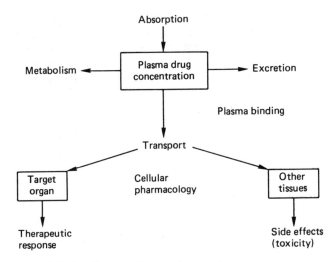

Figure 2.6 Circadian variations in pharmacology

The absorption of drugs from the gastrointestinal tract is affected by a number of variables which are responsible for the wide range of blood concentrations often documented following oral doses of drug. The importance of various foods and fluids, pH, gastric emptying and concomitant therapy are all well-known factors that can affect drug absorption. The absorption of several drugs has also been shown to be affected by time of day of administration. These include indomethacin [11], amitriptyline [12], diazepam [13] and prednisolone [14]. Circadian variations in drug absorption could be caused by circadian variations in a number of gastrointestinal functions, e.g. pH changes, motility, bile salt concentration all of which have been shown to exhibit temporal changes [15].

Hepatic metabolism is a major route of elimination for a wide range of xenobiotics. There are numerous examples in the literature of circadian rhythms in the activity of hepatic enzymes. In one study [16] two hepatic drug-metabolizing enzymes, O-demethylase and hexobarbital oxidase, were shown to have marked diurnal variations in activity. The maximum activity for both enzymes ocurred during the dark period (02:00 and 22:00 h respectively) and the hexobarbital oxidase activity rhythm correlated with hexobarbital sleep time – shortest sleep time occurring at the same time as greatest enzyme-metabolizing activity. The rhythm in enzyme activity could be abolished by continuous exposure to light or darkness indicating that the rhythm was partly exogenous.

In a later paper from another group [17], diurnal rhythms were observed in a number of aspects of hepatic microsomal drug metabolism in the golden hamster. Maximum enzymic activity occurred around the onset of the light phase (04:00–08:00 h) with minimum activity occurring between 16:00 and 18:00 h. The changes in enzyme activity observed were not only due to changes in the amount of enzyme present but were thought to be due to changes in the ability of the enzymes to interact with substrates, e.g. changes in active enzyme centres or substrate binding sites. Significant circadian variations in the activity of the cytochrome P-450 system [18] and in dihydropyrimidine dehydrogenase [19] have been reported.

Glutathione plays an important role in the detoxification of xenobiotics. Concentrations of glutathione display significant circadian fluctuations in several tissues especially the liver [20]. Lipid peroxidation, which is inhibited by glutathione, also varied in a circadian fashion, maximum peroxidation occurring at times of minimum glutathione concentrations. The diurnal rhythm in glutathione concentration may not be entirely caused by endogenous factors since intake of food leads to increased synthesis of glutathione.

For many drugs and their metabolites, renal excretion plays an important role in their elimination from the body. Thus any significant circadian variations in renal mechanisms will cause variations in pharmacological parameters of those drugs primarily eliminated by the kidney. The renal elimination of a compound from the plasma is determined by both the rate of filtration from the bloodstream and by any subsequent reabsorption of the drug in the tubules. Glomerular filtration rate displays a circadian rhythm, being lowest nocturnally (Chapter 6), and whatever the cause of the rhythm, water-soluble drugs will be removed from plasma at a higher rate during the day. Evidence for circadian variations in renal secretory and absorption mechanisms is scarce. However, the well-known circadian rhythm in urinary pH – the 'alkaline tide' [21,22] – will markedly affect the elimination of some drugs, e.g. amphetamine. Other aspects of renal function, for example the excretion of water and electrolytes and the clearance of urea and creatinine from the blood, are highly rhythmic in both animals and man. Circadian variations in renal mechanisms of drug elimination have recently been reviewed [23]. The available evidence suggests that circadian rhythms in drug elimination exist but the extent to which these rhythms are governed by endogenous or exogenous factors remains to be determined. For further discussion see Chapter 6. It is apparent that drugs that are primarily excreted by the kidney, e.g. aminoglycosides, show marked circadian variations in their pharmacokinetics and toxicity. Renal circadian rhythms are important factors to be taken into account in the administration of severely nephrotoxic drugs such as methotrexate and cisplatin.

The extent to which drugs are bound by plasma proteins to some extent determines pharmacodynamic effects since effective blood concentrations and the availability of drug at the end organ receptor are altered. Plasma protein concentrations display a significant circadian rhythm [24,25] reflected in circadian rhythms of plasma binding of, for example, cisplatin [26] and prednisolone [14] in man.

The chronesthesy of drugs may also be determined by variations of transport into cells [27] as well as by variations in target cell susceptibility, e.g. number and/ or quality of receptors, membrane function etc. In cancer chemotherapy, circadian variations in DNA synthesis of both normal and neoplastic cells [28] are important determinants of therapeutic outcome. Optimization of cancer chemotherapy by chronopharmacological principles must ultimately take into account circadian differences in cell proliferation of normal versus neoplastic tissues.

Chronopharmacology in health and disease

Much of our knowledge of chronopharmacokinetics and chronopharmacology in general has been obtained in animal studies or in groups of healthy volunteers or relatively healthy patients. The effects of extremes of age – the newborn and aged – of pregnancy and lactation, of poor nutrition and of polypharmacy on drug metabolism and elimination have been little studied even at single time points. It is conceivable that circadian rhythms in mechanisms of drug disposition may be altered in these groups. For example, circadian rhythms take some time to be established in the newborn, and in old age circadian rhythmicity tends to deteriorate [29]. Likewise, drug disposition in shift workers and after rapid transit across time zones (see Chapter 11) has been virtually unexplored. The implications of circadian rhythms on drug disposition in healthy individuals of all ages and in those undergoing stress, illness or changed lifestyle remain to be investigated.

Conclusions and clinical implications

Chronopharmacology has until recently been a subject of interest to a few dedicated scientists and their clinical colleagues. Its relevance to clinical practice except in a few instances has been largely ignored. One of the first applications of chronopharmacology to clinical medicine was in the timing of steroid therapy to decrease its toxicity and at the same time to increase its efficacy. It was suggested in 1958 [30] that adrenocortical suppression by exogenous steroids could be reduced by administering the drugs in the morning rather than at night or in divided doses. Clinical practice has since shown the benefit of appropriately timed steroid therapy in such diseases as adrenogenital virilism [31]. There can be no doubt now that circadian variations in both the pharmacokinetics and pharmacodynamics of drugs can have a profound clinical effect. This has been most clearly demonstrated in the treatment of malignancy. Anticancer agents are a group of drugs for which the therapeutic index is very narrow and for which any amelioration of toxicity without a concomitant reduction in effectiveness is desirable. The chronotherapy of cancer is comprehensively covered in Chapter 12.

How can our increased knowledge and understanding of chronopharmacology be advantageously applied in clinical practice? Improvements in therapeutic outcome can be achieved by simply altering the time of day of administration. This has been illustrated by steroid therapy and by theophylline treatment of asthma (see Chapter 5). Programmable subcutaneous pumps that automatically deliver drugs according to a predetermined circadian rhythm would eliminate practical problems encountered with night-time administration. Such pumps are also useful for altering the rate of drug infusions (e.g. for anticancer drugs), according to predetermined rhythms of maximum drug tolerance and cell susceptibility (see Chapter 12).

Where optimum timing is clinically inconvenient it may be possible to manipulate or modulate circadian rhythms to improve the therapeutic index of drugs. In our laboratory we have shown [32] that the toxicity of methotrexate in the rat can be modulated by both exogenous corticosteroids and melatonin. In the rat, greatest toxicity following methotrexate administration occurred when the drug was given at 06:00 h. This time not only corresponded to the time of greatest drug exposure but also to the nadir in endogenous corticosterone. The effect of abolishing the normal diurnal rhythm of corticosterone was therefore investigated. In rats fed corticosterone in the diet for 10 days (average dose 250 μg/kg), high corticosterone concentrations were present throughout the 24 h and the toxicity of methotrexate was trivial even when it was administered at 06:00 h – the time normally associated with greatest toxicity and lethality. In contrast, in rats pretreated with dexamethasone (25 μg/kg) and in which corticosterone levels were suppressed throughout the day, methotrexate toxicity was so great that all animals died from toxic effects within 5 days regardless of the time of drug administration.

The circadian rhythm of melatonin production may also influence that of corticosterone: the nadir in plasma corticosterone in rats follows the dark-phase increase in melatonin secretion. The toxicity of methotrexate in the rat could also be modulated by dosing the animals at 15:30 h each day for 6 weeks with melatonin (80 μg/kg). In the melatonin-treated animals, toxicity was not only observed as expected following a dose of methotrexate at 06:00 h but also following the same dose of methotrexate at 24:00 h (100% mortality) and at 18:00 h (33% mortality).

These experiments illustrate that it may be possible to modulate the circadian rhythms in pharmacology in clinical practice by the appropriately timed administration or inhibition of endogenous hormones. Modulation or elimination of the melatonin rhythm may also be possible by the use of appropriate bright lights.

There is increasing evidence that the appropriate timing of drug administration can improve therapeutic outcome and increase the therapeutic index of many drugs. Most of this evidence has been obtained in animal and laboratory experiments where standardized conditions can more easily be achieved. However, the recent success achieved in the clinical environment especially in the field of cancer chemotherapy is evidence that the application of chronopharmacology to drug treatment will be an important consideration of clinicians and pharmacologists in the next few years. Their task will be facilitated by a more complete understanding of the chronopharmacology of drugs. This will be achieved by continued investigation of the circadian variations of pharmacokinetics and pharmacodynamics and their interrelationships as well as by increased understanding of circadian variations in target tissues and those susceptible to toxicity.

Further understanding of the mechanisms governing and maintaining these circadian rhythms will also be required to maximize the improvement in drug use that is possible by applying the principles of chronotherapy.

References

1. Agren, G., Wilander, O. and Jones, E. Cyclic changes in the glycogen content of the liver and muscle of rats and mice. *Biochem. J.*, **25**, 777–785 (1931)
2. Halberg, F. Temporal co-ordination of physiologic functions. *Cold Spring Harbor Symp. Quant. Biol.*, **25**, 289–310 (1960)
3. Reinberg, A. and Smolensky, M.H. Circadian changes of drug disposition in man. *Clin. Pharmacokin.*, **7**, 401–420 (1982)
4. Reinberg, A. Advances in human chronopharmacology. *Chronobiologia*, **3**, 151–166 (1976)
5. Hrushesky, W.J.M., Borch, R. and Levi, F. Circadian time dependence of cisplatin urinary kinetics. *Clin. Pharmacol. Ther.*, **32**, 330–339 (1982)
6. English, J., Aherne, G.W. and Marks, V. The effect of timing of a single injection on the toxicity of methotrexate in the rat. *Cancer Chemother. Pharmacol.*, **9**, 114–117 (1982)
7. Langevin, A.M., Koren, G., Soldin, S.J. and Greenberg, M. Pharmacokinetics case for giving 6-mercaptopurine maintenance doses at night. *Lancet*, **ii**, 505–506 (1987)
8. Rivard, G.E., Hoyoux, C., Infante-Rivarde, C. and Champagne, J. Maintenance chemotherapy for childhood acute lymphoblastic leukaemia: Better in the evening. *Lancet*, **ii**, 1264–1265 (1985)
9. Reinberg, A., Uench, J., Aymard, N. *et al.* Variations circadiennes des effets de l'ethanol et de l'ethanolemie chez l'homme adulte sain (etude chronopharmacologique). *J. Physiol. (Paris)*, **70**, 435–456 (1975)
10. Smolensky, M.H., Reinberg, A. and Queng, J.T. The chronobiology and chronopharmacology of allergy. *Ann. Allergy*, **47**, 234–252 (1981)
11. Clench, J., Reinberg, A., Dziewanowska, Z., Ghata, J. and Smolensky, M. Circadian changes in

the bioavailability and effects of indomethacin in healthy subjects. *Eur. J. Clin. Pharmacol.*, **20**, 359–369 (1981)

12. Nakano, S. and Hollister, L.E. Chronopharmacology of amitriptyline. *Clin. Pharmacol. Ther.*, **33**, 453–459 (1983)

13. Nakano, S., Watanabe, H., Nagai, K. and Ogawa, N. Circadian stage-dependent changes in diazepam kinetics. *Clin. Pharmacol. Ther.*, **36**, 271–277

14. English, J., Dunne, M. and Marks, V. Diurnal variation in prednisolone kinetics. *Clin. Pharmacol. Ther.* **33**, 381–385 (1983)

15. Vener, K. Chronobiological properties of the digestive system affecting xenobiotic absorption. *Annu. Rev. Chronopharmacol..*, **3**, 369–373 (1986)

16. Nair, V. and Casper, R. The influence of light on daily rhythm in hepatic drug metabolizing enzymes in rat. *Life Sci.*, **8**, 1291–8 (1969)

17. Lake, B.G., Tredger, J.M., Burke, M.D., Chakraborty, J. and Bridges, J.W. The circadian variation of hepatic microsomal drug and steroid metabolism in the golden hamster. *Chem.–Biol. Interact.*, **12**, 81–90 (1976)

18. Haen, E. and Golly, I. Circadian variation in the cytochrome *P*-450 system of rat liver. *Annu. Rev. Chronopharmacol.*, **3**, 357–361 (1986)

19. Harris, B.E., Song, R., Ite, Y. and Diasio, R.B. Circadian variation of dihydropyrimidine dehydrogenase activity in rat liver: possible relevance to fluoropyrimidine toxicity with implications for circadian shaping of FP infusion by programmable pumps. *Proc. Amer. Assoc. Cancer*, **29**, Abs. No. 27, p. 7 (1988)

20. Farooqi, N.Y.H. and Ahmed, A.E. Circadian periodicity of tissue glutathione and its relationship with lipid peroxidation in rats. *Life Sci.*, **34**, 2413–2418 (1984)

21. Brunton, C.E. The acid output of the kidney and so-called alkaline tide. *Physiol. Rev.*, **13**, 372–99 (1933)

22. Koopman, M.G., Krechet, R.T. and Arisz, L. Circadian rhythms and the kidney. *Methods J. Med.*, **28**, 416–423 (1985)

23. Waterhouse, J.M. and Minors, D.S. Temporal aspects in renal drug elimination. In *Chronopharmacology, Cellular and Biochemical Interactions* (ed. B. Lemmer), Marcel Dekker, New York, pp. 35–50 (1989)

24. Renbourn, E.T. Variation, diurnal and over longer periods of time, in blood hemoglobin, hematocrit, plasma protein, erythrocyte sedimentation rate and blood chloride. *J. Hyg.*, **45**, 455 (1947)

25. Angeli, A., Frajria, R., Depaoli, R., Fonzo, D. and Ceresa, F. Diurnal variation of prednisolone binding to serum corticosteroid binding globulin in man. *Clin. Pharmacol. Ther.*, **23**, 47–53 (1978)

26. Hecquet, B., Meynadier, J., Bonneterre, J., Adenis, L. and Demaille, A. Time dependency in plasmatic protein binding of cisplatin. *Cancer Treatment Rep.*, **69**, 79–83 (1985)

27. Leszczynska-Bisswanger, A. and Pfulf, E. Diurnal variation of methotrexate transport and accumulation in hepatocytes – a consequence of variations in cellular glutathione. *Biochem. Pharmacol.*, **34**, 1635–1638 (1985)

28. Burns, E.R. and Beland, S.S. Induction by 5-fluorouracil of a major phase difference in the circadian profiles of DNA synthesis between the Ehrlich Ascites Carcinoma and five normal organs. *Cancer Lett.*, **20**, 235–239 (1983)

29. Minors, D.S. and Waterhouse, J.M. *Circadian Rhythms and the Human*, John Wright, Bristol (1981)

30. Di Raimondo, U.C. and Forsham, P.H. Some clinical implications of the spontaneous diurnal variation in adrenal cortical secretory activity. *Amer. J. Med.*, **21**, 321–323 (1958)

31. Nicholas, C.T., Nugent, C.A. and Tyler, F. Diurnal variation in suppression of adrenal function by glucocorticoids. *J. Clin. Endocrinol. Metab.*, **25**, 343–349 (1965)

32. English, J., Aherne, G.W. and Marks, V. The effect of abolition of the endogenous corticosteroid rhythm on the circadian variation in methotrexate toxicity in the rat. *Cancer Chem. Pharmacol.*, **18**, 287–290 (1987)

Part 2

Biological rhythms in practice

Chapter 3

Endocrine rhythms

Eve Van Cauter

Introduction

A prominent feature of the endocrine system is its high degree of temporal
organization. Far from obeying the concept of 'constancy of the internal
environment', which was the dogma of early 20th century endocrinology,
circulating hormone levels spontaneously undergo pronounced oscillations. Typical
examples are shown in Figure 3.1. As is the case for the vast majority of hormones,
plasma levels of adrenocorticotropin (ACTH), growth hormone (GH) and
prolactin (PRL) follow a circadian pattern which repeats itself day after day. PRL
levels decrease rapidly after morning awakening, a time when ACTH release is
close to its maximum and GH secretion is generally quiescent. Both PRL and GH
increase rapidly after sleep onset, a time when ACTH levels are essentially
suppressed. Thus, the release of these three hormones by the pituitary follows a
highly coordinated temporal programme. Pulsatile secretion is evident throughout
the 24-h cycle for ACTH and PRL. In contrast, pulses of GH secretion occur less
frequently and are often confined to the early part of sleep. In addition to the
circadian and pulsatile variations exemplified in Figure 3.1, temporal oscillations
with periods in the range of minutes, as well as with periods in the range of months,
are also present in the endocrine system.

Endocrine rhythms may be classified according to the frequency range of the
oscillation. Presumably because of its ubiquity in living systems, the circadian
periodicity has been used to subdivide the spectrum of biological rhythms in two
ranges: the ultradian range which includes rhythms with periods shorter than 24 h
and the infradian range which includes rhythms with periods longer than 24 h [1].
A variety of ultradian and infradian rhythms occur in the endocrine system. The
ultradian range includes pulsatile release of pituitary and pituitary-dependent
hormones and ultrafast fluctuations with periods of recurrence in the range of
minutes. In man, hormonal pulses generally recur at intervals ranging between 1
and 2 h (i.e. 'hourly'), but this may vary greatly because the pulse frequency of a
given hormone may be modulated by numerous factors, including levels of other
hormones, age, circadian rhythmicity and sleep. When intensified rates of blood
sampling are used and hormonal levels are measured at 1–4 min intervals, ultrafast
fluctuations of low amplitude may appear superimposed on the larger hourly
pulses. Rapid oscillations also appear to characterize beta cell function of the islets
of Langerhans as oscillations with periods in the 10–14 min range have been
observed for both insulin and glucagon. The infradian range of human endocrine

24

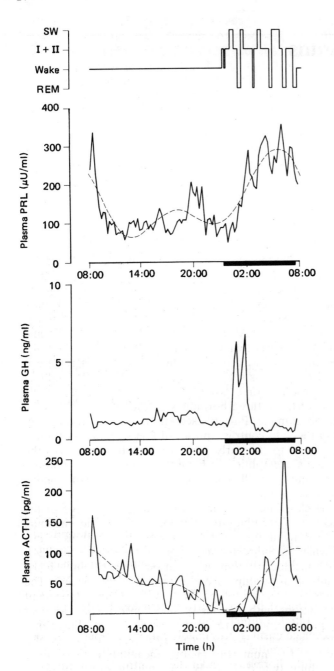

Figure 3.1 Profiles (24 h) of plasma prolactin (PRL), growth hormone (GH) and corticotropin (ACTH) obtained simultaneously in a single subject. The sampling interval is 15 min. Sleep stages are indicated above the hormonal profiles (SW, slow-wave sleep; REM, rapid eye movement). For PRL and ACTH, a best-fit curve quantifying the circadian waveshape is shown in dashed line. The black bars represent the sleep period. Reproduced from ref. [35], with permission

rhythms includes the menstrual cycle and seasonal variations. The latter are still poorly defined and appear to affect primarily the reproductive axis.

From a theoretical standpoint, rhythms may be classified according to the nature of their generating mechanism. If a rhythm is self-sustained and strictly periodic, with an identical pattern recurring at constant intervals, the mechanism generating the rhythm is called a limit-cycle oscillator and necessarily involves highly non-linear processes. The remarkable reproducibility of circadian rhythms during constant conditions is certainly suggestive of the existence of an accurate clock with limit-cycle behaviour. However, other endocrine rhythms, such as hourly pulsatile release, have fairly irregular patterns which could be accounted for by 'sloppy' pacemakers producing pseudoperiodic oscillations, i.e. oscillations for which the time of recurrence is not fixed but varies randomly around a preferred value. Such pseudoperiodic oscillations may be generated from 'noise' or purely random variations by a filtering process which has the effect of concentrating the variability of the random input in a preferred range of frequency. It is very likely that such mechanisms, capable of transforming random variability in pseudoperiodic behaviour, can be realized in the complex circuitry of neural regulatory pathways.

The interest in endocrine rhythms has greatly increased since the recognition of their essential role in maintaining normal endocrine function. Evidence showing that pathological states are associated with abnormal rhythms has accumulated and therapies taking into account the temporal organization of endocrine release have been developed. This chapter provides an overview of the state of knowledge on the most prevalent and most studied hormonal rhythms, circadian rhythmicity and hourly pulsatile release. The first section will focus on the physiological significance and clinical implications of both classes of rhythms. The second section will present quantitative methods for their study. Succinct descriptions of circadian and pulsatile rhythms of hormonal release in each pituitary axis and in pancreatic function will follow.

Physiological significance and clinical implications

Pulsatile hormonal release

For hormones controlled by the hypothalamo–pituitary axis, it is generally accepted that pulsatile variations in plasma levels are caused by intermittent discharge of hypothalamic-releasing (or -inhibiting) factors into the portal circulation. Extensive data support this concept in the case of the pituitary–gonadal axis [2]. In rhesus monkeys, pulses of gonadotropins result from pulses of gonadotropin-releasing hormone (GnRH) obtained by synchronous discharges of GnRH-containing neurones controlled by an hourly pacemaker located in the arcuate nucleus. Although no similar direct evidence exists so far for other hypothalamic factors, a similar mechanism is presumably causing the pulsatility of the other pituitary hormones. Intermittent stimulation by pituitary hormones causes in turn pulsatile release of the hormones under their control. For hormones other than those controlled by the hypothalamo–pituitary axis, the mechanisms causing pulsatile variations in plasma levels remain to be elucidated.

The first demonstration of the physiological importance of pulsatile hormonal release was obtained in experiments showing that normal gonadotropin levels may be restored by pulsatile, but not continuous, administration of exogenous GnRH to primates with lesions of the hypothalamus which had abolished endogenous GnRH production [3]. These findings were rapidly applied to the treatment of a variety of disorders of the pituitary–gonadal axis, using either pulsatile GnRH administration to correct a deficient production of endogenous GnRH [4] or long-acting GnRH analogues to induce pituitary desensitization [5]. Similar therapeutic

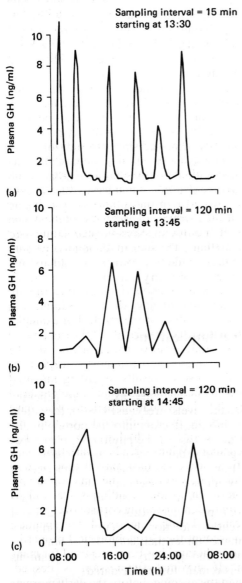

Figure 3.2 Profile (24 h) of plasma growth hormone (GH) obtained at 15-min intervals in a 16-year-old adolescent boy (a), compared to the profiles that would have been obtained if sampling had been performed at 2-h intervals starting either at 13:45 (b) or at 14:45 (c)

advances based on the pulsatile administration of growth hormone-releasing factor (GRF) have been proposed [6].

In clinical practice, the existence of pronounced pulsatile variations of circulating hormonal levels may invalidate evaluations of endocrine function based on samples collected at single time points. Frequent sampling over a prolonged period of time is often necessary to obtain accurate estimations of the amount of hormone secreted. An example is illustrated in Figure 3.2 which compares a 24-h profile of plasma GH levels obtained at 15-min intervals in a normal 16-year-old adolescent boy (Figure 3.2a) to the profiles that would have been observed if sampling had been performed at 120-min intervals, starting either at 13:45 (Figure 3.2b) or at 14:45 (Figure 3.2c). The 120-min sampling schedule totally distorts the GH profile, and does not allow the amount of GH secreted to be correctly estimated. For further discussion, see Chapter 14.

Circadian rhythms

Circadian rhythms have evolved as responses to the enormous fluctuations in the physical environment associated with the alternation of day and night. The acquisition of such temporal programmes, and their proper adjustment to the 24-h environmental cycle, enables the organism to prepare in advance to cope with circumstances as they occur. As exemplified by the profiles illustrated in Figure 3.1, circadian rhythmicity also provides a high degree of temporal organization within the organism, allowing the realization of different states by segregating their times of occurrence. In the reproductive system, circadian rhythms interact with longer-term processes to control the timing of puberty, menstrual cyclicity and pregnancy [7].

The clinical implications of circadian rhythmicity in endocrinology concern both diagnosis and treatment. In many cases, the time of day when the sample was obtained has to be taken into account in the evaluation of the result. For example, a plasma cortisol level of 150 ng/ml at 08:00 h is perfectly normal but the same value obtained 12 h later is a strong indication of some form of hypercortisolism. The glucose response to a standard oral glucose tolerance test is almost twice as large in the evening as in the morning [8]. False positive results regarding impaired glucose control obtained with this test when it is administered late in the day have been referred to as 'afternoon diabetes' [9]. In evaluating patients who have recently travelled across time zones or undergone a shift work rotation, the clinician must keep in mind that many endocrine rhythms do not adapt instantaneously to abrupt changes of schedule. While circadian variations may complicate the interpretation of diagnostic procedures, they may also be used to maximize their discriminant power by adequately selecting the time of sample collection which will best differentiate between various conditions. As will be shown later, this strategy may be very useful in demonstrating cortisol overproduction and establishing its underlying cause. Finally, improved therapeutical protocols may be designed by taking into account the chronobiological properties of the system. In endocrinology, such 'chronotherapy' has been practised for many years for corticosteroid administration. If maximal suppression is desired, exogenous corticosteroids should be given in the evening, before the early morning increase in endogenous ACTH and cortisol secretion. If minimal suppression is desired, a single dose in the morning appears to be optimal.

Quantifying hormonal rhythms

Quantifying the circadian waveshape

The majority of investigations of circadian hormonal rhythms are based on 24-h profiles obtained in a group of individuals following the same protocol. This strategy is obviously dictated by the limitations on the amount of blood volume that can be safely withdrawn. The demonstration of circadian rhythmicity then rests on the observation of consistently reproducible characteristics in the set of 24-h profiles obtained. To validate such an approach, the group of subjects should be as homogeneous as possible, not only in terms of physical parameters such as age, sex and body weight but also in terms of living habits such as bedtimes, meal schedules and indoor/outdoor activities. To maximize interindividual synchronization, the volunteers should comply with a standardized schedule of meals and bedtimes for several days prior to the investigation. Recent research has also

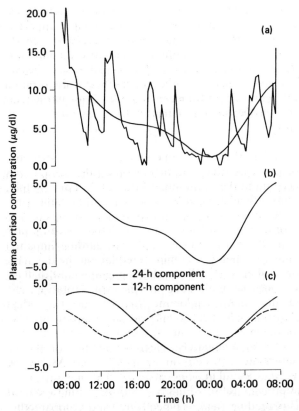

Figure 3.3 Periodogram analysis of a 24-h profile of plasma cortisol obtained at 15-min intervals in a healthy individual. The best-fit curve obtained by periodogram calculations is shown superimposed as a smooth line in (a) and is reproduced, after subtraction of the 24-h mean level, in (b). This best-fit curve was obtained by summing the 24-h and 12-h sine waves shown in (c). A statistical decision procedure determined that these two components of the periodogram contributed significantly to the temporal variation of cortisol levels. Reproduced from ref. [14], with permission.

indicated that, in contrast to previous thinking, human circadian rhythms may be strongly modulated by the light/dark cycle and the timing and duration of the subjects' exposures to bright light should also be controlled to optimize the reliability of circadian estimations. Sampling should be performed at intervals not exceeding 1 h (see also Chapter 14).

The analysis of 24-h hormonal profiles usually involves the fitting of a smooth curve to the data. Because human circadian rhythms are asymmetrical in nature (e.g. the sleep/wake cycle is a 8/16 h, rather than 12/12 h, alternation), procedures based on the fitting of a single sinusoidal curve such as the Cosinor Test [10] provide unreliable estimations of rhythm parameters. A variety of other procedures for the detection and estimation of circadian variation have been based on periodogram calculations (reviewed in ref. [11]). In these approaches, a sum of sinusoidal components is fitted to the series of data and those that contribute significantly to the observed variation are selected. Thus, the asymmetry of the waveshape is described by the inclusion of components other than the 24-h period. This is illustrated in Figure 3.3 which shows the results of periodogram calculations for a 24-h profile of plasma cortisol levels [11]. Both the 24-h and the 12-h components were found significant and added up to obtain the asymmetrical best-fit curve superimposed on the experimental data. Parameters quantifying the circadian waveshape may then be derived from the best-fit curve and used in further analyses. The times of occurrence of the maximum and the minimum of the best-fit curve are often referred to as, respectively, the acrophase and the nadir. The amplitude of the circadian rhythm may be estimated as 50% of the difference between the maximum and the minimum of the best-fit curve. A further extended description of rhythm analysis is to be found in Chapter 14.

Analysing hormonal pulsatility

Santen and Bardin, in their elegant study of gonadotropin pulsatility, proposed the first systematic approach to the analysis of hormonal pulses [12]. They defined a pulse as significant if the increment from nadir to peak exceeded, in relative terms, 20%, i.e. approximately three times the coefficient of variation of their assay. Their criteria did not include a threshold for significance of the declining portion of the pulse. A number of modifications of the Santen and Bardin procedure were subsequently proposed. A detailed review of the characteristics and pros and cons of all available procedures for pulse identification has been recently published [13]. A study aiming at the cross-validation of various programs for hormonal pulse analysis [18] has shown that the performances of three of these algorithms, ULTRA [14,15], DETECT [16] and CLUSTER [17] on large sets of hormonal profiles are essentially similar.

The general principle of the ULTRA algorithm is the elimination of all peaks of plasma concentration for which either the increment or the decrement does not exceed a certain threshold related to measurement error. The increments and decrements are expressed as percentage increase over the preceding nadir and percentage decline from the preceding peak, respectively, and compared to a multiple of the local intra-assay coefficient of variation (CV) in the relevant range of concentration. The peaks that do not meet the threshold criteria are eliminated from the series by an iterative process, leaving a 'clean' series in which all peaks represent significant pulses. Figure 3.4 illustrates, as an example, the application of program ULTRA with a threshold of 2 CV to a 24-h profile of plasma C-peptide

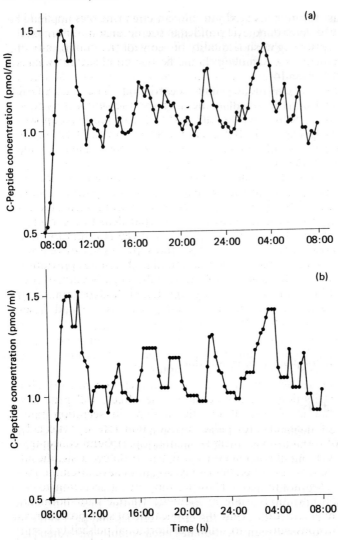

Figure 3.4 Illustration of the output of pulse analysis using algorithm ULTRA for a 24-h profile of plasma C-peptide levels obtained at 15-min intervals in a normal subject. The raw data are shown in (a). (b) shows the 'clean' profile, obtained after eliminating all concentration changes that did not exceed, in relative terms, twice the intra-assay coefficient of variation (i.e. 2 × 4%). In this clean profile, all peaks represent significant pulses. Data source: ref. [19]

levels observed in a normal subject during constant glucose infusion [19]. The intra-assay CV of C-peptide determinations averaged 4% and the threshold for significance of both increases and declines in concentration was thus 8%. The raw data are shown in Figure 3.4(a) and the 'clean' series, which includes only changes in concentration that were found significant by these criteria, is shown in Figure 3.4(b).

The DETECT algorithm is a sophisticated procedure using principles applied in the identification of peaks in electrophoretic profiles to the detection of hormonal pulses [16]. The algorithm provides great flexibility of use with the opportunity of user-selected performance. The program involves the derivation of secretory rates from levels of peripheral concentrations and thus requires the input of initial estimations of parameters for distribution and degradation. The CLUSTER algorithm derives its name from the fact that the user has the option to define peaks and troughs of plasma concentration as 'clusters' of 2, 3 or more data points rather than as isolated time points [17]. The general principle of the CLUSTER program is the comparison by standard t tests of replicate measurements at the peak and at the preceding and following troughs.

So far, the major approach used to evaluate algorithms for pulse identification has been to estimate the false-positive error by analysing series of purely random variations, i.e. 'noise' series [20–22]. Based on the results from such studies, stringent criteria for pulse identification were used to avoid detecting excessive numbers of false-positive pulses. However, we recently showed [15] that the rate of false-positive pulses in noise series greatly overestimates the false-positive error in series of actual hormonal measurements and that the high thresholds previously suggested are often associated with unacceptably large false-negative errors (i.e. failing to detect existing pulses). In particular, with the ULTRA algorithm, using a 2 CV threshold will generally better minimize both false-positive and false-negative errors than using a 3 CV threshold.

Estimating secretion rates from plasma concentrations

Fluctuations in plasma levels reflect not only variations in secretion rate but also the effects of dilution, distribution and degradation. The effects will generally result in a damping of the amplitude of the fluctuations in secretion rate. Furthermore, if the time of recurrence of pulses in secretion rate is noticeably shorter than the half-life of the hormone, measurements of peripheral concentrations, even performed at very frequent intervals, will fail to detect a significant proportion of pulses. In recent years, a number of investigators have attempted to address this problem by designing methods allowing the rate of secretion to be calculated from plasma concentrations using mathematical models for hormone distribution and metabolism [16,23–26]. While the application of such procedures, commonly referred to as 'deconvolution', to studies of hormonal pulsatility is still in its infancy, it is already clear that they will greatly improve the characterization of pulsatile secretion and of its interactions with other processes. A simple example is given in Figure 3.5 where the association between pulsatile GH secretion and sleep stages is studied in a single subject who delayed his sleep until 04:00 h. Figure 3.5(a) represents the plasma levels of GH measured at 15-min intervals. The corresponding profile of GH secretory rates is shown in Figure 3.5(b). The deconvolution calculations used a single-compartment model for GH disappearance with a half-life of 19 min and a volume of distribution of 7% of the body weight [27]. Figures 3.5(c), (d) and (e) illustrate the percentages of each 15-min blood sampling interval spent in stages wake, REM and slow-wave (SW: III + IV), respectively. When the profile of plasma concentrations is compared to the SW profile, it appears that, subsequent to its initiation in concomitance with the beginning of the first SW period, the sleep-onset GH pulse spanned the first 4 h of sleep, without apparent modulation by the succession of non-REM and REM

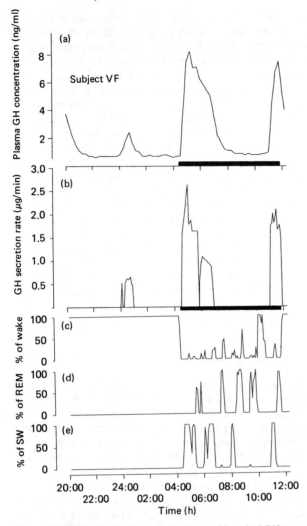

Figure 3.5 Profile (24 h) of plasma GH levels (a) and of GH secretory rates (b) as derived by calculation from the plasma levels using a mathematical model for GH distribution and metabolism. To correlate sleep stages, scored in 20-s epochs, to hormonal data, obtained at 15-min intervals, the percentages of time spent in stages wake, I + II, SW (slow-wave: III + IV) and REM (rapid eye movement) were calculated for each 15-min blood sampling interval. The comparison of the profile of GH secretory rates and of the profile of SW stages illuminates the relationship between GH secretion and SW sleep

stages. However, the profile of secretory rates clearly reveals that GH was preferentially secreted during SW stage, with a brief interruption of secretory activity coinciding with the intervening REM stage.

Rhythms in the corticotropic axis

The 24-h periodicity of pituitary–adrenal secretion is considered as a paradigm for human circadian rhythms. It has been shown to be endogenous in nature, is largely

33

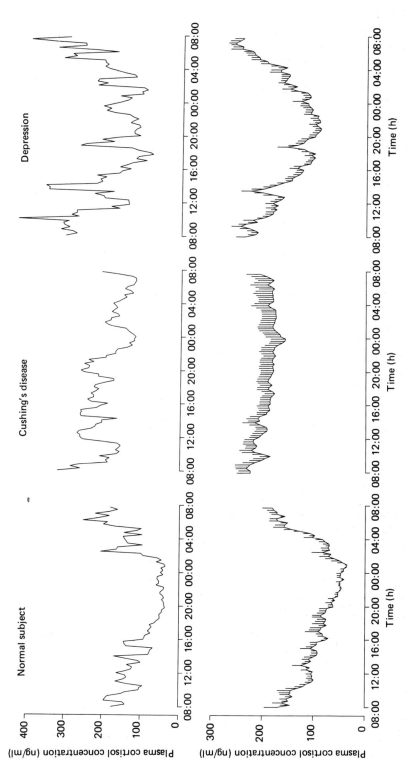

Figure 3.6 Profiles (24 h) of plasma cortisol in normal subjects (left), patients with pituitary Cushing's disease (middle) and patients with major endogenous depression (right). For each condition, a representative example is shown on the upper panel. The mean and s.e.m. of the group is shown on the lower panel. Data sources: refs [33] and [34]

unaffected by short-term manipulations of the sleep/wake cycle, such as sleep reversal and total sleep deprivation, and persists during complete fast or continuous feeding [28]. To cause a rapid shift in the rhythm, critically timed exposure to very bright light is necessary [29]. Transient evoked responses may affect the waveshape of the cortisol rhythm. In particular, the first few hours of sleep have a modest inhibitory effect on cortisol secretion [30] and brief elevations of plasma levels may be associated with meals, especially at lunch time [31].

A typical 24-h profile of ACTH is shown in Figure 3.1. Changes in plasma cortisol occur in parallel to those of ACTH. Their pattern shows an early morning maximum, declining levels throughout daytime, a quiescent period of minimal secretory activity and an abrupt elevation during late sleep (see Figure 3.6, left panels). The amplitude of the circadian variation below and above the mean averages 75% of the 24-h mean [32,33]. With a 15-min sampling rate, approximately 15 pulses of ACTH and cortisol can be detected in a 24-h span [28,34].

The 24-h rhythm of adrenocortical secretion is primarily dependent on the circadian pattern of ACTH release which is amplified by a daily variation in adrenal responsiveness to ACTH. The rhythm in ACTH release results, in turn, from periodic changes in corticotropin-releasing factor (CRF) drive. A circadian variation parallel to that of cortisol has been demonstrated for the plasma levels of all unconjugated adrenal steroids studied so far [35]. The amplitude of the circadian variation is in the same range as that of cortisol for steroids of predominantly or exclusively adrenal origin but is considerably lower for steroids that are only partially controlled by ACTH stimulation [36].

Figure 3.7 shows the adaptation of the 24-h cortisol profile to an 8-h delay shift of the sleep/wake and light/dark cycles performed in the laboratory. Six subjects were studied under baseline conditions and 1 and 3 days after the shift. These results demonstrate some of the remarkable features of the adrenocorticotropic periodicity. On the first day after the shift, the position of the nadir of the rhythm was unchanged as compared to baseline conditions. In contrast, the position of the acrophase was significantly delayed in all subjects. The delays were of variable magnitude, averaging 3 h 6 min, and the resulting lack of interindividual synchronization is one of the causes of the flattening of the mean profile. However, the shift also caused a significant decrease in circadian amplitude in all subjects. Similar, though less marked, disturbances were still present on the third day after the shift. Thus, different mechanisms seem to be responsible for the synchronization of the acrophase, on the one hand, and of the quiescent period on the other hand. The nadir and the end of the quiescent period appear to be robust markers of circadian timing. The timing of the acrophase is more labile and can be influenced by meal timing.

The middle and right panels of Figure 3.6 show the 24-h cortisol profiles in two conditions of hypercortisolism, pituitary Cushing's disease and major endogenous depression [33,34]. In patients with Cushing's syndrome secondary to adrenal adenoma or ectopic ACTH secretion, the circadian variation of plasma cortisol is invariably absent [35]. However, in pituitary-dependent Cushing's disease, a low amplitude circadian variation may persist, suggesting that there is no defect in the neural clock generating the periodicity [37]. Cortisol pulsatility is blunted in about 70% of patients with Cushing's disease, suggesting autonomous tonic secretion of ACTH by a pituitary tumour [34]. In the other patients, the magnitude of the pulses is instead enhanced [34]. These 'hyperpulsatile' patterns could be caused by enhanced hypothalamic release of CRF or by increased pituitary responsiveness to

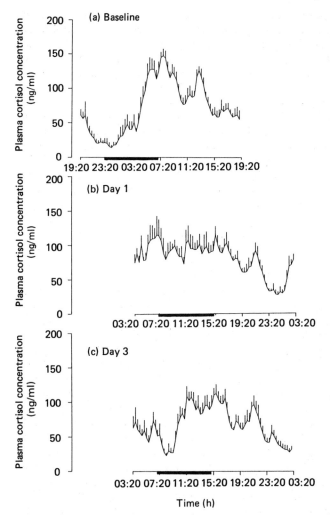

Figure 3.7 Mean cortisol profile (24 h) observed in six normal men before (a) an 8-h delay shift of the sleep/wake and light/dark cycles and 1 day (b) and 3 days (c) after the shift. The vertical bars represent the s.e.m. The black bars represent the sleep period

CRF. Hypercortisolism with persistent circadian rhythmicity and increased pulsatility is found in a majority of acutely depressed patients with primary affective disorder [33]. In these patients, who do not develop the clinical signs of Cushing's syndrome despite the high circulating cortisol levels, the quiescent period of cortisol secretion occurs earlier than in normal subjects of comparable age (compare in Figure 3.6 the positions of the nadir in normal subjects, around 01:00 h, and in depressed patients, around 21:00 h). This 'phase advance' of the rhythm could reflect a decrease in endogenous period of the circadian pacemaker or an alteration in the mechanisms synchronizing the overt rhythm to the central clock. Hypercortisolism and abnormal timing of cortisol secretion in depression are 'state' rather than 'trait' dependent as they disappear when a clinical remission is obtained [38]. For a more in-depth discussion of cortisol secretion in depression, see Chapter 9, which presents a slightly different point of view.

For diagnostic purposes, it is noteworthy that sampling during the expected timing of the quiescent period (20:00–02:00 h) will optimally discriminate normal subjects from patients with hypercortisolism, as well as patients with Cushing's disease from patients with depression (see lower panels of Figure 3.6). In contrast, in the early morning, when it is customary to collect samples in clinical laboratories, there is a wide overlap in the cortisol ranges found in normal subjects, patients with Cushing's disease and depressed patients. Likewise the suppression of cortisol secretion by dexamethasone is time dependent. Suppression is greater after administration at midnight than at other times of the day. This function test is commonly used in endocrinology and psychiatry: care is necessary in the interpretation of results.

Rhythms in the gonadotropic axis

Rhythms in the gonadotropic axis cover a wide range of frequencies, from ultrafast oscillations of plasma lutropin (LH) levels recurring at intervals of a few minutes, to pulsatile release in the hourly range, to circadian rhythmicity and finally menstrual and seasonal cyclicity. These various rhythms interact to provide a coordinated temporal programme for the operation of the reproductive axis at every stage of maturation [7]. The finding that changes in the circadian and pulsatile patterns of gonadotropin secretion are associated with various stages of sexual maturation was the first indication of the physiological significance of the temporal organization of endocrine release [39]. Since then, the modulation and interactions of ultradian, circadian and infradian rhythms in the hypothalamo–pituitary–gonadal axis have been the object of intense study. The current state of knowledge in this field has been reviewed in detail recently [7]. We will limit the present review to the description of 24-h rhythms and their interaction with pulsatile release in normal subjects at various stages of sexual maturation.

In prepubertal children of both sexes, gonadotropins are secreted in pulses of low magnitude throughout the 24-h cycle. A difference between day time and night time becomes apparent when the child approaches puberty. The magnitude of the nocturnal pulses increases progressively in both sexes, resulting in the appearance of a circadian variation with high LH and follitropin (FSH) levels during the night. Studies with shifts or abrupt reversal of the sleep/wake cycle have shown that sleep *per se* induces an elevation of pubertal LH secretion [40]. Figure 3.8 illustrates mean 24-h profiles of plasma LH observed in pubertal children in normal conditions and after a 12-h shift of the sleep/wake cycle. After sleep reversal, an increase in LH release occurs not only during daytime sleep but also at the time when sleep would have occurred under basal conditions, indicating that circadian rhythmicity also influences the temporal pattern of LH release. In pubertal girls, a circadian variation of circulating oestradiol, with daytime levels higher than night-time levels, has been reported. In pubertal boys, the nocturnal rise in testosterone coincides with the elevation of gonadotropin secretion [7].

In males reaching adulthood, the circadian variation of LH and FSH levels is damped and becomes undetectable in the majority of adults. Secretion remains pulsatile, with patterns that vary considerably from one individual to another [41].

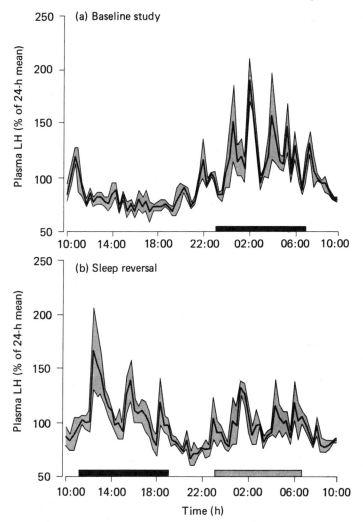

Figure 3.8 Effect of a 12-h shift of the sleep/wake cycle ('sleep reversal') on the 24-h profile of plasma LH in pubertal children. The mean ± S.E.M. of three individual profiles is shown under basal condition (a) and after the shift (b). Data are expressed as percentage of the individual 24-h mean. The black bars represent the sleep times. The shaded bar represents the usual bedtimes on the baseline schedule. Data source: ref. [40]. Reproduced from ref. [47], with permission

Testosterone secretion is also pulsatile and approximately concordant with LH pulses [41,42]. A reproducible circadian rhythm of testosterone, with a nocturnal rise starting shortly before midnight, is present in male adults [36]. This nocturnal increase in testosterone has been shown to be independent of sleep, a fact that further supports the hypothesis of an intrinsic circadian rhythmicity of pituitary–gonadal activity. In young subjects, the amplitude of the circadian rhythm averages 25% of the 24-h mean level [36]. In elderly men, LH and testosterone pulse frequencies decrease and the amplitude of the testosterone rhythm is blunted [43,44].

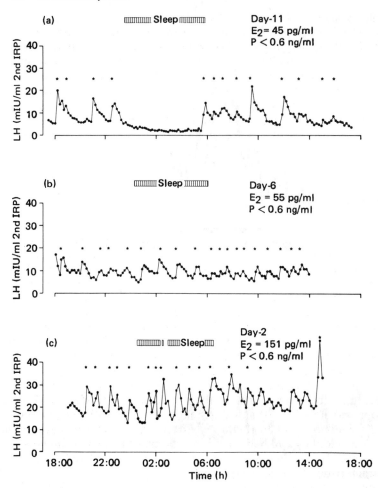

Figure 3.9 Temporal profiles of plasma LH in healthy women studied in the early (a), mid- (b) and late (c) follicular phase of the menstrual cycle. The stage of the follicular phase is indicated from the day of the mid-cycle surge, referred to as day 0. Levels of 17β-oestradiol (E_2) and progesterone (P) represent the mean of samples obtained at 6-h intervals. The hatched bars represent sleep times. The asterisks identify significant LH pulses. 2nd IRP, second International Reference Preparation. Reproduced from ref. [45], with permission

A complex modulation of circadian and pulsatile LH variations by the menstrual cycle occurs in the adult woman [45]. Figure 3.9 illustrates these interactions in a subject studied during the follicular phase. In the early follicular phase (Figure 3.9a), LH pulses are large and infrequent and the overall LH levels decline during sleep because of a slowing of the frequency of secretory pulses. In the mid-follicular phase (Figure 3.9b), pulse amplitude is decreased, pulse frequency increased and the frequency modulation of LH pulsatility by sleep is less apparent. Pulse amplitude increases again by the late follicular phase (Figure 3.9c). No modulation by sleep is apparent until the early luteal phase when nocturnal slowing of pulsatility is again evident. Studies with shifts of the sleep/wake cycle will be needed to determine whether the nocturnal slowing of LH pulsatility is dependent on sleep timing or/and on circadian timing. Towards menopause, gonadotropin levels are elevated with increased pulsatility without consistent circadian pattern. In post-menopausal women, significant pulses of human chorionic gonadotropin, presumably reflecting pituitary secretion, are associated with the large LH and FSH pulses [46]. In normal adult women, a low-amplitude circadian variation of testosterone levels can be detected. Finally, an interaction between the menstrual cycle and circadian rhythmicity appears to be also involved in the timing of the preovulatory LH surge which occurs most often in late sleep or early morning in normal women [7].

Rhythms in growth hormone secretion

In normal subjects, the 24-h profile of plasma GH consists of stable low levels abruptly interrupted by bursts of secretion [47]. A typical example has been shown in Figure 3.1. The most reproducible secretory pulse occurs shortly after sleep onset, in association with the first phase of slow-wave (SW) sleep. Other secretory pulses may occur in later sleep and during wakefulness, in the absence of any identifiable stimulus. Women generally secrete more GH than men of similar age. Because sleep onset will elicit a pulse in GH secretion whether sleep is advanced, delayed, interrupted or fragmented, the 24-h profile of GH secretion in man is often described as entirely dependent on sleep (i.e. exogenous). However, there is also evidence for the existence of a weak endogenous circadian rhythm modulating the occurrence and height of GH secretory pulses [47].

Interestingly, the human is the only species for whom a strong relationship between GH secretion and sleep exists. In the rat, secretory bursts of GH recur at intervals of approximately 3 h without consistent correlation with sleep episodes. The existence of a similar ultradian rhythm of GH release has been suggested in the dog, goat, rhesus monkey and baboon. It may be that the association between sleep and GH secretion in the human is the result of the consolidated sleep/wake cycle that is characteristic of our species.

The total amount of GH secretion is strongly dependent on age. Figure 3.10 illustrates the ontogeny of the 24-h GH profile in male subjects [48]. In children, the amount of GH secreted reaches a maximum in late puberty. Adult men typically present a single GH pulse, occurring in synchrony with the first SW stage in sleep. In older subjects, the 24-h GH secretion is drastically diminished but sleep-related pulses may still be identified. In women, the effects of age on GH secretion correlate with the decline in circulating oestradiol concentrations [49].

There is an inverse relationship between adiposity and GH release which results in a suppression of GH levels throughout the 24-h span in obese subjects [35]. A normal pattern can be restored after prolonged fasting. Non-obese diabetics hypersecrete GH throughout the 24-h span. This abnormality disappears when blood sugar levels are strictly controlled. In anorexia nervosa with severe weight loss, the sleep-onset GH pulse is absent. In normal subjects, prolonged fasting results in an overall increase in GH secretion, due to an increase in both number and amplitude of pulses [50].

In acromegaly, high amplitude episodic pulses of GH occur over elevated basal levels throughout the 24-h span. After trans-sphenoidal surgery, a normal temporal profile can be restored [35]. In narcoleptic subjects, two types of GH profiles have

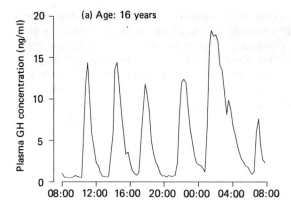

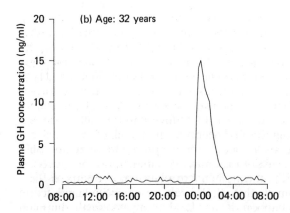

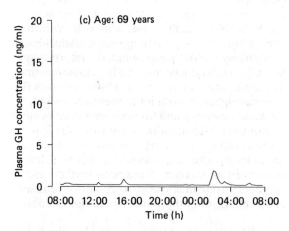

Figure 3.10 Ontogeny of the 24-h profile of plasma growth hormone (GH). Profiles obtained at 15-min intervals are shown for three healthy male subjects, ages 16 (a), 32 (b) and 69 (c). Bedtimes were 23:00–07:00 h. Data source: ref. [48]

been observed: one with low, and one with high, GH concentrations [35]. In both cases, there was no consistent association between GH release and SW sleep. Patients with major endogenous depression, especially those with the unipolar form of the illness, hypersecrete GH during the daytime [48]. Moreover, the major nocturnal pulse frequently occurs before, rather than after, sleep onset. This early timing of the nocturnal GH pulse could reflect a 'phase advance' of a circadian component underlying the temporal organization of GH release. After successful treatment, a normalization of GH profiles is observed but a tendency for persistent daytime hypersecretion is still present [38]. The possible role of a chronic reduction of food intake in causing the daytime hypersecretion of GH in depressed subjects remains to be evaluated.

Rhythms in the thyrotropic axis

The recent availability of ultrasensitive thyrotropin (TSH) assays has contributed significantly to the quantitative characterization of circadian and pulsatile TSH variations. In normal adult men, TSH levels are low throughout the daytime and increase abruptly around 20:00 h. Elevated levels are observed throughout the night and are followed by a sharp decrease in the morning hours (Figure 3.11). Studies involving sleep deprivation and reversal of the sleep/wake cycle have consistently indicated that an inhibitory influence is exerted on TSH secretion during sleep [51]. In some, but not all, individuals, this inhibitory influence is reflected in declining levels throughout the sleep period. The timing of the evening rise seems to be controlled by circadian rhythmicity. Sex appears to be one of the factors influencing the timing of the daily maximum of circulating TSH levels. Indeed, in women, early studies have indicated that this maximum occurs in the early morning hours, before awakening [52]. In both sexes, low-amplitude pulsatile fluctuations of plasma TSH occur throughout the 24-h span. A small diurnal variation of serum total thyroxine (T_4) and tri-iodothyronine (T_3), with slightly lower levels during the night, can be detected in normal conditions and has been shown to be related to the posture-dependent daily variation of total plasma proteins. Serum free T_3 appears to vary in parallel with TSH. Because of the known negative feedback of glucocorticoids on TSH secretion, the temporal relationships between the circadian variation of cortisol and TSH are particularly interesting (Figure 3.11). The major increase in TSH concentrations is indeed concomitant with the beginning of the quiescent period of cortisol secretion. However, in the early morning and during most of the daytime period, both hormones vary roughly in parallel. Studies using low-dose dexamethasone administration (3 mg over 24 h) have concluded that corticosteroids do not affect the circadian profile of TSH [53]. When larger doses were used (8 mg over a 3-h period), TSH secretion was totally suppressed, without evidence of a circadian pattern [54]. However, the fact that the evening rise may be blocked by corticosteroids given in pharmacological dosage does not prove that, under physiological circumstances, the late evening suppression of adrenal output is the physiological stimulus allowing the rise in TSH secretion.

Alterations in the 24-h profile of plasma TSH have only been studied in a limited number of pathological conditions. A normal pattern is preserved in patients with mild or moderate hypothyroidism as well as in patients treated with thyroxine. The

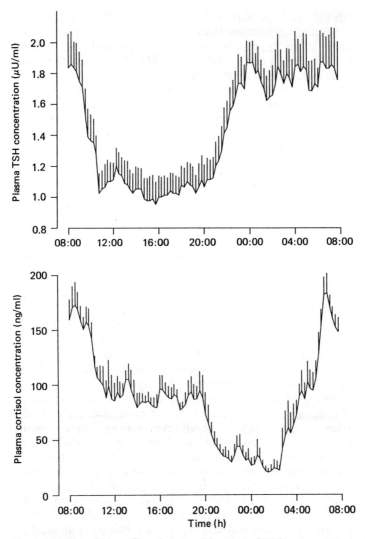

Figure 3.11 Mean 24-h profiles of plasma thyrotropin (TSH) and cortisol obtained simultaneously at 15-min intervals in eight normal men, aged 20–27 years. The vertical bars represent the s.e.m. Data source: refs [33] and [66]

diurnal variation is abolished in untreated patients with severe hypothyroidism [55].

Rhythms in prolactin (PRL) secretion

Under normal conditions, the 24-h profile of plasma PRL levels follows a bimodal pattern, with minimal concentrations around noon, an afternoon phase of augmented secretion and a major nocturnal elevation starting shortly after sleep

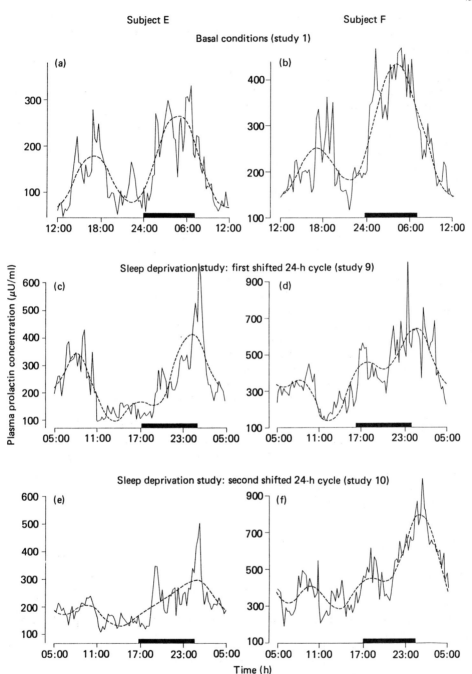

Figure 3.12 Profiles (24 h) of plasma prolactin (PRL) obtained at 15-min intervals in two normal men before (a,b), 24 h after (c,d) and 48 h after (e,f) a 33-h period of sleep deprivation, resulting in a 7-h advance of the sleep/wake cycle. The dashed lines represent a best-fit curve obtained by periodogram calculations. The black bars represent the polygraphically monitored sleep times. Note the shift in clock times reported on the abscissa between the top panels and the lower panels. Data source: ref. [57]

onset and culminating around mid-sleep [56]. Examples are shown in Figure 3.12(a) and (b). Episodic pulses occur throughout the 24-h span. Studies on PRL during daytime naps or after shifts of the sleep period have demonstrated that sleep onset is invariably associated with an increase in prolactin secretion [47]. However, studies on the effects of 'jet lag' or sleep deprivation have shown that the temporal organization of PRL release is not entirely dependent on sleep but has also an inherent circadian rhythmicity [47]. The results of such a study are illustrated in Figure 3.12(c), (d), (e) and (f) [57]. After having slept in the study unit from 23:00 to 07:00 h, two healthy male volunteers were kept continuously awake for 33 h and were then allowed to sleep from 16:00 to 24:00 h. This manipulation resulted in a 7-h advance of the sleep/wake cycle. The subjects were then kept awake and active for 16 h and went back to bed for a second shifted 'night' from 16:00 to 24:00 h. Only modest elevations of prolactin occurred after sleep onset during the first and second shifted nights. Sustained maximum levels were reached only after awakening, at the time of the anticipated sleep onset before the imposed time shift. These results clearly indicate that the 24-h profile of PRL secretion includes a circadian component which is expressed as a secretory rise synchronized, under normal conditions, with the early part of sleep.

Absence or blunting of the nocturnal increase of PRL has been reported in a variety of pathological states, including uraemia, breast cancer in post-menopausal women, diabetes mellitus, anorexia nervosa and Cushing's disease [35]. In hyperprolactinaemia associated with prolactinomas, the nocturnal elevation is absent in the majority of cases. Normal patterns have, however, been reported in patients with microadenomas, suggesting that there is no defect in the CNS control of the temporal programme of normal PRL release. This hypothesis is further supported by the fact that selective removal of prolactinomas can result in the normalization of the 24-h profile. In women with galactorrhoea but normal PRL levels, the circadian pattern is unaltered. In patients with the unipolar form of major depressive illness, the nocturnal rise in prolactin secretion generally occurs prior to, rather than after, sleep onset [58]. Taken together with the findings of early timing of the cortisol rise and of the nocturnal GH secretion as well as of a reduction in REM latency, this observation indicates that a chronobiological disorder, consisting of a phase advance of events timed by the circadian clock, may underlie certain forms of the illness [59].

Rhythms of insulin and glucose

A number of studies have indicated that time of day influences the normal regulation of glucose levels by insulin. Following oral or intravenous glucose administration, as well as in response to meals, glucose tolerance has been shown to be decreased in the afternoon or evening, as compared to the morning [8]. The term 'afternoon diabetes' has been used to describe this phenomenon [9]. Recent studies have indicated that 'afternoon diabetes' actually reflects a progressive decrease in glucose tolerance which reaches its minimum around mid-sleep in normal subjects [19]. Figure 3.13 shows the mean glucose profiles observed in nine normal non-obese fasted subjects who were given a constant glucose infusion for 30 h. Blood was sampled at 15-min intervals for the last 24 h of the infusion. A nocturnal maximum of blood glucose levels was present in all individual profiles. This variation was not a direct reflection of the rest/activity cycle since it was

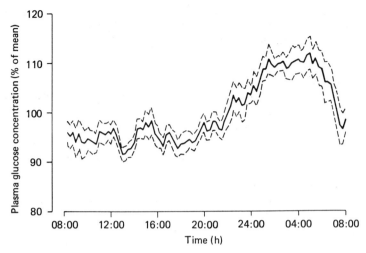

Figure 3.13 Mean 24-h glucose profile obtained in nine normal subjects studied during constant glucose infusion at either 5 g/kg per 24 h or 8 g/kg per 24 h. Because similar waveshapes were observed with both infusion rates, the data were pooled after expressing each individual profile as a percentage of the corresponding 24-h mean. The subjects remained fasted and recumbent throughout the study. From 23:00 to 07:00 h, the lights were turned off and the subjects slept. Blood was sampled at 15-min intervals. The nocturnal elevation apparent in the mean profile was present in each individual profile. Data source: ref. [67]

observed during continuous bed rest. The amplitude of the variation is a function of the size of the stimulus, i.e. the rate of glucose infusion. In the absence of a stimulus, previous studies have generally failed to observe a diurnal variation in glucose levels in fasted subjects [8]. Decreased glucose uptake by cells seems to be the immediate cause of the decreased nocturnal glucose tolerance. The relative roles of insulin secretion and/or insulin resistance remain to be elucidated. The finding of a diurnal variation in insulin-induced hypoglycaemia with blood glucose levels more than twofold higher in the late evening (20:00–24:00 h) than in the morning (08:00–12:00 h) suggests that some degree of insulin resistance may develop as the day progresses [60].

In insulin-dependent as well as non-insulin-dependent diabetic subjects, insulin requirements and/or glucose levels reach a maximum in the early morning hours, between 06:00 and 09:00 h [61]. A number of studies have indicated that sleep-related secretion of the counter-regulatory hormone GH is involved in causing this 'dawn phenomenon'. It remains to be determined whether the dawn phenomenon in diabetes represents a delay of the nocturnal maximum observed in normal subjects.

Extensive studies in dogs, monkeys and human subjects have shown the existence of oscillations in insulin secretion with periodicities in the 10–14 min range (reviewed in ref. [62]). The physiological significance of these ultrafast oscillations has been indicated by studies showing that the oscillations increase the efficiency of the hypoglycaemic action of insulin, presumably because the intermittent nature of the stimulus avoids the down-regulation of receptors and enhances hormone action [62]. More recently, slower oscillations of insulin secretion and glucose levels of larger amplitude than the ultrafast pulsations have

46

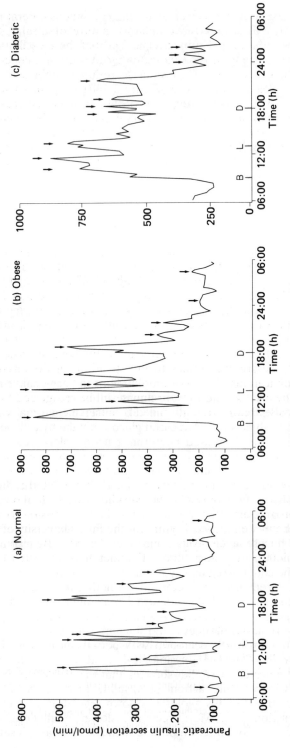

Figure 3.14 Profile (24 h) of insulin secretory rates in one normal subject (a), one obese subject (b) and one patient with non-insulin-dependent diabetes (c). Three mixed meals were served over the daytime period (B: breakfast; L: lunch; D: dinner). Pancreatic insulin secretory rates were derived from peripheral C-peptide concentrations using a mathematical model for C-peptide distribution and metabolism. The arrows identify significant pulses of insulin secretion. Data source: refs [24 and 65].

been observed in response to meals as well as during continuous enteral nutrition [24,63,64]. Figure 3.14(a) illustrates the oscillatory nature of insulin secretion following meal ingestion in a normal subject. The fact that these oscillations may also be observed during constant infusion indicate that they are not dependent on food ingestion [19]. In obese subjects, insulin secretion is enhanced but the pulsatile nature of the release is preserved (Figure 3.14b). In patients with non-insulin-dependent diabetes, profound alterations of the normal oscillatory pattern of post-meal insulin secretion are observed (Figure 3.14c). The abnormalities are more pronounced after dinner, when pre-meal glucose levels are elevated, then after breakfast, when the patients are in better glycaemic control [65]. These observations suggest that the lack of coordinated oscillatory output of insulin may play a role in the pathophysiology of diabetes.

Conclusions

The present review, which is far from exhaustive, has served to demonstrate the diversity and importance of rhythms in endocrinology. Essentially all hormonal secretions undergo pronounced oscillations, resulting in a high degree of temporal organization of the endocrine system. Three different types of mechanisms seem to interact to produce the complex patterns of hormonal release during the 24-h cycle: pulsatility, circadian rhythmicity and intrinsic effects of sleep. Longer-term processes, such as the menstrual cycle and seasonal variations, may exert additional modulatory effects. Over the last decade, research in the field of endocrine rhythms has moved from purely descriptive studies to investigations of the physiological function and clinical implications of temporal oscillations in hormonal release and we have now reached the exciting stage where timing will be recognized as a major element in the diagnosis, treatment and clinical management of a variety of endocrine disorders.

Acknowledgements

Figures 3.5, 3.7, 3.10 and 3.11 include unpublished data obtained in collaborative studies with Drs D. Bosson, G. Copinschi, M. Kerkhofs and P. Linkowski (Free University of Brussels, Belgium). I am grateful for their permission to illustrate these data. Studies on human endocrine rhythms at the Free University of Brussels are partially supported by a grant 'Actions Concertées' from the Belgian Ministere de la Politique Scientifique and by the APMO Foundation.

References

1. Halberg, F. and Reinberg, A. Rythmes circadiens et rythmes de basses frequences en physiologie humaine. *J. Physiol.*, **59**, 117–200 (1967)
2. Pohl, C.R. and Knobil, E. The role of the central nervous system in the control of ovarian function in higher primates. *Annu. Rev. Physiol.*, **44**, 583–593 (1982)
3. Belchetz, P.E., Plant, T.M., Nakai, Y., Keogh, E.J. and Knobil, E. Hypophyseal responses to continuous and intermittent delivery of hypothalamic gonadotropin releasing hormone. *Science*, **202**, 631–632 (1978)
4. Hoffman, A.R. and Crowley, Jr. W.F. Induction of puberty in men by long-term pulsatile administration of low-dose gonadotropin-releasing hormone. *N. Engl. J. Med.*, **307**, 1237–1241 (1982)

5. Comite, F., Cutler, G.B.Jr., Rivier, J., Vale, W.W., Loriaux, D.L. and Crowley, W.F.Jr. Short-term treatment of idiopathic precocious puberty with a long-acting analogue of luteinizing hormone-releasing hormone. *N. Engl. J. Med.*, **305**, 1546–1550 (1981)

6. Borges, J.L.C., Blizzard, R.M., Evans, W.S., Furlanetto, R., Rogol, A.D., Kaiser, D.L., Rivier, J., Vale, W. and Thorner, M.O. Stimulation of growth hormone (GH) and somatomedin C in idiopathic GH-deficient subjects by intermittent pulsatile administration of synthetic human pancreatic tumor GH-releasing factor. *J. Clin. Endocrinol. Metab.*, **59**, 1–6 (1984)

7. Turek, F.W. and Van Cauter, E. Biological rhythms in reproduction. In *Physiology of Reproduction* (eds E. Knobil and J. O'Neill), Raven Press, New York (1988)

8. Jarrett, R.J. Rhythms in insulin and glucose. In *Endocrine Rhythms* (ed. D.T. Krieger), Raven Press, New York, pp. 247–258 (1979)

9. Jarrett, R.J., Viberti, G.E. and Al Sayegh, H. Does 'afternoon diabetes' predict diabetes? *Brit. Med. J.*, **1**, 548–549 (1978)

10. Halberg, F., Tong, Y.L. and Johnson, E.A. Circadian system phase – An aspect of temporal morphology; Procedures and illustrative examples. In *Cellular Aspects of Biorhythms*, Springer Verlag, Berlin, pp. 20–48 (1965)

11. Van Cauter, E. Method for the characterization of 24-hour temporal variations of blood components. *Amer. J. Physiol.*, **237**, E255–E264 (1979)

12. Santen, R.J. and Bardin, C.W. Episodic luteinizing hormone secretion in man. *J. Clin. Invest.*, **52**, 2617–2628 (1973)

13. Urban, R.J., Evans, W.S., Rogol, A.D., Kaiser, D.L., Johnson, M.L. and Veldhuis, J.D. Contemporary aspects of discrete peak-detection algorithms. I. The paradigm of the luteinizing hormone pulse signal in man. *Endocrine Rev.*, **9**, 3–37 (1988)

14. Van Cauter, E. Quantitative methods for the analysis of circadian and episodic hormone fluctuations. In *Human Pituitary Hormones: Circadian and Episodic Variations* (eds E. Van Cauter and G. Copinschi), Nijhoff, The Hague, pp. 1–25 (1981)

15. Van Cauter, E. Estimating false-positive and false-negative errors in analyses of hormonal pulsatility. *Amer. J. Physiol.*, **254**, E786–794 (1988)

16. Oerter, K.E., Guardabasso, V. and Rodbard, D. Detection and characterization of peaks and estimation of instantaneous secretory rate for episodic pulsatile hormone secretion. *Comput. Biomed. Res.*, **19**, 170–191 (1986)

17. Veldhuis, J.D. and Johnson, M.L. Cluster analysis: a simple versatile, and robust algorithm for endocrine pulse detection. *Amer. J. Physiol.*, **250**, E486–E493 (1986)

18. Urban, R.J., Kaiser, D.L., Van Cauter, E., Johnson, M.L. and Veldhuis, J.D. Comparative assessments of objective peak-detection algorithms. II. Studies in men. *Amer. J. Physiol.*, **254**, E113–E119 (1988)

19. Shapiro, E.T., Tillil, H., Polonsky, K.S., Fang, V.S., Rubenstein, A.H. and Van Cauter, E. Oscillations in insulin secretion during constant glucose infusion in normal man: relationship to changes in plasma glucose. *J. Clin. Endocrinol. Metab.*, **67**, 307–314 (1988)

20. Ross, L.E., Barnes, K.M., Brody, S., Merriam, G.R., Loriaux, D.L. and Cutler, G.B. Jr. A comparison of two methods for detecting hormone peaks: the effect of sampling interval on gonadotropin peak frequency. *J. Clin. Endocrinol. Metab.*, **59**, 159–163 (1984)

21. Veldhuis, J.D., Evans, W.S., Rogol, A.D., Drake, C.R., Thorner, M.O., Merriam, G.R. and Johnson, M.L. Performance of LH pulse-detection algorithms at rapid rates of venous sampling in humans. *Amer. J. Physiol.*, **247**, E554–E563 (1984)

22. Veldhuis, J.D., Rogol, A.D. and Johnson, M.L. Minimizing false-positive errors in hormonal pulse detection. *Amer. J. Physiol.*, **248**, E475–E481 (1985)

23. Eaton, R.P., Allen, R.C., Schade, D.S., Erickson, K.M. and Standefer, J. Prehepatic insulin production in man: kinetic analysis using peripheral connecting peptide behaviour. *J. Clin. Endocrinol. Metab.*, **51**, 520–528 (1980)

24. Polonsky, K.S., Given, B.D. and Van Cauter, E. Twenty-four hour profiles and pulsatile patterns of insulin secretion in normal and obese subjects. *J. Clin. Invest.*, **81**, 442–448 (1988)

25. Van Cauter, E. and Honinckx, E. The pulsatility of pituitary hormones. In *Ultradian Rhythms in Physiology and Behavior* (eds H. Schulz and P. Lavie), Springer-Verlag, Berlin, pp. 41–60 (1985)

26. Veldhuis, J.D., Carlson, M.L. and Johnson, M.L. The pituitary gland secretes in bursts: Appraising the nature of glandular secretory impulses by simultaneous multiple-parameter deconvolution of

plasma hormone concentrations. *Proc. Natl Acad. Sci. USA*, **84**, 7686–7690 (1987)

27. Golstein, J., Van Cauter, E., Desir, D., Noel, P., Spire, J.-P.. Refetoff, S. and Copinschi, G. Effects of 'jet lag' on hormonal patterns. IV. Time shifts increase growth hormone release. *J. Clin. Endocrinol. Metab.*, **56**, 443–440 (1983)

28. Krieger, D.T. Rhythms in CRF, ACTH and corticosteroids. In *Endocrine Rhythms* (ed. D.T. Krieger), Raven Press, New York, p.123 (1979)

29. Czeisler, C.A., Allan, J.S., Strogatz, S.H., Ronda, J.M., Sanchez, R., Rios, C.D., Freitag, W.O., Richardson, G.S. and Kronauer, R.E. Bright light resets the human circadian pacemaker independent of the timing of the sleep–wake cycle. *Science*, **233**, 667–671 (1986)

30. Weitzman, E.D., Zimmerman, J.C., Czeisler, C.A. and Ronda, J. Cortisol secretion is inhibited during sleep in normal man. *J. Clin. Endocrinol. Metab.*, **56**, 352–358 (1983)

31. Follenius, M., Brandenburger, G., Simeoni, M. and Reinhardt, B. Diurnal cortisol peaks and their relationships to meals. *J. Clin. Endocrinol. Metab.*, **55**, 757–761 (1982)

32. Desir, D., Van Cauter, E., Fang, V., Martino, E., Jadot, C., Spire, J.-P., Noel, P., Refetoff, S., Copinschi, G. and Golstein, J. Effects of 'jet lag' on hormonal pattern. I. Procedures, variations in total plasma proteins and disruption of adrenocorticotropin-cortisol periodicity. *J. Clin. Endocrinol. Metab.*, **52**, 628–641 (1981)

33. Linkowski, P., Mendlewicz, J., Leclercq, R., Brasseur, M., Hubain, P., Golstein, J., Copinschi, G. and Van Cauter, E. The 24-hour profile of adrenocorticotropin and cortisol in major depressive illness. *J. Clin. Endocrinol. Metab.*, **61**, 429–438 (1985)

34. Van Cauter, E. and Refetoff, S. Evidence for two subtypes of Cushing's disease based on the analysis of episodic cortisol secretion. *N. Engl. J. Med.*, **312**, 1343–1344 (1985)

35. Van Cauter, E. and Aschoff, J. Endocrine and other biological rhythms. In *Endocrinology* (ed. L.J. DeGroot), W.B. Saunders, Philadelphia, Vol. 3, pp. 2658–2705 (1989)

36. Lejeune-Lenain, C., Van Cauter, E., Desir, D., Beyloos, M. and Franckson, J.R.M. Control of circadian and episodic variations of adrenal androgens secretion in man. *J. Endocrinol. Invest.*, **10**, 267–275 (1987)

37. Refetoff, S., Van Cauter, E., Fang, V.S., Laderman, C., Graybeal, M.L. and Landau, R.L. The effect of dexamethasone on the 24-hour profiles of adrenocorticotropin and cortisol in Cushing's syndrome. *J. Clin. Endocrinol. Metab.*, **60**, 527–535 (1985)

38. Linkowski, P., Mendlewicz, J., Kerkhofs, M., Leclercq, R., Golstein, J., Brasseur, M., Copinschi, G. and Van Cauter, E. 24-hour profiles of adrenocorticotropin, cortisol and growth hormone in major depressive illness: Effect of antidepressant treatment. *J. Clin. Endocrinol. Metab.*, **65**, 141–152 (1987)

39. Boyar, R., Finkelstein, J., Roffwarg, H., Kapen, S., Weitzman, E. and Hellman, L. Synchronization of augmented luteinizing hormone secretion with sleep during puberty. *N. Engl. J. Med.*, **287**, 582–586 (1972)

40. Kapen, S., Boyar, R.M., Finkelstein, J.W., Hellman, L. and Weitzman, E.D. Effect of sleep-wake cycle reversal on luteinizing hormone secretory pattern in puberty. *J. Clin. Endocrinol. Metab.*, **39**, 293–299 (1974)

41. Spratt, D.I., O'Dea, L.St.L., Schoenfeld, D., Butler, J.P., Rao, P.N. and Crowley, W.F. Jr. Neuroendocrine-gonadal axis in men: frequent sampling of LF, FSH and testosterone. *Amer. J. Physiol.*, **254**, E658–E666 (1988)

42. Veldhuis, J.D., King, J.C., Urban, R.J., Rogol, A.D., Evans, W.S., Kolp, L.A. and Johnson, M.L. Operating characteristics of the male hypothalamo-pituitary-gonadal-axis: Pulsatile release of testosterone and follicle-stimulating hormone and their temporal coupling with luteinizing hormone. *J. Clin. Endocrinol. Metab.*, **65**, 929–941 (1987)

43. Deslypere, J.P., Kaufman, J.M., Vermeulen, T., Vogelaers, D., Vandalem, J.L. and Vermeulen, A. Influence of age on pulsatile luteinizing hormone release and responsiveness of the gonadotrophs to sex hormone feedback in men. *J. Clin. Endocrinol. Metab.*, **64**, 68–73 (1987)

44. Bremner, W.J., Vitiello, M.V. and Prinz, P.N. Loss of circadian rhythmicity in blood testosterone levels with aging in normal men. *J. Clin. Endocrinol. Metab.*, **56**, 1278 (1983)

45. Filicori, M., Santoro, N., Merriam, G.R. and Crowley, W.F. Jr. Characterization of the physiological pattern of episodic gonadotropin secretion throughout the human menstrual cycle. *J. Clin. Endocrinol. Metab.*, **62**, 1136–1144 (1986)

46. Odell, W.D. and Griffin, J. Pulsatile secretion of human chronic gonadotrophin in normal adults. *N. Engl. J. Med.*, **317**, 1688–1691 (1987)

47. Van Cauter, E. and Refetoff, S. Multifactorial control of the 24-hour secretory profiles of pituitary hormones. *J. Clin. Endocrinol. Metab.*, **8**, 381–389 (1985)
48. Mendlewicz, J., Linkowski, P., Kerkhofs, M., Desmedt, D., Golstein, J., Copinschi, G. and Van Cauter, E. Diurnal hypersecretion of growth hormone in depression. *J. Clin. Endocrinol. Metab.*, **60**, 505–512 (1985)
49. Ho, K.Y., Evans, W.S., Blizzard, R.M., Veldhuis, J.D., Merriam, G.R., Samojlik, E., Furnaletto, R., Rogol, A.D., Kaiser, D.L. and Thorner, M.O. Effects of sex and age on the 24-hour profile of growth hormone in man: Importance of endogenous estradiol concentrations. *J. Clin. Endocrinol. Metab.*, **64**, 51–58 (1987)
50. Ho, K.Y., Veldhuis, J.D., Johnson, M.L., Furlanetto, R., Evans, W.S., Alberti, K.G.M.M. and Thorner, M.O. Fasting enhances growth hormone secretion and amplifies the complex rhythms of growth hormone secretion in man. *J. Clin. Invest.*, **81**, 968–975 (1988)
51. Parker, D.C., Rossman, L.G., Pekary, A.E. and Hershman, J.M. Effect of 64-hour sleep deprivation on the circadian waveform of thyrotropin (TSH): further evidence of sleep-related inhibition of TSH release. *J. Clin. Endocrinol. Metab.*, **64**, 157–161 (1987)
52. Vanhaelst, L., Van Cauter, E., Degaute, J.P. and Golstein, J. Circadian variations of serum thyrotropin levels in man. *J. Clin. Endocrinol. Metab.*, **35**, 479 (1972)
53. Chan, V., Jones, A., Liendoch, P., McNeilly, A., Landon, J. and Besser, B.M. The relationship between circadian variations in circulating thyrotropin, thyroid hormones and prolactin. *Clin. Endocrinol.*, **9**, 337–349 (1979)
54. Brabant, G., Brabant, A., Ranft, V., Ocran, K., Kohrle, J., Hesch, R.D. and von zur Mulhen, A. Circadian and pulsatile thyrotropin secretion in euthyroid man under the influences of thyroid hormone and glucocorticoid administration. *J. Clin. Endocrinol. Metab.*, **65**, 83–88 (1987)
55. Caron, P.J., Nieman, L.K., Rose, S.R. and Nisula, B.C. Deficient nocturnal surge of thyrotropin in central hypothyroidism. *J. Clin. Endocrinol. Metab.*, **62**, 960–964 (1986)
56. Van Cauter, E., L'Hermite, M., Copinschi, G., Refetoff, S., Desir, D. and Robyn, C. Quantitative analysis of spontaneous variations of plasma prolactin in normal men. *Amer. J. Physiol.*, **241**, E355–E363 (1981)
57. Desir, D., Van Cauter, E., L'Hermite, M., Refetoff, S., Jadot, C., Caufriez, A., Copinschi, G. and Robyn, C. Effects of 'jet lag' on hormonal patterns. III. Demonstration of an intrinsic circadian rhythmicity in plasma prolactin. *J. Clin. Endocrinol. Metab.*, **55**, 849–857 (1982)
58. Halbreich, U., Grunhaus, L. and Ben-David, M. 24-hour rhythm of prolactin in depressive patients. *Arch. Gen. Psychiat.*, **36**, 1183–1186 (1979)
59. Van Cauter, E. and Turek, F.W. Depression: a disorder of time-keeping? *Perspect. Biol. Med.*, **29**, 510–519 (1986)
60. Sensi, S. and Capani, F. Circadian rhythm of insulin-induced hypoglycemia in man. *J. Clin. Endocrinol. Metab.*, **43**, 462 (1976)
61. Bolli, G.B. and Gerich, J.E. The 'dawn phenomenon' – a common occurrence in both non-insulin-dependent and insulin-dependent diabetes mellitus. *N. Engl. J. Med.*, **310**, 746–750 (1984)
62. Lefebvre, P.J., Paolisso, G., Scheen, A.J. and Henquin, J.C. Pulsatility of insulin and glucagon release: physiological significance and pharmacological implications. *Diabetologia*, **30**, 443–452 (1987)
63. Simon, C., Follenius, M. and Brandenburger, G. Postprandial oscillations of plasma glucose, insulin and C-peptide in man. *Diabetologia*, **30**, 769–773 (1987)
64. Simon, C., Brandenburger, G. and Follenius, M. Ultradian oscillations of plasma glucose, insulin, C-peptide in man during continuous enteral nutrition. *J. Clin. Endocrinol. Metab.*, **64**, 669–674 (1987)
65. Polonsky, K.S., Given, B.D., Hirsch, L.J., Tillil, H., Shapiro, E.T., Beebe, C., Frank, B.H., Galloway, J.A. and Van Cauter, E. Abnormal patterns of insulin secretion in non-insulin-dependent diabetes mellitus. *N. Engl. J. Med.*, **318**, 1231–1240 (1988)
66. Van Coevorden, A., Laurent, E., Decoster, C., Kerkhofs, M., Neve, P., Van Cauter, E. and Mockel, J. Decreased basal and stimulated thyrotropin secretion in healthy elderly men. *J. Clin. Endocrinol. Metab.*, in press
67. Van Cauter, E., Desir, D., Decoster, C., Fery, F. and Balasse, E.O. Nocturnal decrease of glucose tolerance during constant glucose infusion. *J. Clin. Endocrinol. Metab.*, in press

Chapter 4

Circadian rhythms in the cardiovascular system

Björn Lemmer

Introduction

Chronobiology of the cardiovascular system

There is a growing body of evidence demonstrating 24-h or circadian rhythms in cardiovascular functions in experimental animals and in man. In fact, biological rhythms in heart rate (HR) and blood pressure (BP) were already described in the 19th century. In 1801 Autenrieth reported in his *Handbuch der empirischen menschlichen Physiologie* that the pulse was slower in the morning than in the evening and that daily changes also occurred in body temperature [1]. Zadek in 1881 reported a within-day variability in blood pressure, observing that it increased during the afternoon and tended to fall at night with daily variations in peak value in the range 8–15 mmHg [2]. A prominent fall in blood pressure in healthy subjects during the night was also reported by Hill in 1898 [3]. Following these early observations, numerous more sophisticated studies have provided additional convincing evidence for a circadian rhythm in heart rate and in systolic and diastolic blood pressure in both healthy subjects and in patients suffering from cardiovascular disease (for reviews see [4–6]). Figure 4.1 demonstrates that this rhythm in blood pressure can even be demonstrated in recumbent normotensive controls and patients with essential hypertension [7]. The question of separate autonomic control mechanisms for blood pressure and heart rate has been the subject of controversy. Recent findings from patients dependent on ventricular-demand pacemakers show that the circadian rhythm of blood pressure continues to persist, indicating separate autonomic control mechanisms for heart rate and blood pressure circadian rhythms [8]. This hypothesis is further supported by the observation of a circadian variation in heart rate, but not in blood pressure after heart transplantation [9].

A great deal of research on the mechanisms of action of cardiovascular active drugs has been performed in rodents. In order to compare adequately animal data with findings in human beings, it is important to take into account the fact that rodents such as rats and mice are night-active animals in contrast to day-active human beings. In consequence the acrophases of the circadian rhythms in heart rate and blood pressure in rats occur during the night.

Whilst the rhythms in heart rate and blood pressure are the best-known periodic functions in the cardiovascular system, other parameters have been shown to

52

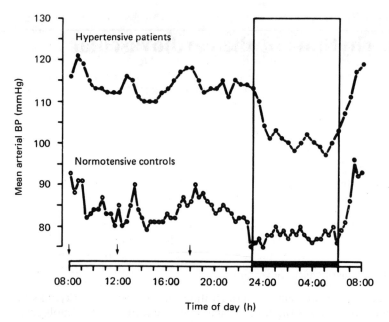

Figure 4.1 Circadian rhythm in mean arterial blood pressure in recumbent normotensives and in hypertensive patients. Arrows indicate meal times, sleep is indicated by a bar. Redrawn from ref. [7]

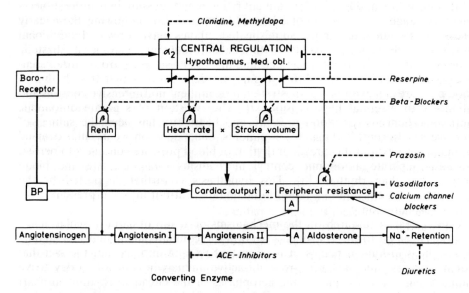

Figure 4.2 Simplified scheme of main mechanisms involved in the regulation of the blood pressure and main sites of action of antihypertensive drugs. Drug-induced blockade is indicated by ⊢------, and drug-induced stimulation by ◄-----

exhibit circadian variations as well. Some of these, pertinent for an understanding of the chronopathology of cardiovascular disease and the chrono-pharmacokinetics and -dynamics of cardiovascular active drugs, will be mentioned here (if not otherwise stated, references are compiled in the review articles mentioned above).

Figure 4.2 shows some basic mechanisms involved in the regulation of the cardiovascular system which are subject to daily variations.

Cardiovascular functions with daily variations

Blood volume in humans increases during the evening and falls at midnight. An explanation for the circadian rhythm in blood volume is not readily apparent. Blood volume is controlled by a balance between the influx and efflux of water, electrolytes, plasma proteins and red blood cells as well as by haemodynamic factors. Circadian rhythms are present in renal water and electrolyte excretion, renal plasma flow and glomerular filtration rate, with peak values during the daytime and trough values during the night (see Chapter 6). Total plasma protein, haematocrit and blood viscosity, for example, also manifest circadian rhythms with trough values late at night (see below). These may also contribute to the rhythm in blood volume. Similar findings have been obtained in rats, where the cerebral blood volume was highest at the onset of the resting period during the light phase.

Circadian rhythm in blood flow (e.g. forearm, calf) in humans peaks around the early afternoon hours with trough values at night. In rats the hepatic flow is greatest at the early activity period at night. Stroke volume and cardiac output are higher during the activity phase in humans. Capillary resistance has also been shown to vary over 24 h. A circadian rhythm in adrenergic vascular response, monitored by an increase in arterial blood pressure due to the infusion of noradrenaline, has been demonstrated in humans [10]. A dose-dependent blood pressure increase was found throughout a 24-h period. The effect, however, was more marked during the daytime and greatly reduced during the night [10]. An early morning increase in vascular reactivity, around 03:00–04:00 h, was prominent. This is of interest because an early morning rise in blood pressure has been described frequently in normotensive and hypertensive patients (see below).

Various parameters obtained from ECG recordings and cardiac functions in humans may also vary with time of day, such as PQ-, QRS-, QT-intervals, systolic time interval (STI), corrected pre-ejection period (PEPI), left ventricular ejection time (LVETI), etc. QT-intervals for example were larger during sleep than during waking hours and diurnal variations blunted in transplanted patients. Recently, no diurnal variations were found in LVETI and external isovolumic contraction time (EICT) in five normal subjects. In patients with coronary heart disease, the EICT was, however, significantly prolonged from 00:00 to 04:00 h, suggesting a decrease in left ventricular contractility in these patients [11].

Urinary and more importantly plasma or serum concentrations of noradrenaline or adrenaline in man exhibit higher values during early daytime hours than during the night, indicating a daily variation in sympathetic tone. This rhythm continued whether subjects had a normal activity/rest cycle or were recumbent over a 24-h period [7].

In agreement with these findings, plasma levels of the second messenger cyclic AMP (cAMP) in normal adults were higher during daytime activity than during nocturnal sleep. Similarly, the turnover of noradrenaline in the rat heart was significantly higher in the dark than in the light span, indicating that sympathetic tone is higher in the activity period during darkness than in the resting period during light ([12], see also [5]).

Significant daily rhythms are also present in the plasma concentrations of renin, angiotensin and aldosterone as well as in atrial natriuretic hormone [13]. The renin–angiotensin–aldosterone system constitutes another regulator of the cardiovascular system (see Figure 4.2). A circadian rhythm in plasma renin and aldosterone with peak values at, or just before, the usual time of awaking from night rest was described in subjects who remained recumbent throughout 24 h, as well as in subjects who were investigated while adhering to a normal activity/rest cycle. In night-active rats, pineal angiotensin converting enzyme (ACE) exhibited a pronounced circadian rhythm with a peak at the end of the rest period, during the daytime. If this phase relationship is true also for humans, the occurrence of increased ACE activity would be expected to coincide with peak values in angiotensin II and aldosterone, before or at the onset of the human activity cycle (see above). Thus, there is at least a coincidence in the occurrence of circadian peak values of pressor hormones, such as the catecholamines, renin, aldosterone and angiotensin II, although this coincidence might not represent a causal relationship!

Blood viscosity, haemoglobin and haematocrit as well as adrenaline or ADP-induced platelet aggregation in man display significant daily variations which are greatest during the morning hours. Red blood cell count and plasma protein concentrations are also circadian-phase-dependent. Recently it has been shown that the fibrinolytic activity is greatly reduced during early morning hours which is related to increased plasminogen activator inhibition [14] (Figure 4.3).

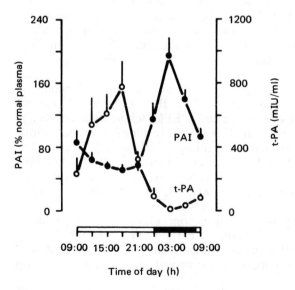

Figure 4.3 Daily variations in the plasma activities of t-PA (tissue-type plasminogen activator, ○) and PAI (plasminogen activator inhibitor, ●) over 24 h. Values are means ± s.e.m. Redrawn from ref. [14]

In rat tissues (heart, brain) significant daily rhythms are present at the level of the beta-adrenoceptor–adenylate cyclase–cAMP–phosphodiesterase system ([15] see also [36]).

These findings clearly demonstrate a pronounced rhythmic circadian organization of both the cardiovascular system and the mechanisms involved in its regulation (see Figure 4.2). This holds true for overt functions such as blood pressure and heart rate, but can be traced down to the cellular and subcellular level of the organism.

Chronopathology of the cardiovascular system

In addition to circadian rhythms in physiological functions of the cardiovascular system, various clinical reports clearly indicate that the onset of cardiovascular diseases and symptoms exhibits pronounced temporal dependency. It has already been mentioned that the circadian rhythm in blood pressure is not only conserved but is even more pronounced in most patients suffering from essential hypertension (see Figure 4.1). In patients with coronary heart disease the onset and/or number of vasospastic angina attacks as well as ECG abnormalities (ST-segment elevation, T-wave pseudonormalization) are more frequent during the night (around 04:00 h) than at other times of day (Figure 4.4). These findings in patients with Prinzmetal (vasospastic) angina pectoris have been confirmed by several groups. Moreover, the ergonovine threshold for provoking ST-segment elevation is lower at 04:00 h than at 16:00 h [16] (see Table 4.1). As already mentioned patients with coronary heart disease, but not normal subjects, are reported to show a decrease in left ventricular contractility between midnight and 04:00 h [11]. On the other hand, ST-segment depressions are registered more often during the daytime (Figure 4.4), indicating that the pathophysiological mechanisms underlying ST elevation and ST depression follow different time courses [17].

Cardiac morbidity also may be circadian-phase-dependent. Several groups have provided sound evidence that the onset of myocardial infarction, as verified by ECG recordings, blood enzymes or the MB-creatine kinase method, displays a circadian rhythm. In all of these studies a prominent peak in myocardial infarction was found around 10:00 h and sometimes an additional but smaller peak was observed around 20:00–22:00 h (Figure 4.4).

Finally, a circadian rhythm has been reported in the occurrence of cerebral infarction with a peak around 03:00 h and a trough around 15:00 h (Figure 4.4). Thus, the highest incidence of cerebral infarction coincides with the fall in blood pressure at night.

Chronopharmacology

These physiological and pathophysiological findings of circadian changes in the regulatory mechanisms and functions of the cardiovascular system clearly indicate that the effects (desired and undesired) as well as the pharmacokinetics of drugs used in the treatment of cardiovascular disorders are likely to exhibit circadian temporal dependencies as well. This has been convincingly demonstrated not only

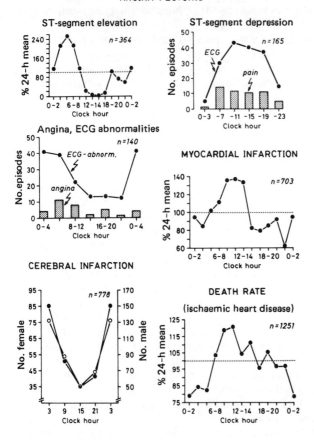

Figure 4.4 Summary of circadian-stage-dependent pathophysiological findings in cardiovascular diseases. *Angina pectoris:* ST-segment elevation in 25 patients with variant angina [18]; angina attacks and ECG abnormalities such as ST-segment elevation, T-wave pseudonormalization in 13 patients with variant angina [16]; ST-segment depression and painful episodes (*n*=165) during ambulatory monitoring in patients subsequently undergoing coronary angiography [17]. *Myocardial infarction:* Onset evaluated by the MB-creatinase method in 703 patients [19]. *Cerebral infarction:* Evaluated in 778 male (●) and female (○) patients [21]. *Death rate:* Evaluated in 1251 patients on ischaemic heart disease [20]. Figures were redrawn according to the references mentioned

in animal experiments but in human chronopharmacological studies. The references for the observations mentioned in this chapter are compiled in review articles [4–6], if not mentioned otherwise.

Beta-adrenoceptor-blocking drugs

Beta-receptor-blocking drugs are of great therapeutic value in treating various cardiovascular disorders, e.g. coronary heart disease, hypertension and arrhythmias. This group of drugs has been intensively studied in animal experiments as well as in patients in relation to circadian time. It is important to note that the various beta-receptor-blocking drugs differ not only in their specific effects (receptor affinity and selectivity, intrinsic sympathomimetic activity), but also in their non-specific effects, which are related to the lipophilicity of the various compounds. Whereas beta-adrenoceptor-blocking activity is about 100-fold greater for the (−)-isomer than for the (+)-isomer, no stereospecificity is present for the non-specific effects of these drugs. Furthermore, the beta-receptor-blocking drugs differ greatly in their main routes of elimination; lipophilic compounds are mainly biotransformed in the liver, whereas the hydrophilic ones are eliminated mainly in unchanged form by the kidney. Since both these organs exhibit 24 h bioperiodicities, differences in the pharmacokinetics of beta-receptor-blocking drugs should be studied in relation to circadian time.

The chronopharmacokinetics of various beta-receptor blocking drugs have been studied extensively only in rats. In these night-active animals the elimination half-lives in plasma, heart, lung, muscle and brain of both the lipophilic (propranolol and metoprolol) and the hydrophilic (atenolol and sotalol) beta-blockers were shorter when administered during the dark than the light span [22]. The increased elimination of the hydrophilic compounds atenolol and sotalol during the activity span is compatible with increased renal function in rats then. The increased elimination of the lipophilic compounds propranolol and metoprolol during the active period of rats, on the other hand, can be explained by an increased liver

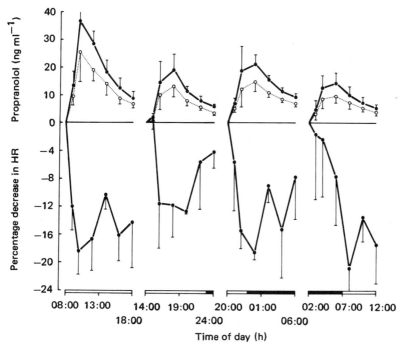

Figure 4.5 Circadian-phase-dependency in the plasma concentrations of (−)-propranolol (●—●) and (+)-propranolol (○·····○) and in heart rate decrease as % of circadian control values after oral intake of 80 mg of racemic propranolol at 08:00, 14:00, 20:00 or 02:00 h local time by four healthy volunteers. Mean values ± s.e.m. Data from ref. [24]

Table 4.1 Chronopharmacodynamics on blood pressure (BP) and heart rate (HR) of cardiovascular active drugs in man

Drug	Subjects (number of studies/subjects)	Major observation
Beta-blockers		
Atenolol[c]	Hypertensives (3/26)	Reduction in BP and HR throughout 24 h or less effective in late night and early morning
Atenolol[s]	Stable angina pectoris (1/15)	Reduction in HR throughout 24 h, rhythm preserved
Acebutolol[c]	Hypertensives (1/10)	Reduction in BP and HR, less effective at night
Labetalol[c]	Hypertensives (1/14)	Reduction in BP and HR, not significant at night
Mepindolol[c]	Hypertensives (1/20)	Reduction in BP and HR, circadian rhythm preserved
Metoprolol[c]	Hypertensives (2/17)	Reduction in BP and HR, diastolic BP less or BP not significantly reduced at night
Nadolol[c]	Hypertensives (2/23)	Reduction in BP and HR throughout 24 h or less effective during early morning
Oxprenolol[c]	Hypertensives (1/20)	Reduction in BP and HR, less effective at night and early morning
Pindolol[c]	Hypertensives (1/9)	Reduction in BP mainly during daytime, HR only reduced during early daytime, no effect at night
Pindolol[s]	Stable angina pectoris (1/15)	Reduction in HR only during daytime, HR increased at late night
Propranolol[c]	Hypertensives (2/23)	Decrease in BP and HR, rhythm preserved
Propranolol[c]	Stable angina pectoris (1/30)	HR and ST-segment displacement during exercise significantly greater at 16:00 h than at 08:00 h and 12:00 h
Propranolol[a]	Healthy (2/10)	BP decrease longer lasting at 02:00 h; T_{max} decrease in HR shortest at 08:00 h, longest after R_x at 20:00 h (Figure 4.5)
Pindolol + clopamide[c]	Hypertensives (1/16)	BP and HR reduction throughout 24 h
Timolol + hydrochloro- thiazide + amiloride[c]	Hypertensives (1/18)	BP and HR reduction throughout 24 h
Calcium channel blockers		
Verapamil[c]	Hypertensives (1/16)	BP and HR decrease, particularly during day
Nifedipine[c]	Hypertensives (1/16)	Constant decrease in BP over 24 h, most marked during day, HR unaffected
Nitrendipine[c]	Hypertensives (1/22)	BP not reduced during sleep, HR increase during early morning and no effect at other times
Other antihypertensives		
Clonidine[c]	Hypertensive children (1/15)	No significant effects on 24-h rhythms in LH, FSH, prolactin, cortisol, aldosterone, testosterone
Clonidine[c] (transdermal disk)	Hypertensives (1/7)	BP reduction during day, not investigated at night
Indoramine[c]	Hypertensives (1/12)	BP and HR reduction over 24 h, less significant at night, circadian rhythm preserved
Prazosin[c]	Hypertensives (2/25)	BP reduction during day and early night, no effect on early morning rise; or nearly no effect on BP and HR circadian rhythms

Drug	Subjects (number of studies/subjects)	Major observation
Methyldopa + cyclopen- thiazide[c]	Hypertensives (1/15)	Decrease in BP, circadian rhythm preserved
Captopril[c]	Healthy (1/4)	Plasma aldosterone rhythm not altered
Xipamide[c]	Hypertensives (1/18)	BP reduction over 24 h, circadian rhythm preserved
Antianginal drugs		
Glyceryl trinitrate[a]	Variant angina (1/13)	At 06:00 h exercise-induced attacks and ST-segment elevation prevented by drug; no effect at 15:00 h; increase in coronary artery diameter by drug at 06:00 h but not at 15:00 h
Isosorbide dinitrate[a]	Healthy (1/6)	Decrease in standing systolic BP and HR increase most pronounced at R_x at 02:00 h than at 08:00 h, 14:00 h, 20:00 h
Isosorbide 5- mononitrate (immediate release)[a]	Healthy (1/8)	Decrease in standing BP and increase in HR more pronounced at R_x at 06:30 h than 18:30 h; at 18:30 h peak effects before peak drug concentration
Isosorbide 5- mononitrate (retard)[a]	Healthy (1/10)	T_{max} in standing BP decrease and HR increase shorter after R_x at 20:00 h than at 08:00 h; at 20:00 h peak effects before peak drug concentration
Others		
Ergonovine[c]	Variant angina pectoris (1/13)	Ergonovine threshold at which attacks occurred lower in morning than afternoon
Heparin[s] (48 h infusion)[s]	Thrombo- embolism (1/6)	Significant rhythms in thromboplastin time, thrombin time, Factor Xa inhibition assay (Figure 4.10)
Potassium chloride (infusion)[a]	Healthy (1/5)	ST-segment elevation greater after R_x at 24:00 h than at 12:00 h
Phenylpro- panolamine[s]	Healthy (1/18)	No pressor effects on circadian rhythms in systolic and diastolic BP, HR increased at night

[c]Chronic drug application
[a]Acute drug application
[s]Subacute drug application
References for data: [5,6,24,26,28–33]

blood flow during this period thus leading to their more rapid hepatic metabolism in the dark phase.

In man, only the pharmacokinetics of propranolol have been studied in relation to time of day [23,24]. Significant daily variations in peak drug concentration (C_{max}), area under the curve (AUC) and elimination half-life have been reported when racemic propranolol was administered at four circadian times (08:00, 14:00, 20:00, 02:00 h) to healthy subjects. As shown in Figure 4.5 trough values in C_{max} and AUC were found after drug application at 02:00 h and peak values in C_{max} and AUC were obtained with R_x at 08:00 h [24]. As has been shown for other lipophilic drugs [25], the absorption of propranolol was clearly circadian-stage-dependent, being greatest when ingested at 08:00 h [24] (Figure 4.5). At any time of drug intake the ratio of the plasma concentrations of (−)- to (+)-propranolol was about

1.5 [24] (see Figure 4.5). Thus, the stereospecific metabolism of propranolol did not display a circadian-phase-dependency. Interestingly, in man shorter elimination half-lives of either (−)- or (+)-propranolol were found when the drug was given at 08:00 h rather than at 20:00 h (Figure 4.5). Taking into consideration the phase difference in the activity/rest cycle of rat and man, the chronopharmacokinetic data obtained in humans are in excellent accordance with all those found in rodents.

Considerably more data are available on the circadian-stage-dependent cardiovascular effects of beta-receptor-blocking drugs (Table 4.1). These drugs decrease cardiac output by reducing both heart rate and stroke volume and antagonize the release of renin (see Figure 4.2). In addition, they may reset the baroreceptor reflex and have central antisympathotonic effects. Various groups have convincingly demonstrated that beta-receptor-blocking drugs reduce high blood pressure and heart rate in hypertensive patients more profoundly during the day than during the night when taken regularly (Table 4.1). However, the early morning rise in blood pressure seems either to be not affected, or only slightly reduced, by chronic beta-receptor blockade. Results of a representative study obtained with the beta-blocker oxprenolol in hypertensive patients are shown in Figure 4.6. This pattern in the circadian-stage-dependent effects was, in general,

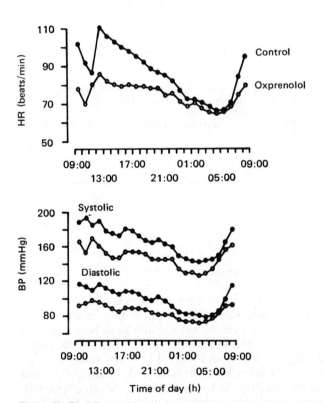

Figure 4.6 Circadian rhythms in heart rate and blood pressure in 20 hypertensive patients before and after 6 weeks of chronic treatment with the beta-blocker oxprenolol. Redrawn from ref. [26]

observed with all the different beta-blockers studied (Table 4.1). The pattern was found regardless of whether lipophilic (e.g. propranolol, oxprenolol) or hydrophilic (e.g. atenolol), non-selective (e.g. propranolol, oxprenolol, pindolol) or relative β_1-selective (e.g. atenolol, metoprolol) compounds were applied, or whether the drugs are known to be eliminated mainly by hepatic metabolism (lipophilic ones) or by renal excretion (hydrophilic ones). However, it is interesting to note that a beta-blocker with intrinsic sympathomimetic activity, pindolol, did not only not reduce, but even increased heart rate at night (Table 4.1), at a time at which sympathetic tone is low. Quite a similar effect on heart rate at night has been described for the sympathomimetic drug phenylpropanolamine [29], which is used as an anorectic drug (see Table 4.1). These data already indicate that the circadian rhythm in sympathetic tone may be of utmost importance in influencing the magnitude of beta-receptor blockade in the course of 24 h. Furthermore, Table 4.1 suggests that the combination of a beta-blocker and a diuretic, the latter having a different site of action, see Figure 4.2, reduces high blood pressure and heart rate throughout 24 h.

Circadian-stage-dependent effects of propranolol have also been described after a single oral drug application to healthy subjects. Figure 4.5 illustrates the changes in heart rate in relation to corresponding circadian control values. These changes were markedly different depending on the time of propranolol ingestion (Table 4.1). The most interesting finding of this study was that after administration of propranolol at 02:00 h the heart rate was only slightly affected for about 6 h. However, 2 h later, at the onset of the activity span when sympathetic tone is high, the effect of propranolol on the heart rate was more pronounced and with a time course about equal to that found after drug application at 08:00 h [24]. Plasma concentrations of propranolol at these two time points, on the other hand, differed by a factor of about three (Figure 4.5).

The results found in humans with propranolol are in good agreement with those obtained on the heart rate of conscious rats [12,22]. In this species beta-receptor blockade by propranolol also reduced heart rate more effectively when administered in a dose-dependent way during the activity period at night compared with during rest in the light phase [22]. In view of these findings it is evident that the reactivity of the sympathetic nervous system to beta-receptor blockade is comparable in man and rats taking into consideration the phase difference between these two species in the activity/rest cycle as well as in sympathetic tone.

In view of the above findings, it is evident that the chronopharmacokinetics of beta-receptor blockers do not explain the more pronounced cardiovascular effects that occur during the activity period of both man and rat. In consequence, it has been assumed that the day/night variation in drug effects may be due to temporal changes in the sensitivity of the target organs to beta-receptor blockade. There is evidence for a daily variation in vascular reactivity (see above), and the circadian-phase-dependency in the effects of the beta-blockers is also in favour of this hypothesis. In further support of this assumption are a number of observations in rats concerning daily rhythms in sympathetic function at the cellular and subcellular level [5,12,15,22]. Biochemical studies in rat heart ventricles and in rat forebrain have shown pronounced temporal variation in the basal level of the second messenger cAMP as well as in the activities of the enzymes involved in its formation (adenylate cyclase) and hydrolysis (phosphodiesterase). Beta-receptor affinity and/or number either did not vary or changed only slightly with time of day [15].

All these examples demonstrate that both the pharmacokinetics and the effects of a drug (chronesthesy) can vary clearly with time of the day. The data also suggest that the extent of beta-receptor blockade by propranolol at different times of day is related more to the circadian rhythm in sympathetic tone and cardiovascular responsiveness than to the drug's chronopharmacokinetics (see also, Chapter 12).

It is of interest to note that even seasonal variations in blood pressure of hypertensive patients were maintained during chronic administration with the beta-blocker propranolol or the diuretic bendrofluazide (Figure 4.7), indirectly indicating seasonal variations in sympathetic tone.

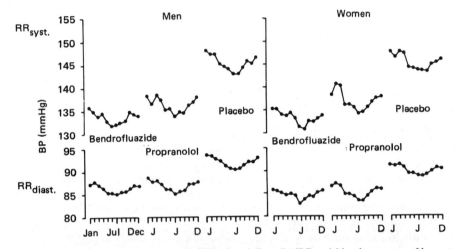

Figure 4.7 Seasonal variation in systolic (RR_{sys}) and diastolic (RR_{diast}) blood pressures of hypertensive men and women after placebo or treatment with either propanolol or bendrofluazide. Redrawn from ref. [27]

Circadian-stage-dependent effects of propranolol have also been described in patients with stable angina pectoris [28]. In 30 male Caucasian patients, exercise-limited effects on heart rate and ST-segment depression in the ECG have been studied at three different times of day with and without propranolol treatment (Table 4.1). Under control conditions as well as under treatment with propranolol, maximum increases in heart rate and ST-segment depression occurred when exercise was scheduled at 16:00 h rather than at 08:00 h and 12:00 h (Figure 4.8), indicating that exercise is better tolerated in the afternoon than in the early morning.

A relative imbalance in myocardial oxygen demand and supply in the early morning hours [31] may be due to the interaction of various factors already mentioned, such as circadian rhythms in blood pressure and heart rate (see Figures 4.1 and 4.6), plasma noradrenaline, blood viscosity, platelet aggregability and inhibition of fibrinolytic activity (see Figure 4.3). These factors could contribute to a lower threshold for the development of myocardial ischaemia leading to myocardial infarction and sudden death [31] (Figure 4.4) more often in the early morning than at other times of day.

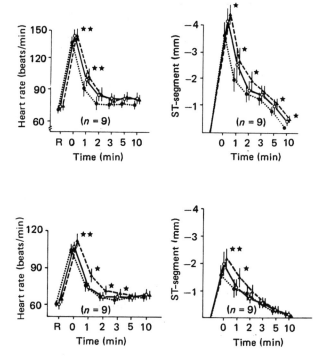

Figure 4.8 Circadian-stage-dependency in exercise-limited increase in heart rate and ST-segment depression in nine Caucasian patients with stable angina pectoris without (upper part) or with chronic therapy with propranolol (lower part). Exercise was performed at 08:00 (●), 12:00 (○) or 16:00 h (▲). *$P<0.05$, **$P<0.025$ for difference between exercise at 16:00 and 08:00 h. Redrawn from ref. [28]

Calcium channel blockers

Calcium channel blockers (calcium antagonists) are used in the treatment of coronary heart disease and in the treatment of hypertension. Drugs like verapamil, diltiazem, nifedipine and nitrendipine decrease the free intracellular calcium concentration in the heart leading to a reduction in oxygen demand. They also have a relaxing effect on vascular smooth muscle. Calcium channel blockers of the verapamil-type and diltiazem have a more prominent cardiac effect (i.e. negative chronotropic effect), whereas those of the dihydropyridine-type (nifedipine, nitrendipine) have a more dominant vasodilating effect. With the latter compounds it is even possible to observe a reflex-induced increase in heart rate. Chronopharmacological studies in hypertensive patients have shown that, in general, the blood-pressure-lowering effect of these drugs is more marked during daytime than during night (Table 4.1). During sleep, nitrendipine had no effect on blood pressure. More interestingly, however, the difference in the predominant site of action of the two groups of calcium channel blockers (cardiac versus vascular) can clearly be observed in their effects on the circadian rhythm in heart rate. Whereas verapamil reduced heart rate (slightly more pronounced during day), nifedipine had no effect on heart rate and nitrendipine even increased heart rate during the early morning hours (Table 4.1).

Other antihypertensives

Clonidine is known to reduce high blood pressure by decreasing centrally mediated sympathetic tone mainly via stimulation of central alpha-2-adrenoceptors (Figure 4.2). Chronic treatment of hypertensive patients with clonidine applied by a transdermal disk reduced blood pressure during the daytime (Table 4.1): no measurements were reported at night. Clonidine did not affect the rhythms of various hormones in hypertensive children (Table 4.1).

After a combined treatment with methyldopa (see Figure 4.2) and a diuretic, the circadian rhythm in blood pressure was maintained, although the 24-h level was reduced relative to the pretreatment value (Table 4.1). Alpha-adrenoceptor-blocking drugs such as indoramine and prazosin (see Figure 4.2) had quite similar effects on the circadian rhythms in blood pressure and heart rate to those already described for beta-blockers (Table 4.1). In one study, however, prazosin did not have any effect on these rhythms (Table 4.1). Thus, at least these data do not provide convincing evidence for a crucial role of alpha-adrenoceptors in the regulation of the early rise in blood pressure.

Diuretics are among the drugs of first choice in the treatment of hypertension. They are known to decrease peripheral vascular resistance by inhibiting sodium retention (Figure 4.3). Hydrochlorothiazide-induced diuresis and electrolyte excretion were more pronounced in healthy subjects, if the drug was administered during the daytime hours rather than during the night. A higher sodium/potassium ratio after dosing late in the afternoon indicates minimal potassium loss after drug application at this time of the day [6]. The antihypertensive effects of the diuretic xipamide have been studied after chronic dosing in hypertensive patients. Xipamide reduced the level of elevated blood pressure throughout 24 h (Table 4.1). The fact that this diuretic also reduced the early morning rise in blood pressure may explain why a consistent 24-h decrease in high blood pressure has been described for combined treatment with beta-blocking drugs and diuretics as already mentioned above (see Table 4.1).

Antianginal drugs

As already described, the onset of angina pectoris and the frequency of angina attacks exhibit a circadian rhythm (Figure 4.4), a finding that has been confirmed by many authors [5,6]. It is therefore not surprising that antianginal drugs may also exert circadian-phase-dependent effects in patients with variant (Prinzmetal) or stable angina pectoris. The first evidence for this was provided by the classical paper of Yasue et al. [34]: in this study 13 patients with Prinzmetal's variant angina performed treadmill exercise tests in the early morning (05:00–08:00 h) and again in the afternoon (13:00–16:00 h). Exercise-induced angina attacks as well as ECG abnormalities occurred in all patients in the morning, but in only two patients in the afternoon. Interestingly, glyceryl trinitrate administration in the morning prevented the angina attacks and had a greater dilating effect on the coronary vessel than when given in the afternoon (Figure 4.9, Table 4.1), indicating temporal variations in vasomotor tone. Essentially the same results were obtained with the calcium channel blocker diltiazem, whereas propranolol aggravated the symptoms when given in the early morning. This study clearly demonstrated for the first time that exercise-induced coronary spasm was dependent on the time of the day at which the exercise challenge was performed. Supporting this hypothesis and the

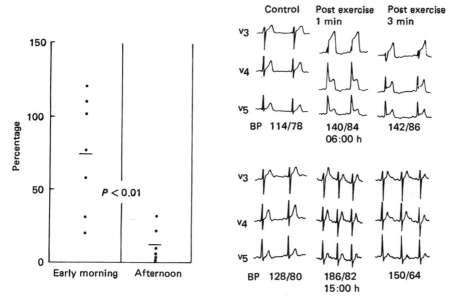

Figure 4.9 Circadian-stage-dependency in exercise ECG (right; one patient) and glyceryl trinitrate-induced percentage increase in coronary artery diameter (left; 13 patients) in patients with Prinzmetal angina pectoris. Redrawn from ref. [34]

time-dependency of medication, the authors of the glyceryl trinitrate study demonstrated an increase in patency of the great coronary arteries, induced by this drug when taken in the morning but not when taken in the afternoon (Figure 4.9). Similar findings in patients with stable angina pectoris without and with treatment by propranolol were mentioned above (see Figure 4.8). Further support for a daily variation in arterial hyper-reactivity comes from the study on patients with variant angina pectoris in whom the threshold of ergonovine (an alpha-adrenoceptor-stimulating secale alkaloid)-provoked angina attacks was lower in the morning than in the afternoon [16] (Table 4.1).

The chronopharmacology of the oral nitrates isosorbide dinitrate (ISDN) and isosorbide 5-mononitrate (IS-5-MN) has been investigated only in preliminary studies after acute dosing in healthy subjects ([6] and unpublished results). ISDN-induced decreases in blood pressure and increases in heart rate (standing position) were found after night-time dosing, even though peak concentrations of ISDN occurred after the morning dosing. Recently, daily variations were also seen in the pharmacokinetics of an immediate-release preparation of IS-5-MN with T_{max} being 0.9 and 2.1 h at R_x of 06:30 h and 18:30 h respectively. A decrease in standing blood pressure and increase in heart rate occurred at about 0.6–1.0 h after drug ingestion at either dosing time, thus providing evidence for a dissociation in time between peak drug concentrations and peak effects during the evening hours. Similar results were obtained after oral dosing of a IS-5-MN retard formulation at either 08:00 h or 20:00 h. The maximum decrease in standing blood pressure and increase in heart rate occurred about 3 h, after drug intake at 20:00 h but about 5–6 h after drug intake at 08:00 h. Most interestingly, no circadian-phase-dependency was observed in the pharmacokinetics of this retard preparation; at either dosing time peak drug concentrations were found after about 6 h. These data clearly demonstrate that the drug formulation may influence the pharmacokinetic profile of a drug when taken at different times of day. Studies are in progress to investigate the pharmacokinetics and cardiovascular effects of these oral nitrates at different circadian stages in patients with coronary heart disease.

Other drugs

Inhibitors of angiotensin-converting enzyme (ACE, see Figure 4.2) are also used in the treatment of hypertension. Captopril and enalapril were recently shown to affect the circadian rhythm in blood pressure of hypertensive patients similarly [38,39] to that shown for the beta-blockers. The ACE-inhibitor captopril was reported not to influence the circadian rhythm of plasma aldosterone in healthy subjects (Table 4.1). In humans there are no data concerning the possible circadian-phase-dependency of the antihypertensive effects of reserpine. In studies in rats, noradrenaline depletion due to reserpine was more pronounced in the period of increased sympathetic tone during the nocturnal activity span. Reserpine-induced decreases in heart rate in conscious rats were also more pronounced in the dark than in the light phase ([5,36] and unpublished results).

Recently, a significantly higher bioavailability and higher C_{max} values of oral digoxin have been described after morning (07:00 h) than after evening (19:00 h) application to elderly male subjects [40].

A circadian-stage-dependent variation in the pharmacokinetics and cardiac effect of intravenously infused potassium chloride has been reported in healthy subjects (Table 4.1). Plasma potassium concentration was about 40% higher after infusion at midnight than at noon. Since the urinary potassium excretion was less at midnight than at noon, plasma potassium levels apparently reflect a 24-h fluctuation in renal potassium excretion. Thus it was not surprising that the ST-segment elevation in the ECG resulting from potassium infusion at midnight was more than twice that found at noon [35]. Certainly, in the case of infused potassium chloride the circadian-stage-dependent pharmacokinetics of the drug greatly contributes to the circadian variation in its side effects.

Clinical implications

There is virtually no system other than the cardiovascular, in which so much evidence indicates that all its functions display a pronounced circadian variation. Furthermore, pathophysiological events in cardiovascular diseases are circadian-phase-dependent as well. Such knowledge is pertinent to the diagnosis and drug treatment of cardiovascular disease. This circadian rhythmicity also has implications for the evaluation of drugs used in the treatment of cardiovascular diseases [6,36].

Since blood pressure in hypertensive patients varies markedly with time of day, the time at which blood pressure measurements are taken has to be controlled by the patient as well as by the medical staff, whether or not the patient is under antihypertensive treatment. Similarly, a careful evaluation of the circadian time structure of angina attacks has to precede any kind of drug treatment.

The published data on the chronopharmacology of cardiovascular active drugs may have clinical implications: it is quite evident that the pharmacokinetics as well

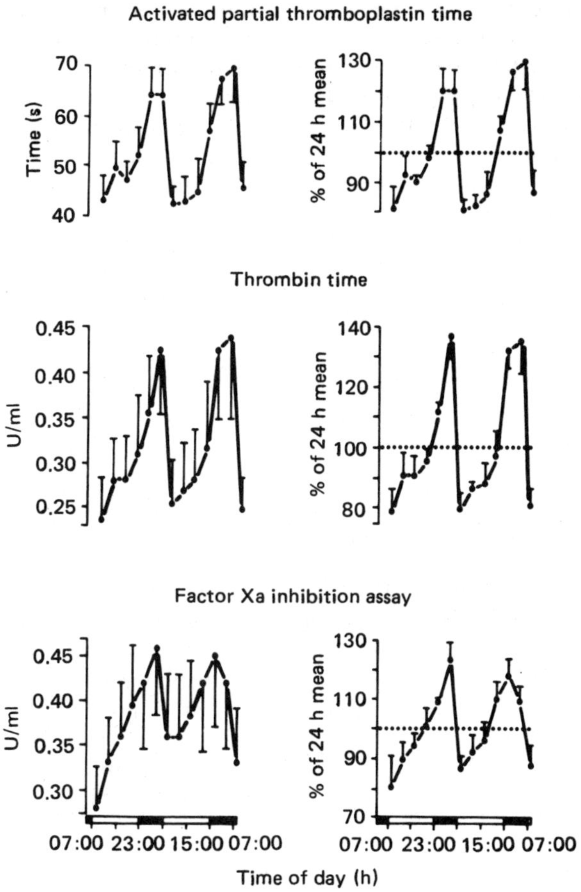

Figure 4.10 Circadian rhythms in anticoagulant effects of heparin infused at a constant rate over 48 h in patients suffering from thromboembolism. Redrawn from ref. [37]

as the effects of these drugs display within-day variability in both healthy subjects and patients. These data call for a careful re-evaluation of conventional regimens of drug treatment. First of all, these findings, together with the rhythmic organization of all functions of the cardiovascular system, make the assumption unlikely that 'therapeutic ranges' really do exist in drug treatment. Recently published findings for heparin in patients with thromboembolism [37] clearly demonstrate that treatment designed to achieve a constant drug level throughout 24 h may be unwise. In this study heparin was infused at a constant rate over 48 h, and thromboplastin time, thrombin time and Factor Xa inhibition were evaluated at 4-h intervals (Table 4.1). Significant circadian rhythms in the effects of heparin were found; the peak-to-trough variation in thromboplastin time for the individual patient, for example, was in the range 40–60% of the respective 24-h mean (Figure 4.10). Most importantly, the greatest anticoagulant effect consistently occurred early in the night during each day of the 48-h infusion (Figure 4.10); this was the time when bleeding was most often observed. Since heparin and other anticoagulants are used in the prophylaxis and treatment of thromboembolic occlusive vascular disease, such as venous thrombosis and myocardial infarction, these chronopharmacological findings are of great clinical importance.

There is further evidence disproving the hypothesis that constant drug levels will result in constant effects at different times: in patients with coronary heart disease continuous transdermal application of ISDN may rapidly induce nitrate tolerance. Since this phenomenon has important therapeutic implications, it is of interest to evaluate the chronophysiological and chronopathophysiological features of these patients together with the chronopharmacology of organic nitrates in order better to understand the mechanisms of nitrate tolerance and to treat patients more efficiently.

In the drug treatment of hypertension it seems reasonable to assume that beta-receptor-blocking drugs and calcium channel blockers are of less value when applied in late afternoon or at night. Elevated blood pressure has to be treated when it is high. Nightly application of antihypertensive drugs may lead to too great a reduction in cerebral blood pressure and cerebral infarction may occur (Figure 4.4). On the other hand, there are some indications that a combination of beta-blockers and diuretics may reduce the early morning increase in blood pressure.

In conclusion, the data already published on the chronopharmacology of cardiovascular active drugs indicate that a constant drug delivery over 24 h is not what the diseased patient needs. First of all, it cannot be assumed that a constant drug supply really leads to constant drug levels, unless this has been shown convincingly. Secondly, even if the drug level is maintained throughout 24 h, it cannot be assumed that this will also result in constant drug effects. Thus, in order to improve drug therapy, future developments of drug delivery systems, including retard formulations, transdermal applications and even mechanical pumps, must take into consideration the pronounced rhythmic organization of biological functions.

References

1. Autenrieth, J.H.F. *Handbuch der empirischen Physiologie*, Teil 1. Jakob Friedrich Heerbrandt, Tübingen (1801)
2. Zadek, J. Die Messung des Blutdrucks des Menschen mittels des Bach'schen Apparates. *Z. Klin. Med.*, **2**, 509–551 (1881)
3. Hill, L. On rest, sleep and work and the concomitant changes in the circulation of the blood. *Lancet, i*, 282–285 (1898)
4. Smolensky, M.H., Tatar, S.E., Bergmann, S.A., Losmann, J.G., Barnard, C.N., Dacso, C.C. and Kraft, I.A. Circadian rhythmic aspects of human cardiovascular function: a review by chronobiologic statistical methods. *Chronobiologia*, **3**, 337–371 (1976)
5. Lemmer, B. The chronopharmacology of cardiovascular medications. *Annu. Rev. Chronopharmacol.*, **2**, 199–258 (1986)
6. Lemmer, B. Cardiovascular medications. In *Klinische Pharmakologie* (eds H.-P. Kuemmerle, G. Hitzenberger and K.H. Spitzy), *Landsberg München, ecomed Verlagsgesellschaft*, **4**, Auflage – 12. Erg. Lfg. 11/87, pp. 1–14 (1987)
7. Tuck, M.L., Stern, N. and Sowers, J.R. Enhanced 24-h norepinephrine and renin secretion in young patients with essential hypertension: relation with the circadian pattern of arterial blood pressure. *Amer. J. Cardiol.*, **55**, 112–115 (1985)
8. Davies, A.B., Gould, B.A., Cashman, P.M.M. and Raftery, E.B. Circadian rhythm of blood pressure in patients dependent on ventricular demand pacemaker. *Brit. Heart J.*, **52**, 93–98 (1984)

9. Wenting, G.J., von der Meiracker, A.H., Simoons, M.L., Bos, E., Ritsema von Eck, H.J. and Schalekamp, M.A.D.H. Circadian variation of heart rate but not of blood pressure after heart transplantation. *Transplant. Proc.*, **19**, 2554–2555 (1987)

10. Hossmann, V., FitzGerald, G.A. and Dollery, C.T. Circadian rhythm of baroreflex reactivity and adrenergic vascular response. *Cardiovasc. Res.*, **14**, 125–129 (1980)

11. Aronow, W.S., Harding, P.R., ·DeQuattro, V. and Isbell, M. Diurnal variation of plasma catecholamines and systolic time intervals. *Chest*, **63**, 722–726 (1973)

12. Lemmer, B., Bathe, K., Lang, P.-H., Neumann, G. and Winkler, H. Chronopharmacology of β-adrenoceptor blocking drugs: Pharmacokinetic and pharmacodynamic studies in rats. *J. Amer. Coll. Toxicol.*, **2**, 347–358 (1983)

13. Donicker, J., Anderson, J.V., Yeo, T. and Bloom, S.R. Diurnal rhythm in the plasma concentration of atrial natriuretic peptide. *N. Engl. J. Med.*, **315**, 710–711 (1986)

14. Andreotti, F., Davies, G.J., Hackett, D.R., Khan, M.I., De Bart, A.C.W., Aber, V.R., Maseri, A. and Kluft, C. Major circadian fluctuations in fibrinolytic factors and possible relevance to time of onset of myocardial infarction, sudden cardiac death and stroke. *Amer. J. Cardiol.*, **62**, 635–637 (1988)

15. Lemmer, B., Bärmeier, H., Schmidt, S. and Lang, P.-H. On the daily variation in the beta-receptor – adenylate cyclase – cAMP – phosphodiesterase – system in rat forebrain. *Chronobiol. Int.*, **4**, 469–475 (1987)

16. Waters, D.D., Miller, D.D., Bouchard, A., Bosch, X. and Theroux, P. Circadian variation in variant angina. *Amer. J. Cardiol.*, **54**, 61–64 (1984)

17. von Arnim, T., Höfling, B. and Schreiber, M. Characteristics of episodes of ST elevation or ST depression during ambulatory monitoring in patients subsequently undergoing coronary angiography. *Brit. Heart J.*, **54**, 484–488 (1985)

18. Araki, H., Koiwaya, Y., Nakagaki, O. and Nakamura, M. Diurnal distribution of ST-segment elevation and related arrhythmias in patients with variant angina: a study by ambulatory ECG monitoring. *Circulation*, **67**, 995–1000 (1983)

19. Muller, J.E., Stone, P.H., Turin, Z.G., Rutherford, J.G., Czeisler, C.A., Parkers, C., Poole, W.K., Passamani, E., Roberts, R., Robertson, T., Sobel, B.E., Willerson, J.T. and Braunwald, E. The Milis study group: Circadian variation in the frequency of onset of acute myocardial infarction. *N. Engl. J. Med.*, **313**, 1315–1322 (1985)

20. Mitler, M.M., Hajdukovic, R.M., Shafor, R., Hahn, P.M. and Kripke, D.F. When people die. Cause of death versus time of death. *Amer. J. Med.*, **82**, 266–274 (1987)

21. Marshall, J., Diurnal variation in occurrence of strokes. *Stroke*, **8**, 230–231 (1977)

22. Lemmer, B., Winkler, H., Ohm, T. and Fink, M. Chronopharmacokinetics of beta-receptor blocking drugs of different lipophilicity (propranolol, metoprolol, sotalol, atenolol) in plasma and tissues after single and multiple dosing in the rat. *Naunyn-Schmiedeberg's Arch. Pharmacol.*, **330**, 42–49 (1985)

23. Semenowicz-Siuda, K., Markiewicz, A. and Korczynska-Wardecka, J. Circadian bioavailability and some effects of propranolol in healthy subjects and liver cirrhosis. *Int. J. Clin. Pharmacol. Ther. Toxicol.*, **22**, 653–658 (1984)

24. Langner, B. and Lemmer, B. Circadian changes in the pharmacokinetics and cardiovascular effects of oral propranolol in healthy subjects. *Eur. J. Clin. Pharmacol.*, **33**, 619–624 (1988)

25. Lemmer, B. *Chronopharmakologie – Tagesrhythmen und Arzneimittelwirkung*, 2nd edn, Wiss. Verlagsges., Stuttgart (1984)

26. Raftery, E.B., Millar-Craig, M.W., Mann, S. and Balasubramanian, V. Effects of treatment on circadian rhythms of blood pressure. *Biotelem. Pat. Monitor.*, **8**, 113–120 (1981)

27. Brennan, P.J., Greenberg, G., Miall, W.E. and Thompson, S.G. Seasonal variation in arterial blood pressure. *Brit. Med. J.*, **285**, 919–923 (1982)

28. Joy, M., Pollard, C.M. and Nunan, T.O. Diurnal variation in exercise in angina pectoris. *Br. Heart J.*, **48**, 156–160 (1982)

29. Goodman, R.P., Wright, J.T., Barlascini, C.O., McKenney, J.M. and Lambert, C.M. The effect of phenylpropanolamine on ambulatory blood pressure. *Clin. Pharmacol. Ther.*, **40**, 144–147 (1986)

30. Magometschnigg, D. and Hitzenberger, G. (eds) *Blutdruckvariabilität*, Uhlen Verlagsgesellschaft, Wien (1983)

31. Rocco, M.B., Nabel, E.G. and Selwyn, A.P. Circadian rhythms and coronary artery disease. *Amer. J. Cardiol.*, **59**, 13C–17C (1987)
32. White, W.B., Smith, V.E., McCabe, E.J. and Meeran, M.K. Effects of chronic nitrendipine on casual (office) and 24-h ambulatory blood pressure. *Clin. Pharmacol. Ther.*, **38**, 60–64 (1985)
33. Mancia, G., Ferrari, A., Pomidossi, G., Parati, G., Bertinieri, G., Grassi, G., Gregorini, L., diRienzo, M. and Zanchetti, A. Twenty-four-hour blood pressure profile and blood pressure variability in untreated hypertension and during antihypertensive treatment by once-a-day nadolol. *Amer. Heart J.*, **108**, 1078–1083 (1984)
34. Yasue, H., Omote, S., Takizawa, A., Nagao, M., Miwa, K. and Tanaka, S. Circadian variation of exercise capacity in patients with Prinzmetal's variant angina: role of exercise-induced coronary arterial spasm. *Circulation*, **59**, 938–948 (1979)
35. Moore-Ede, M.C., Meguid, M.M., FitzPatrick, G.F., Boyden, C.M. and Ball, M.R. Circadian variation in response to potassium infusion. *Clin. Pharmacol. Ther.*, **23**, 218–227 (1978)
36. Lemmer, B. (ed). *Chronopharmacology – Cellular and Biochemical Interactions.* Marcel Dekker, New York, Basel (1989)
37. Decousos, H.A., Croze, M., Levi, F.A., Jaubert, J.G., Perpoint, B.M., DeBonadonna, J.F., Reinberg, A. and Queneau, P.M. Circadian changes in anticoagulant effect of heparin infused at constant rate. *Brit. Med. J.*, **290**, 341–344 (1985)
38. Boxho, G. Twenty-four-hour blood pressure recording during treatment with captopril twice daily. *Curr. Ther. Res.*, **44**, 361-366 (1988)
39. Blankenstijn, P.J., Wenting, G.J. and Schalekamp, M.A.D.H. 24-Hour blood pressure profiles during ACE inhibition. A comparative study of twice daily captopril versus once daily enalapril. *International Symposium on ACE Inhibition*, London, Abstr. F164 (1989)
40. Bruguerolle, B., Bouvenot, G., Bartolin, R. and Manolis, J. Chronopharmacocinétique de la digoxine chez le sujet de plus de soixante-dix ans. *Therapie*, **43**, 251–253 (1988)

Chapter 5

Circadian rhythms in the respiratory system

Peter J. Barnes

Introduction

Recently there has been considerable interest in circadian rhythms in respiratory medicine, since this provides an explanation for the worsening of lung function at night in patients with asthma and, to a lesser extent, chronic bronchitis. Nocturnal and early morning wheezing have been recognized since the first known descriptions of asthma. Dr John Floyer, in 1698, clearly described his own attacks of asthma, which occurred exclusively at night over a period of 7 years [1]. Nocturnal asthma is a common and troublesome symptom; one survey showed that approximately 75% of all asthmatics attending a hospital clinic admitted to nocturnal wheeze and cough [2], and a more recent survey in general practice demonstrated that as many as 85% of 8000 patients continued to report nocturnal symptoms, despite therapy, and over 50% woke with asthma at night more than once a week [3]. Because some asthmatics may have no symptoms during the day, the diagnosis is often overlooked. The clinical importance of this symptom is emphasized by the finding that many sudden deaths and episodes of ventilatory arrest occur at night [4], and in a prospective study of high-risk asthmatics two deaths occurred in patients with marked early morning bronchoconstriction [5].

Despite the common occurrence of nocturnal asthma it is only recently that the underlying mechanisms have become better understood. Three hundred years ago Thomas Willis suggested that wheezing at night might be explained by overheating of the blood by the bedclothes and, since then, many explanations for nocturnal wheezing have been proposed [6,7] (Table 5.1).

Table 5.1 Possible mechanisms of nocturnal asthma

Allergen exposure – allergens in bedding
                     – late-reaction
                     – bronchial hyper-responsiveness
Supine posture
Sleep
Timing of bronchodilator administration
Gastro-oesophageal reflux
Impaired mucociliary clearance
Airway cooling
Circadian rhythms

Proposed mechanisms of nocturnal asthma

Allergens

Many years ago it was suggested that exposure to allergens, such as house dust mite and feathers in bedding, might precipitate wheezing at night, yet allergen avoidance provided little benefit. Recently, more rigorous exclusion of house dust mite allergen has been shown to decrease bronchial reactivity and early morning wheeze [8]. Nocturnal asthma could represent a late reaction to allergens inhaled during the day. Experimental inhalation of antigen can cause nocturnal wheezing which may persist over several days [9]. Although allergen-induced bronchocon-striction, particularly the induced hyper-responsiveness, may contribute to nocturnal wheezing it is unlikely to be the major cause since nocturnal asthma is as frequent in intrinsic asthmatics [2]. It is more likely to be the non-specific hyper-responsiveness *per se* that is the critical factor, as discussed below (see also Chapters 7 and 13).

Sleep

The supine posture is not responsible since nocturnal wheeze also develops when patients sleep seated [10]. The relationship between nocturnal wheeze and sleep is uncertain. Studies in shift workers have demonstrated that the pattern of bronchoconstriction takes several days to reverse, suggesting that it is not dependent on sleep, but may be associated with a sleep-related circadian rhythm [10]. Sleep interruption and deprivation studies have also shown that the bronchoconstriction at night may occur independently of sleep, since its time course may be preserved even in the absence of sleep [11]. Several studies have investigated the relationship between bronchoconstriction and the different stages of sleep, with conflicting results. No relationship has been found between asthmatic attacks which cause awakening and the stage of sleep in either adults or children, and there is no obvious relationship to REM sleep [12]. However, these studies suffer from the defect that the threshold from awakening from bronchoconstriction may vary in different stages of sleep. Studies of bronchial tone in asthmatics during undisturbed sleep are required before the relationship between sleep stage and bronchoconstriction can be determined.

Bronchodilator withdrawal

Inhaled bronchodilators do not have a length of action that will cover the period of sleep, and the waning of bronchodilator effect overnight might, therefore, be the cause of nocturnal and early morning wheeze. However, even when patients are treated at regular intervals during the 24 h, nocturnal bronchoconstriction persists and is, of course, present in the absence of treatment [10].

Oesophageal reflux

In some asthmatics aspiration of gastric contents has been demonstrated and it has been suggested that inhalation of gastric contents at night may produce broncho-spasm. It seems unlikely that this would account for many of the cases of nocturnal bronchoconstriction and it is more likely that reflux of acid into the oesophagus might initiate reflex bronchoconstriction. A high incidence of gastro-oesophageal reflux has been found in asthmatics, possibly as a result of the spasmolytic effect of bronchodilators on the gastro-oesophageal junction. Oesophageal challenge with acid causes bronchoconstriction in asthmatic but not in normal patients, particularly those who are symptomatic of acid reflux [13]. There is a significant relationship between the severity and the incidence of nocturnal wheeze. Recent studies have shown that oesophageal challenge with dilute acid, while having no effect on airway tone, may greatly increase bronchial hyper-reactivity to histamine [14]. It is unlikely that this mechanism would explain all nocturnal asthma, but this mechanism is worthy of further investigation, as it may lead to specific treatment with histamine H2-blockers, such as cimetidine or ranitidine.

Mucus retention

It is well known that mucus plugging may contribute to airway narrowing in asthma, and it has been shown that mucociliary clearance, measured by radioaerosol, may be impaired in normal subjects at night [15]. While this may certainly contribute to nocturnal wheeze, it is unlikely to be the major component as the bronchoconstriction is so rapidly relieved by inhaled beta agonists.

Airway cooling

There is considerable evidence that cooling of the upper airways may lead to bronchospasm. It has recently been suggested that the fall in body temperature at night may, therefore, underlie nocturnal wheezing. However, the fall in core temperature at night is very small. Nevertheless, the breathing of warmed humidified air overnight has been shown to reduce the amount of bronchoconstriction [16].

Circadian rhythms relevant to respiratory disease

While several of the external factors mentioned above may contribute to bronchospasm at night in individual patients, they do not provide a universal explanation for the exacerbation of asthma at night. Many biological functions show a variability over a 24-h period and airway function is no exception. With recent advances in the understanding and analysis of endogenous biological rhythms, there is increasing evidence that circadian rhythms may underlie nocturnal asthma [17–19]. There are several circadian rhythms that may be relevant to asthma (Table 5.2).

Table 5.2 Circadian rhythms that may be relevant to asthma

Airway calibre: FEV, peak flow, airway resistance
Bronchial reactivity to histamine, allergen
Mast cell inflammatory cell mediator release
Circulating eosinophils, neutrophils
Adrenergic responsiveness
Plasma cortisol
Circulating catecholamines
Cholinergic tone

Airway tone

In normal subjects there is a diurnal variation in FEV1 (forced expiratory volume in 1 s) of about 5% [20], in peak expiratory flow of about 8% [21], and in specific airway conductance of about 25% [22]. The recognition that there is a diurnal variation in airway calibre in normal subjects has suggested that the nocturnal wheezing in asthma may represent an exaggeration of this normal rhythm (Figure

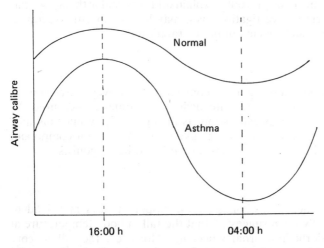

Figure 5.1 Circadian rhythms in bronchomotor tone. Nocturnal asthma may represent an amplification of the normal diurnal rhythm in airway calibre. Reproduced from ref. [23] with permission

5.1). In support of this, the amplitude of peak flow change in asthmatics is greater than 50% of the 24-h mean with an identical time course to that seen in normal subjects [6]. Furthermore, there is a significant association between non-specific bronchial hyper-responsiveness measured by response to inhaled histamine, and the amplitude of diurnal variation in peak flow [23]. This is convincing evidence that nocturnal bronchospasm represents an amplification of the normal rhythm because of increased bronchial reactivity in asthma, and that the pathogenesis of nocturnal asthma may be understood by investigating circadian changes in airway control.

Bronchial responsiveness

Bronchial responsiveness to inhaled constrictors, such as histamine and acetylcholine, is markedly increased in asthmatics at night [24,25], suggesting that airway smooth muscle may be more sensitive to constrictor influences at night (see also Chapters 7 and 14). Reactivity to inhaled allergen is also greater at night [26]. These studies are difficult to interpret because changes in baseline lung function themselves will change reactivity because of the altered geometry. There is some evidence for increased cutaneous sensitivity to histamine and the polyamine histamine liberator 48/80 [27,28], suggesting that there may be a circadian rhythm in mast cell releasability.

Other cells that may be relevant to asthma also show a circadian variation. Thus, eosinophil counts are highest at 04:00 h, although the plasma concentration of eosinophil cationic protein is not increased, indicating that they may not be releasing their products in the airways [29]. The increase in eosinophil count at night might result from the fall in plasma cortisol at night (see below).

Adrenoceptor function

There is considerable evidence that adrenergic responsiveness may be abnormal in asthma, with impairment of beta adrenoceptor function and exaggeration of alpha receptor function [30]. In animals, circadian fluctuations in brain adrenoceptor density have been reported [31]. It is therefore attractive to speculate that altered airway adrenoceptor function at night may be a mechanism of increased bronchoconstrictor responses. This has been investigated by measuring responses to incremental infusions of the endogenous beta$_2$-agonist, adrenaline, at different times during a 24-h period. There is no evidence that airway responses to infused or to inhaled adrenaline are impaired at night [32]. Similarly, the increase in plasma cyclic AMP (mediated by beta$_2$-receptors) and in cardiovascular responses (mediated by a combination of alpha and beta receptors) are no different at night compared with the day. This argues against a significant change in adrenergic receptor function accounting for nocturnal wheezing.

Cortisol

Circulating rhythms in the plasma concentration of hormones and mediators may be relevant to the pathogenesis of asthma. One of the best studied circadian rhythms is that of plasma cortisol, and because of the effectiveness of steroids in treating asthma it was logical to suggest that the circadian rhythm in endogenous cortisol might be responsible for nocturnal asthma. Although plasma cortisol is lowest at night (Figure 5.2), there is no close temporal relationship between bronchoconstriction and plasma concentration [33]; however, if the phase is advanced by 4 h the correlation does become significant [34]. Since the actions of corticosteroids are delayed in onset and decay slowly, it is possible that the delayed effect of the fall in endogenous cortisol might contribute to nocturnal bronchoconstriction. An infusion of hydrocortisone at night, which is sufficient to compensate for the nocturnal fall in plasma cortisol, fails to abolish nocturnal asthma however [33], suggesting that the fall in endogenous cortisol at night is unlikely to be the primary cause of nocturnal asthma, although it may be important in conjunction with coincident rhythms. Recently the importance of microvascular leakage and airway oedema have been emphasized in asthma [35]. Endogenous steroids may be important in regulation of microvascular leakage, and adrenalectomy in rats leads to increased cutaneous microvascular leakage with inflammatory mediators [36]. The fall in endogenous cortisol at night may therefore predispose to airway oedema.

Endogenous catecholamines

There is a circadian variation in catecholamine excretion in normal subjects, being lowest between 01:00 and 05:00 h [37]. A similar pattern is seen in asthmatics and

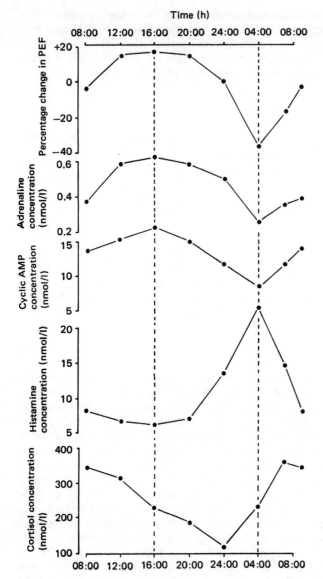

Figure 5.2 Daily variations in peak expiratory flow, together with plasma levels of adrenaline, cyclic AMP, histamine and cortisol, in asthmatic patients. PEF, peak expiratory flow

there is a significant correlation between the fall in excretion of adrenaline and noradrenaline and the fall in peak flow at night [38]. Circulating adrenaline is an important protective mechanism against bronchoconstriction in asthma [39], in the absence of functional sympathetic innervation of human airways [30]. There is a circadian rhythm in plasma adrenaline which is lowest at 04:00 h and highest at 16:00 h in normal subjects, and the rhythm is identical in asthmatics (Figure 5.2)

[34]. The fall in endogenous adrenaline at night is due to reduced secretion from the adrenal medulla, since plasma clearance is unchanged [39]. Secretion of adrenaline is regulated by the hypothalamus, which is involved in the control of several circadian rhythms and appears to be the site of the central 'clock'. The fall in adrenaline at night closely correlates with the fall in peak flow, suggesting that the withdrawal of the protective influence of adrenaline may be the cause of bronchoconstriction at night, in the same way that beta adrenoceptor antagonists produce increased bronchoconstriction in asthmatics, by blocking the effect of endogenous adrenaline [39]. However, the coincidence of these rhythms for airway tone and circulating adrenaline does not prove cause and effect, and studies in which the phase relationship of the two rhythms is changed are required for such confirmation.

Adrenaline may produce bronchodilation directly by stimulating beta receptors on airway smooth muscle, but also indirectly by inhibiting the release of inflammatory mediators from pulmonary mast cells, and by modulation of cholinergic neurotransmission. Thus, the reduced circulating adrenaline concentrations at night may lead to bronchoconstriction by a permissive action on pulmonary mast cell mediator release. In support of this, plasma histamine concentrations, used as an indicator of mediator secretion, rise at night in asthmatics, and the plasma concentration is inversely correlated with the peak flow and plasma adrenaline. Infusion of adrenaline in low concentration (0.01 µg/kg per min) to reverse the fall in endogenous adrenaline reduces the elevated plasma histamine at night [34]. In normal subjects, no significant variation in plasma histamine concentration is seen, suggesting that the increased secretion of bronchoconstrictor mediators from the sensitized mast cells of asthmatic airways may amplify the nocturnal changes in airway tone. The source of histamine in plasma is uncertain, and more recent evidence suggests that it is more likely to be derived from basophils than from airway mast cells. Nevertheless, basophils may reflect the behaviour of mast cells in the lung.

An additional mechanism that may contribute to worsening of asthma with a fall in plasma adrenaline might be an effect on microvascular leakage in airways. Adrenaline is very effective in preventing microvascular leakage due to inflammatory mediators in airways [40], and thus a fall in endogenous adrenaline concentration may result in increased leakage and airway oedema, particularly in combination with the preceding fall in endogenous cortisol.

Cholinergic reflex mechanisms

Human airway smooth muscle is densely innervated by the vagus nerve, and stimulation of the vagus causes bronchoconstriction which is mediated by cholinergic receptors and can be blocked by atropine [30]. It is possible that vagal tone might increase at night, resulting in bronchoconstriction, and several mechanisms may be involved (Figures 5.3 and 5.4). An increase in vagal tone at night is the most likely explanation for the increase in airway resistance in normal subjects at night, since vagal tone is the only reversible mechanism. In asthmatics there are several mechanisms that may increase vagal tone [30].

Inflammatory mediators, such as histamine, secreted at night by the mechanisms described above, might stimulate airway irritant receptors leading to reflex bronchoconstriction. In addition, gastro-oesophageal reflux may initiate vagal

78

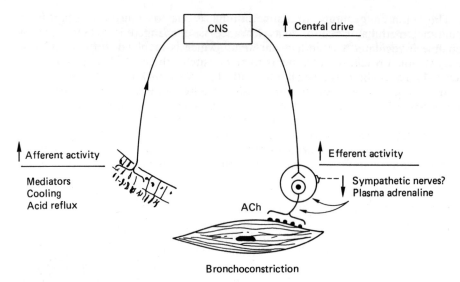

Figure 5.3 Several mechanisms are possible for an increase in cholinergic bronchoconstriction at night. CNS, central nervous system; ACh, acetylcholine

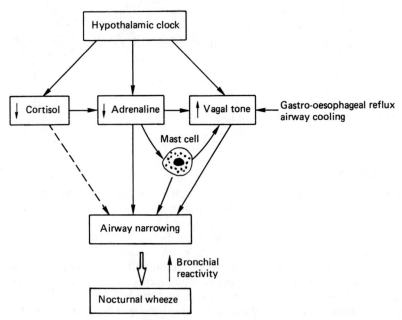

Figure 5.4 Nocturnal asthma may be explained by interacting circadian rhythms resulting in airway narrowing which is greatly amplified by bronchial hyper-reactivity in asthmatic patients

reflex bronchoconstriction. The fall in plasma adrenaline may lead to increased cholinergic neurotransmission, since beta agonists inhibit acetylcholine release from cholinergic nerves in human airways [41]. It has not yet been possible to directly measure vagal tone in the airways at night, but recordings of heart rate, which may reflect general vagal tone, have demonstrated a fall in heart rate overnight [42], the time course of which is similar to that of peak flow [32]. Measurement of the sinus arrhythmia gap, which more closely reflects cardiac vagal tone, has been shown to be related to nocturnal asthma in some subjects [43]. Anticholinergic drugs may reduce nocturnal wheeze in some subjects [44], and have a greater effect in the early morning than in the afternoon, indicating that increased vagal tone may contribute to morning dipping [45].

Coincidence of rhythms

It seems likely that nocturnal asthma is best undestood in terms of endogenous circadian rhythms, with an exaggeration of the normal 24 h change in airway tone. A plausible explanation is that several different rhythms coincide (Figure 5.4). Thus, the fall in circulating adrenaline may occur at the same time as an increase in vagal tone, and both may be regulated by a central hypothalamic clock. In addition, the delayed effects of the fall in plasma cortisol (which precedes that of adrenaline by some 4 h) may also contribute. There may indeed be complex interactions between the different rhythms. Thus the fall in cortisol may contribute to the fall in adrenaline secretion, since glucocorticoids are required for adrenaline synthesis in the adrenal gland [46]. In normal subjects these rhythms have only a small effect on airway function, which is clinically insignificant. In asthmatic subjects, however, bronchial hyper-responsiveness magnifies this change, resulting in a large reduction in airway calibre, which may be sufficient to awaken the patient. The effect of these rhythms may be further exaggerated in asthmatic subjects by mediator release from 'leaky' mast cells, and by the tendency to develop airway oedema as part of the inflammatory response. Of course, external factors, such as acid reflux and airway cooling, may also contribute in individual patients to the exaggerated bronchoconstriction at night.

Implications for therapy

Because the underlying mechanisms of nocturnal asthma are complex and inter-related, it follows that treating only one factor, such as the fall in adrenaline, will not necessarily be effective. If the proposed hypothesis is accepted there are four logical strategies for treating nocturnal asthma.

(1) Removal of trigger factors
It is important to remove any obvious triggering factors, such as allergens in the bedding, and to treat gastric reflux with an H2 antagonist.

(2) Adjust central clock
Interfering with the central clock, which drives the rhythms underlying nocturnal asthma, is neither feasible nor desirable.

(3) Reduce bronchial hyper-responsiveness
A third possibility is to reduce bronchial hyper-reactivity, which is the mechanism whereby the normally small amplitude in variability of bronchial tone becomes exaggerated. Treating asthmatic patients with regular inhaled corticosteroids is effective in controlling nocturnal symptoms in many patients [47].

(4) Long-acting bronchodilators
The fourth strategy is the administration of a long-acting bronchodilator. At present the most effective treatment for nocturnal asthma is slow-release theophylline (see also Chapter 13). When used as a single dose at night, slow-release formulations of theophylline provide therapeutic plasma concentrations for the duration of sleep, and usually control nocturnal asthma [48–50]. Circadian rhythms may underlie nocturnal asthma, but are also important in considering therapy. Thus, the pharmacokinetics and pharmacodynamics of many drugs may show important circadian rhythmicity and this must be borne in mind when considering therapy for nocturnal asthma [17]. This is particularly important with theophylline, and patients require a higher dose at night, since absorption is delayed, possibly because of the supine posture [51] (see also Chapters 2, 7 and 13).

Slow-release beta agonists appear to be less effective as therapy [52], possibly because of poor formulation of beta agonists. More recent studies with slow-release terbutaline show that it is effective in some patients, however [53], and some patients with marked nocturnal asthma, and who are resistant to all other therapies, respond to infusion of a beta agonist overnight [54]. Long-acting inhaled beta agonists, such as salmeterol, may prove to be particularly effective in nocturnal asthma.

Anticholinergic drugs are also useful in some patients, as discussed above [44].

Conclusions

It now seems likely that nocturnal asthma can be explained by an interaction of circadian rhythms against a background of hyper-responsive airways. The circadian variation in bronchomotor tone in normal individuals is probably explained entirely by cholinergic tone, which becomes exaggerated by airway inflammation. In addition, the effects of a fall in circulating adrenaline and the delayed effects of a fall in plasma cortisol may contribute to this exaggeration by increased release of inflammatory mediators, by further enhancement of cholinergic tone and by increasing airway microvascular leakage and mucosal oedema. Treatment of nocturnal asthma should be directed at reducing the inflammatory component by inhaled steroids, by giving a long-acting bronchodilator (theophylline or beta agonist) or by an inhaled anticholinergic agent (in some patients).

References

1. Floyer, J. *A Treatise of the Asthma*, R. Wilkins and W. Innis, London (1698)
2. Turner-Warwick, M. Definition and recognition of nocturnal asthma. In *Nocturnal Asthma* (eds P.J. Barnes and J. Levy), Oxford University Press, Oxford, pp. 3–5 (1984)
3. Turner-Warwick, M. Management of chronic asthma. In *Asthma: Basic Mechanisms and Clinical Management* (eds P.J. Barnes, N.C. Thomson and I. Rodger), Academic Press, pp. 731-742 (1988)

4. Editorial. Asthma at night. *Lancet*, **i**, 220–222 (1983)
5. Bateman, J.R.M. and Clarke, S.W. Sudden death in asthma. *Thorax*, **34**, 40–44 (1979)
6. Hetzel, M.R. The pulmonary clock. *Thorax*, **36**, 481–486 (1981)
7. Barnes, P.J. Nocturnal asthma: mechanisms and treatment. *Brit. Med. J.*, **288**, 1397–1398 (1984)
8. Platts-Mills, T.A.E., Mitchell, E.B., Nock, P., Tovey, E.R., Moszoro, H. and Wilkins, S.R. Reduction of bronchial hyperreactivity during prolonged allergen avoidance. *Lancet*, **ii**, 675–677 (1982)
9. Newman-Taylor, A.J., Davies, R.J., Hendrick, D.J. and Pepys, J. Recurrent nocturnal asthmatic reactions to bronchial-provocation tests. *Clin. Allergy*, **9**, 213–219 (1979)
10. Clark, T.J.H. and Hetzel, M.R. Diurnal variation of asthma. *Brit. J. Dis. Chest*, **71**, 87–92 (1977)
11. Hetzel, M.R. and Clark, T.J.H. Does sleep cause nocturnal asthma? *Thorax*, **34**, 749–754 (1979)
12. Montplasir, J., Walsh, J. and Malo, J.L. Nocturnal asthma: features of attacks, sleep and breathing patterns. *Amer. Rev. Respir. Dis.*, **125**, 18–22 (1982)
13. Spaulding, M.S., Mansfield, L.E., Stein, M.R., Sellner, S.C. and Gremillion, D.E. Further investigation of the association between gastroesophageal reflex and bronchoconstriction. *J. Allergy Clin. Immunol.*, **69**, 516–521 (1982)
14. Wilson, N.M., Charette, L., Thomson, A.H. and Silverman, M. Gastro-oesophageal reflux and childhood asthma: the acid test. *Thorax*, **40**, 592–597 (1985)
15. Bateman, J.R.M., Pavia, D. and Clarke, S.W. The retention of lung secretions during the night in normal subjects. *Clin. Sci.*, **55**, 523–527 (1978)
16. Chen, W.Y. and Chai, H. Airway cooling and nocturnal asthma. *Chest*, **81**, 675–680 (1982)
17. Smolensky, M.H., Reinberg, A. and Queng, J.T. The chronobiology and chronopharmacology of allergy. *Ann. Allergy*, **47**, 234–252 (1981)
18. Barnes, P.J. Circadian variation in airway function. *Amer. J. Med.*, **79**, Suppl. 6A, 5–9 (1985)
19. Smolensky, M.H., Barnes, P.J., Jonkman, J.H.G. and Scott, A.H. The chronopharmacology and chronotherapy of bronchodilator medications. *Annu. Rev. Chronopharmacol.*, **2**, 229–273 (1986)
20. Guberan, E., Williams, M.K., Walford, J. and Smith, M.M. Circadian variation in FEV1 in shift workers. *Brit. J. Ind. Med.*, **26**, 121–125 (1969)
21. Hetzel, M.R. and Clark, T.J.H. Comparison of normal and asthmatic rhythms in peak expiratory flow rate. *Thorax*, **35**, 732–738 (1980)
22. Kerr, H.D. Diurnal variation of respiratory function independent of air quality. *Arch. Environ. Hlth*, **26**, 144–152 (1973)
23. Ryan, G., Latimer, K.M., Dolovich, J. and Hargreave, F.E. Bronchial responsiveness to histamine: Relationship to diurnal variation of peak flow rate, improvement after bronchodilator and airway calibre. *Thorax*, **37**, 423–439 (1982)
24. De Vries, K., Goei, J.T., Booij-Noord, H. and Orie, N.G.M. Changes during 24 hours in the lung function and histamine hyperreactivity of the bronchial tree in asthmatic and bronchitic patients. *Int. Arch. Allergy*, **20**, 93–101 (1962)
25. Liu, Y.-N., Sasaki, H., Ishil, M., Sekizawa, K., Hida, W., Ichinose, M. and Takashima, T. Effect of circadian rhythm on bronchomotor tone after deep inspiration in normal and in asthmatic subjects. *Amer. Rev. Respir. Dis.*, **132**, 278–282 (1985)
26. Gervais, P., Reinberg, A., Gervais, C., Smolensky, M. and DeFrance, O. Twenty-four hour rhythms in the bronchial hyperreactivity to house dust in asthmatics. *J. Allergy Clin. Immunol.*, **59**, 207–213 (1977)
27. Lee, R.E., Smolensky, M.H., Leach, C.S. and McGovern, J.P. Circadian rhythms in the cutaneous reactivity to histamine and selected antigens including phase relationship to urinary cortisol excretion. *Ann. Allergy*, **38**, 231–236 (1977)
28. Reinberg, A., Sidi, E. and Ghata, J. Circadian reactivity rhythms of human skin to histamine or allergen and the adrenal cycle. *J. Allergy*, **36**, 273–283 (1965)
29. Dahl, R. Diurnal variation in the number of circulating eosinophil leukocytes in normal controls and asthmatics. *Acta Allergol*, **32**, 301–303 (1977)
30. Barnes, P.J. Neural control of human airways in health and disease. *Amer. Rev. Respir. Dis.*, **134**, 1289–1314 (1986)
31. Wirz-Justice, A., Krauchi, K., Campbell, I.C. and Feer, H. Adrenoceptor changes in spontaneously hypertensive rats: a circadian approach. *Brain Res.*, **262**, 238–242 (1983)

32. Barnes, P.J., FitzGerald, G.A. and Dollery, C.T. Circadian variation in adrenergic responses in asthmatic subjects. *Clin. Sci., 62,* 349–354 (1982)
33. Soutar, C.A., Costello, J., Ijaduola, O. and Turner-Warwick, M. Nocturnal and morning asthma: relationship to plasma corticosteroids and response to cortisol infusion. *Thorax, 30,* 436–440 (1975)
34. Barnes, P., FitzGerald, G., Brown, M. and Dollery, C. Nocturnal asthma and changes in circulating epinephrine, histamine and cortisol. *N. Engl. J. Med., 303,* 263–267 (1980)
35. Persson, C.G.A. Role of plasma exudation in asthmatic airways. *Lancet,* ii, 1126–1128 (1986)
36. Leme, G.J. and Wilhelm, D.L. The effects of adrenalectomy and corticosterone on vascular permeability responses in the skin of the rat. *Brit. J. Exp. Pathol., 56,* 402–407 (1975)
37. Townshend, M.M. and Smith, A.J. Factors influencing the urinary excretion of free catecholamines in man. *Clin. Sci., 44,* 253–265 (1973)
38. Soutar, C.A., Carruthers, M. and Pickering, C.A.C. Nocturnal asthma and urinary adrenaline and noradrenaline excretion. *Thorax, 32,* 677–683 (1977)
39. Barnes, P.J. Endogenous catecholamines and asthma. *J. Allergy Clin. Immunol., 77,* 791–795 (1986)
40. Barnes, P.J. Autonomic control of the airways and nocturnal asthma. In *Nocturnal Asthma* (eds P.J. Barnes and J. Levy), Oxford University Press, Oxford, pp. 69–75 (1984)
41. Boschetto, P., Roberts, N.M., Rogers, D.F. and Barnes, P.J. Adrenaline, but not salbutamol, inhibits airway microvascular leakage in guinea-pigs. *Clin. Sci., 74,* 46–47P (1988)
42. Rhoden, K.J., Meldrum, L.A. and Barnes, P.J. β-Adrenergic modulation of cholinergic neurotransmission in human airways. *Amer. Rev. respir. Dis., 135,* A91 (1987)
43. Clarke, J.M., Hamer, J., Shelton, J.R., Taylor, S. and Venning, G.R. The rhythm of the normal human heart. *Lancet,* ii, 508–512 (1976)
44. Postma, D.S., Keyzer, J.J., Koeter, G.H., Sluiter, H.J. and De Vries, K. Influence of the parasympathetic and sympathetic nervous systems on nocturnal bronchial obstruction. *Clin. Sci., 69,* 251–258 (1985)
45. Coe, C.I. and Barnes, P.J. Reduction of nocturnal asthma by an inhaled anticholinergic drug. *Chest, 90,* 485–488 (1986)
46. Pohorecky, L.A. and Wurtman, R.J. Adrenocortical control of epinephrine synthesis. *Pharmacol. Rev., 23,* 1–35 (1971)
47. Gaultier, C., Reinberg, A., Gerbeaux, J. and Girard, F. Circadian changes in lung resistance and dynamic compliance in healthy and asthmatic children. Effects of two bronchodilators. *Resp. Physiol., 31,* 169–182 (1975)
48. Horn, C.R., Clark, T.J.H. and Cochrane, G.M. Inhaled therapy reduces morning dips in asthma. *Lancet,* i, 1143–1145 (1984)
49. Barnes, P.J., Greening, A.P., Neville, L., Timmers, J. and Poole, G.W. Single dose slow-release aminophylline at night prevents nocturnal asthma. *Lancet,* i, 299–301 (1982)
50. Neuenkirchen, H., Wilkens, J.H., Oellerich, M. and Sybrecht, G.W. Nocturnal asthma and sustained release theophylline. *Eur. J. Respir. Dis., 66,* 196–204 (1985)
51. Warren, J.B., Cuss, F. and Barnes, P.J. Posture and theophylline kinetics. *Brit. J. Clin. Pharmacol., 19,* 707–709 (1985)
52. Fairfax, A.J., McNabb, W.R., Davies, H.J. and Spiro, S.G. Slow-release oral salbutamol and aminophylline in nocturnal asthma: relation of overnight changes in lung function and plasma drug levels. *Thorax, 35,* 526–530 (1980)
53. Koeter, G.H., Postma, D.S., Keyzer, J.J. and Meurs, H. The effects of oral slow-release terbutaline on early morning dyspnoea. *Eur. J. Clin. Pharmacol., 28,* 159 (1985)
54. Ayers, J., Fish, D.R., Wheeler, D.C., Wiggins, J., Cochrane, G.M. and Skinner, C. Subcutaneous terbutaline and control of brittle asthma on appreciable morning dipping. *Br. Med. J., 288,* 1715–1716 (1984)

Chapter 6

Urinary and renal circadian rhythms

M.G. Koopman, D.S. Minors and J.M. Waterhouse

An alternative to blood sampling

Biochemical reactions that are catalysed by enzymes take place in an aqueous environment. Total body water can be divided into several compartments: of these, blood is by far the most direct to sample and it can be separated into plasma and cells by centrifugation. As other chapters have shown, examination of the constituents of blood (cells, ions, foodstuffs, hormones and plasma proteins) can give valuable information to the clinician.

There are occasions when an alternative means of sampling body fluids is required. Such occasions might be:

1. With babies or patients when invasive methods are undesirable.
2. When repetitive sampling is required and this would be too intrusive or the total volume of samples would be unacceptably high.
3. In difficult circumstances, e.g. subjects isolated or in an inclement climate.

In such circumstances, urine collection can be a useful alternative to blood sampling. In addition, provided that the sampling is frequent enough, information on circadian changes can be obtained; these rhythms are influenced not only by the composition of the blood but also by the activity of the kidneys and their blood supply.

When healthy subjects drink very large amounts of fluid, high urinary flow rates can be achieved and samples can be obtained by spontaneous voiding with intervals of 20–30 min. This procedure is often used in short-term experiments. However, to study circadian rhythms in urine, sampling has to be performed over a longer period. Collecting urine every 20–30 min during one or more days is too heavy a burden for healthy subjects as well as patients, even if the large amounts of fluid, necessary to obtain high urine flow, are administered intravenously. In practice, collection periods of 2–4h can be achieved over the course of several days with comparative ease, provided that the subject is taking orally about 2.5 litres of fluid divided over the day. This length of sampling period will limit the frequency of changes that can be assessed in, for example, hormone rhythms (see Chapter 14) and short episodes of secretion can be missed.

Urine samples are integrated samples, collected in the bladder since the last time of micturition. This could be a major advantage for those substances whose concentration in blood fluctuates rapidly over a substantial range; as a result of this, a blood sample taken at a single point in time would be meaningless. Provided the bladder is emptied completely and the time of micturition is accurately recorded, urine samples provide the opportunity to calculate excretion rates of several solutes over successive collection periods during the day. Inability to empty the bladder completely can sometimes be a problem, especially when healthy subjects or patients are kept recumbent during the study. This is one of the main disadvantages of urine sampling in comparison with blood sampling. It could be overcome by using an indwelling bladder catheter. However, this is invasive and bears the risk of infection, thereby removing one of the reasons for choosing urinary rather than blood sampling in the first place.

Urine formation

The kidneys are the main route by which excess water-soluble substances are removed from the body. Towards this end the kidneys receive a large proportion of the cardiac output and, due to the anatomical arrangement of the capillaries and adjacent blood vessels, filter about 20% of the plasma at the glomeruli. Further removal from the vascular compartment can occur for certain organic acids and bases, amongst which are several drugs. This removal takes place by active secretion into the tubular lumen by the proximal tubular cells. Removal of a substance from the bloodstream can be completed during a single passage through the kidney; that is, the clearance is limited in such cases by the renal blood flow. In health, most water-soluble substances up to a molecular weight of 30000 are filtered at the glomeruli with little restriction; above this molecular weight the substance experiences restricted passage into the ultrafiltrate. Therefore, the filtration of plasma proteins into the luminal fluid is normally small. If abnormal cells produce water-soluble substances that are not too large, these substances, after filtration at the glomeruli, will also appear in the urine, where they can be used as a marker for the disease process (see later).

Under normal circumstances there is a very large reabsorption of filtered materials by the proximal convoluted tubule. This essentially clears the luminal fluid of glucose, fatty acids and amino acids and of proteins. Further, approximately 80% of electrolytes are reabsorbed, with water following osmotically. Subsequent changes to the water and electrolytes in the luminal fluid are, to a large extent, under hormonal control, the result in health being that most (>95%) of the filtered load is reabsorbed. The implication of this is that a large concentration gradient exists for waste materials and this tends to promote passive reabsorption. The amount of reabsorption of these that takes place depends upon how easily any material passes from the tubular lumen into the blood. This in turn depends upon the permeability of different parts of the nephron to each individual substance.

It is very likely that at least some of the processes show circadian variation and contribute to circadian changes in the composition of urine.

Circadian rhythms in urinary excretion in healthy adults

The rhythmic excretion of a wide variety of electrolytes has been described [1]. In most cases peak excretion occurs diurnally though common exceptions are phosphate and titratable acid which are excreted nocturnally in greater amounts.

Some rhythms, for example those of flow and the excretion of sodium, potassium, chloride and urate, are of considerable amplitude, nocturnal rates being less than 50% of those during the daytime. The phasing of rhythms of flow, sodium, chloride and potassium are similar but not identical [2]. Thus chloride and potassium tend to peak earlier than sodium; also the day-by-day variation in the difference in times of peaks of sodium and chloride is less than that between sodium and potassium [3]. This implies that the mechanisms for sodium and chloride reabsorption are linked more closely than those for sodium and potassium; this is in agreement with what is known of tubule function.

Undoubtedly, dietary factors and postural changes are important exogenous influences, though the mechanisms by which these effects are exerted (do postural changes act through mechanical, neural and/or humoral factors?) are unknown. Postural and dietary changes are not wholly responsible for renal circadian rhythms since the rhythms continue when diet and posture are controlled, although sometimes with a reduction in amplitude [4]. This means that these rhythms also have an endogenous component. This is quite large in the case of potassium, and smaller (though still appreciable) for sodium and chloride. It is also noteworthy that the ability of the kidney to deal with imposed water and saline loads varies circadianly, changes in the daytime being more brisk than those at night [5]. This has important implications for the clinician who is treating his patients with continuous intravenous infusions; there is more likelihood of iatrogenic oedema in the night. With potassium and cortisol infusions also there are circadian differences in the changes they produce. Potassium infusion produces a larger rise of plasma potassium at night than during the daytime even though aldosterone levels change by equal amounts [6]. Thus the body is less able to remove potassium (as well as, to a lesser extent, water and sodium) during the night. Similarly, a high dose of cortisol at night produces a smaller increase in the reabsorption of sodium at the level of the distal tubule than a similar dose during the day [7].

Mechanism causing circadian rhythmicity

To attempt an explanation of the mechanisms of circadian rhythms in renal excretion is horrendous! Several factors are responsible for this difficulty. First, the amount of material lost in the urine is often a very small percentage of that initially filtered. Second, the amount of substance appearing in the urine is determined by many factors, some or all of which might show circadian rhythmicity. These factors can be summarized as:

Amount in urine = amount filtered + amount secreted − amount reabsorbed

The amount filtered (the filtered load) is, in turn, the product of the glomerular filtration rate (GFR) and the plasma concentration of the substance under consideration.

In the following sections we will deal with the several factors that might contribute to the circadian rhythms.

Plasma concentration
Circadian changes in plasma concentration of most substances are generally small, though phosphate (with peak values during the evening with sharp falls towards the end of sleep) and urea (gradual rise throughout the daytime) are exceptions [8]. However, a circadian rhythm in filtered load that could account for a circadian

rhythm in urinary excretion (assuming no changes in reabsorption) could be due to circadian changes in plasma concentration that were too small to detect by present methods.

Glomerular filtration rate

GFR is measured by the clearance of inulin or, less accurately, creatinine; it equals 125 ml/min in an average adult. There is a circadian rhythm in GFR as measured by these techniques; GFR is generally lowest during sleep at night and shows an amplitude (maximum minus minimum) of about 20% of the daily mean (see ref. [9] for a review). The extent to which this rhythmicity is due to day–night differences in lifestyle (posture, activity, protein intake) rather than the expression of some endogenous oscillator is not known in any detail; both components are likely to play some part since the rhythm does not disappear during constant bedrest and identical meals every 3 h [10,11]. Whatever the detailed explanation, the implication of the finding is that removal of a water-soluble substance from the plasma by glomerular ultrafiltration will be higher diurnally than nocturnally.

Single-nephron GFR in rats is determined by several factors and these have been reviewed recently by Brenner et al. [12]. Their equations direct attention to those factors that might account for the circadian variation in overall GFR, assuming that such equations apply to humans and to the kidneys as a whole. For many of the factors, information about circadian changes is not available but there are two exceptions: the concentration of plasma proteins and renal plasma flow.

Plasma proteins are more concentrated diurnally than nocturnally. An explanation might be that this results from increased tissue fluid formation during the daytime as a consequence of a raised blood pressure and cardiac output. The amplitude of the rhythm of plasma protein concentration is about 10% of the 24-h mean.

For measurement of renal plasma flow, the clearance of p-aminohippurate (PAH) is used. PAH is partly filtered in the glomeruli and the remainder is actively secreted from the peritubular blood vessels into the urine by the proximal tubular cells. In healthy subjects, PAH is almost totally (91%) extracted from the blood by these mechanisms during one passage through the kidney: accordingly, the clearance of PAH can be used as an indirect measure of the effective renal plasma flow (ERPF). A circadian rhythm in PAH clearance has been reported by some, but not all, investigators (see ref. [9] for a review). The rhythm has a tendency to be in phase with the better-documented rhythm for blood pressure [13–15]. In this rhythm, nocturnal values are lower than those measured diurnally even in subjects on constant bedrest; normally, blood pressure shows a rapid rise at the time of waking and a marked fall on retiring. It has been found that the phase of the GFR rhythm is not identical to that of the ERPF rhythm [11] (Figure 6.1). The meaning of this phenomenon is not clear. One has to bear in mind that circadian variations in PAH clearance are the net result of circadian fluctuations in GFR (which are known and can accurately be measured) and unknown variations in tubular secretion over the 24 h. As the filtration fraction (FF) is nothing more than the ratio of GFR to PAH clearance, it is even more difficult to comment on any circadian variation in this variable.

A hormone such as angiotensin II can alter glomerular ultrafiltration via its influence on K_f (the ultrafiltration coefficient) through action upon mesangial cells [16]. Although plasma renin activity has a definite circadian rhythm in humans, this rhythm has a different phase in subjects living a normal lifestyle when

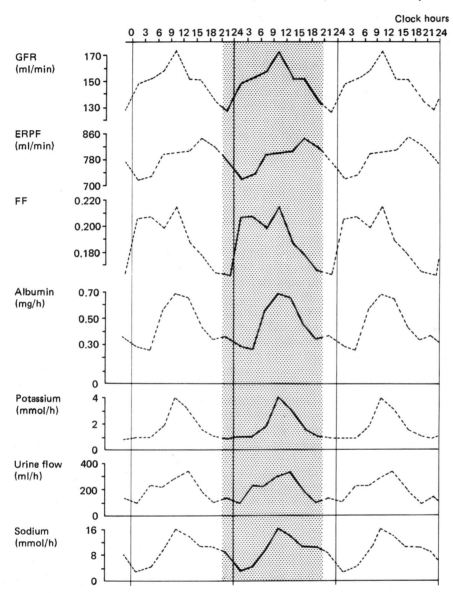

Figure 6.1 Healthy male, age 32 years; urine and blood sampling every 3 h during 1 day of continuous bedrest and equally spaced identical meals. GFR (inulin clearance) and ERPF (PAH clearance), uncorrected for body surface. FF, filtration factor. The data are repeated twice for a better impression of the circadian rhythms

compared with subjects undergoing constant bedrest [17]. Also other hormones, such as prostaglandins, atrial natriuretic peptide, vasopressin and cortisol, are reported to influence (single nephron) GFR and to show circadian rhythmicity as well [18–20]. All these hormones interact and some of them (angiotensin, prostaglandins) are locally produced in the kidney too. Therefore, it is not clear yet whether, and, if so, how, rhythmic changes in the activity of these hormones in blood and urine have an influence upon the circadian rhythm of GFR and of PAH clearance.

When these factors are considered together, a circadian rhythm of filtered load, with maximum values in the daytime and minimum values during nocturnal sleep, is found. Its relative amplitude is not high, with peak and trough values differing from the 24-h mean by 20% or less. However, since, in absolute quantities, day/night differences in the filtered load of electrolytes are enormous, they are more than ample to account for any observed circadian changes, even when other factors remain constant over the 24 h.

Secretion and reabsorption

The majority of most substances that are filtered at the glomeruli is reabsorbed during subsequent passage through the renal tubules; in addition, material that has not been filtered at the glomeruli can be removed from the peritubular fluid and actively secreted into the tubular lumina. In the case of many drugs that are organic acids or bases, this mechanism is of particular importance in the proximal convoluted tubule. For substances such as amino acids, many drugs and the major ions, considerable detail is known with regard to the specificity and kinetics of the carriers involved, together with the size of gradients that can be set up. However, circadian changes in these parameters do not seem to have been measured.

Passive reabsorption of many molecules takes place along the length of the tubule. It requires a concentration or electrochemical gradient to exist between the tubular lumen, the tubular cell and the peritubular fluid; a concentration gradient arises because of the water reabsorption that has taken place down an osmotic gradient, itself a consequence of prior reabsorptive activity by the tubule. In the presence of such a concentration gradient, the amount of substance that is reabsorbed will depend upon two factors. These are the permeability of the segment to the substance and the speed at which the luminal fluid is flowing through that part of the tubule; this latter, in turn, depends upon the amount of water reabsorption that has taken place. The permeability of the cortical and medullary collecting duct is controlled by antidiuretic hormone; this hormone increases the permeability of parts of the collecting duct to urea also. For many water-soluble drugs their ease of passage out of the distal nephron back into the blood is determined by their degree of ionization and the pH of the luminal fluid.

Neural factors

The participation of the nervous system in generating renal rhythmicity in health remains obscure; similarly, the role of renal nerves in maintaining sodium and water balance is not clear. Several, but not all, animal experiments [21] indicate that renal denervation leads to a significant increase in sodium excretion [22–24], especially during a sodium-restricted diet [25]. The mechanisms by which renal nerves alter renal sodium handling appear to be multiple. The tone of both afferent and efferent arterioles (and thus GFR, ERPF and filtration fraction) can be influenced by sympathetic nerves either as a result of direct innervation [26] or through changes in activity of the renin–angiotensin system [27]. Other studies show a direct influence of renal nerves on proximal tubular sodium reabsorption [22].

A transplanted kidney is denervated. Although in many patients the function of the transplant is normal, as a model to study the participation of nerves in renal rhythms it is far from ideal. All renal transplant patients are given immunosuppressive drugs, although after 1 year only a low dose is used. Corticosteroids are known to modify the urinary potassium rhythm, and cyclosporin influences renal tubular function. One finding in patients with transplanted kidneys taking corticosteroids and azathioprine is that the circadian rhythms for urinary water and sodium excretion are inverted in those who are ambulant but not in those undergoing continuous bedrest [28,29]. This is also found in many patients with renal and cardiovascular disease, especially when accompanied by oedema, and will be commented upon later. In addition, patients with autonomic failure are reported to have abnormal or inverted rhythms for urinary water and sodium excretion [30–32].

Hormones

Cortisol, aldosterone, renin, angiotensin, antidiuretic hormone, several prostaglandins and atrial natriuretic peptide are all reported to have a circadian rhythm in humans [9,17–20,33,34].

The phase and amplitude of these rhythms may be variable, depending on the conditions during the study of the subjects (bedrest, activity, sodium chloride intake, etc.). Some of these hormones probably influence glomerular filtration rate (and its circadian rhythm); all of them directly or indirectly act on tubular function, especially in the distal parts of the nephron. It is likely that they have a considerable influence on the circadian changes in the excretion of water and electrolytes in the urine. Bearing in mind the various interactions of these hormones and the complicated handling of water and electrolytes by the kidney, we will now discuss the circadian changes in some electrolytes, water, urea and acid excretion and the possible influence of hormones on these processes.

Sodium reabsorption is at least partly dependent on aldosterone but the role of aldosterone in the circadian rhythm of urinary sodium loss is not clear. Aldosterone itself has a circadian rhythm that is strongly affected by posture; some investigators could not detect this rhythm in recumbency on a normal diet. Williams *et al.* [35] found a rhythm for aldosterone during recumbency with a peak in the early morning (06:00 h); this was at the same time as plasma renin activity (PRA) and cortisol had their peak values. However, the position is complicated by the view [36] that the aldosterone rhythm is controlled more by that of PRA when body sodium levels are low (and PRA is high) but more by that of adrenocorticotropin when the body is replete with sodium (and PRA is low). The peaks of PRA and aldosterone shift several hours later when the subject rises to an upright position in the morning and starts his daily activities. The peak of the atrial natriuretic hormone (ANP) rhythm is, perhaps surprisingly, during the night in healthy subjects during a regimen of sleep at night and normal daily activities [19]. Urinary prostaglandin E_2 (PGE_2) has its maximum excretion in the evening in recumbent healthy women [18]. Both ANP and PGE_2 produce natriuresis. Although the hormones that have an influence on urinary sodium excretion have different phases and shift easily under different conditions, the circadian rhythm of urinary sodium excretion is, by contrast, rather stable in healthy individuals with a peak in the afternoon [2].

The rhythm of urinary excretion of potassium is remarkable for an even higher endogenous component than that possessed by the sodium rhythm; it is little affected by the immediate effects of diet and posture. One of the hormones that influences the rhythm is cortisol. Administration of corticosteroids in divided doses over the day will make the rhythm undetectable or will reverse it after a few days. Potassium shifts from the intracellular to the extracellular compartment under the influence of cortisol and so potassium and cortisol rhythms are linked to some extent [6]. However, the urinary potassium rhythm is not wholly the result of the circadian changes in plasma potassium (amplitude 10% of the mean) caused by this mechanism. Thus, potassium infusion during the night, with a concomitant rise in plasma potassium, does not lead to an increase in urinary potassium excretion, although a normal reactive rise in plasma aldosterone is observed [6]. It is likely that cortisol and aldosterone play some role in the increase in urinary potassium excretion in the morning by their influence on the secretion of potassium by the distal part of the tubule.

The clearance of urea from the circulation is dependent on urine flow. When urine flow rates are low – in the presence of high plasma antidiuretic hormone (ADH) – more time exists for equilibration between the plasma and the fluid in the distal nephron. Water absorption will concentrate the urea which will in turn pass back into the blood by diffusion. This process is aided by the fact that ADH also increases the permeability of the collecting duct to urea. In contrast to plasma cortisol, the circadian rhythms of urine flow and plasma ADH concentration are much influenced by changes in diet and posture. In subjects living a normal lifestyle, urine flow shows a marked circadian rhythm with peak values during the daytime and the concentration of plasma ADH shows an equally marked rhythm with diurnal values lower than nocturnal ones. These two rhythms are inter-related and reflect the normal behavioural pattern of drinking during the daytime but not at night. They possess an endogenous component insofar as urine flow is less nocturnally, and ADH concentrations are highest at about 06:00 h, in healthy subjects in whom posture and fluid intake have been controlled. However, the endogenous component is small since, in these circumstances, the amplitude of the rhythms is considerably less [9]. In addition, it is likely that the nocturnal decreases in cardiac output and GFR (see earlier) will promote nocturnal oliguria.

The circadian rhythms of acid secretion by the tubule and of urinary pH are of considerable importance as far as the elimination of drugs and their metabolites are concerned. The implications of these circadian changes are considered elsewhere. Hydrogen ion handling by the kidney is complicated but, in general, the circadian rhythm in hydrogen ion excretion shows an inverse relationship to urinary potassium excretion [37]. Thus, the hours after rising are associated with a rapid rise in potassium excretion and a fall in acid secretion such that the urine might even verge on alkaline; the declining excretion of potassium from the late afternoon onwards is coupled with an increasing acidification of urine, nocturnal urine being lowest in potassium and highest in acid.

Urine rhythms in individuals other than healthy adults

So far in this chapter we have dealt with renal circadian rhythms in the 'standard man', a creature beloved of research workers! Clearly the position might be different, and in some critical way, in an unhealthy patient, a newborn child, an aged person or an expectant mother. These groups would differ from the 'standard man' also if they were receiving drugs; since drugs are removed from the circulation mainly by the kidneys, abnormalities in renal circadian rhythms might be an important consideration in these cases.

Expectant mothers

There are hardly any data available that deal with circadian rhythms in renal function in expectant mothers. It is known that GFR and renal plasma flow increase during pregnancy [38] and this will raise the rate at which drugs and other substances, e.g. urea, can be removed from the body either by filtration or by active secretion. Whether there are changes in the amplitude or timing of circadian rhythms is not known. Moreover we are ignorant as to any changes in the circadian rhythms of urine flow or acidity and any differences in drug elimination by the kidneys that these changes might produce.

Newborn babies

Circadian rhythms and renal function are immature at birth and take months or even years to develop fully. Renal immaturity manifests itself as a lower GFR and renal plasma flow (in relation to body size), a poorer ability to concentrate urine and decreased reabsorptive and secretory abilities. Bicarbonate reabsorption and ammonia secretion are underdeveloped also [39] and this is particularly important when the phenomenon of 'diffusion trapping' of drugs is considered. These factors will contribute to a decreased renal elimination of drugs and decreased abilities to eliminate excesses, or conserve deficits of water and electrolytes. 'Corrections' of drug dosage and intravenous infusion rates for neonates take into account the neonates' decreased size and their limitations in renal function. They have to take into account also the observation that fluid compartments in a neonate are a different proportion of total body weight when compared with adults. All these factors will affect the half-life of a drug in the body. This is illustrated in Table 6.1.

Table 6.1 Effect of age upon renal function and the renal elimination of a drug

	Infant	Youth	Aged subject
Weight (kg)	3.5	70	70
Body water (%)	75	60	60
Volume of body water (ml)	2625	42000	42000
GFR (ml/min per kg)	0.90	1.80	1.00
GFR (ml/min)	3.15	126	70
$t_{1/2}$	577	231	416

The drug is assumed to be distributed throughout the body water and to be lost by glomerular filtration without further secretion or reabsorption. $t_{1/2}$, half-life of a drug in the plasma. (After ref. [40]).

There is also a diminished amplitude of renal circadian rhythms, or such rhythms might even be completely absent [41]. This is a result of at least two factors – the immaturity of the endogenous circadian system and an underdeveloped lifestyle insofar as day–night differences in sleeping, activity and mealtimes are considered.

These differences, which might vary widely between individuals at differing stages of maturity, mean that the regimen for any neonate requiring drugs or intravenous infusions must be assessed individually and with particular care.

The aged

In old age too circadian rhythmicity and renal function deteriorate [33,42]. Some glomeruli become functionless and renal blood flow falls; GFR will be decreased to about 60% of young adult values by the age of 70 years. Some implications of this are considered in Table 6.1 where the half-life of a drug in the circulation has been calculated for an aged subject. There are further implications for drug excretion. Thus the ability to concentrate urine and mechanisms for active reabsorption and secretion (including that responsible for urine acidification) all decline with age [42].

Circadian rhythmicity deteriorates with age [33]; this decline can be seen as another example of 'senescence' of the body. One implication is that, with a decline in the amplitudes of circadian rhythms, there will be a fall in any day/night differences in the processes of renal elimination of substances. There is also a report [43] that indicates that reflex changes in urine flow in response to postural changes over-ride circadian effects in aged subjects, as is found with transplanted kidneys and in some renal disorders (below).

In summary, as with infants, particular care must be exercised and the dosing and infusion regimens adjusted for each individual.

Renal rhythms in clinical disorders

In patients with renal disorders, ERPF, GFR and the tubular secretion of organic acids and bases can all be depressed to some extent. For all drugs and their metabolites that depend upon the kidney for their elimination, these changes would increase their half-life in the circulation and the risk of toxicity. Knowledge of circadian rhythms in healthy subjects, together with possible changes in various disease states, can be useful in the understanding and treatment of clinical problems.

In patients with chronic renal failure the relative amplitude (amplitude/mean) of the circadian rhythm in urinary excretion of several electrolytes is usually diminished. The rhythms for sodium excretion and, especially, urine flow are often reduced or absent (Figure 6.2). Alternatively, the excretion rate during the night is higher than during the day [9,44–46]. The circadian rhythm for urinary potassium excretion is more stable and less often phased abnormally.

Patients with glomerulopathies may lose large amounts of protein in the urine (Figure 6.2). GFR in these patients can vary from being normal to severely reduced. Particularly in patients with normal or only slightly reduced renal function, there is a marked circadian rhythm for proteinuria, with a maximum protein excretion in the daytime and a minimum excretion during the night [47]. This rhythm is present even when the patients are kept in bed and consume identical amounts of protein every 3 h. The relative amplitude of the proteinuria rhythm (50–70% of the 24-h mean) is much higher than those for GFR and ERPF. In many patients with glomerular disease and nephrotic syndrome, the circadian rhythm for urine flow and sodium excretion are absent or reversed, even when the subjects are studied during bedrest (sitting in bed during the day, strictly recumbent during the night) and when GFR is normal [9]. The circadian rhythm for potassium excretion is usually normal, although often with a lower relative amplitude than in healthy individuals during similar conditions. In patients with marked proteinuria and severe renal insufficiency, the circadian rhythm for urinary

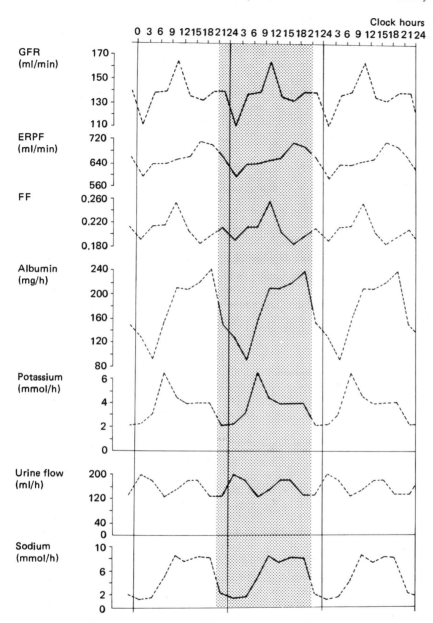

Figure 6.2 Male, age 18 years; nephrotic syndrome. Same protocol and presentation of data as in Figure 6.1

protein excretion can be absent; if present, the relative amplitude is often low [10].

Abnormal, absent or inverted rhythms – especially for urine flow and sodium excretion – are also reported for patients suffering from cirrhosis of the liver with ascites [48,49], cardiac failure and oedema [1,48,50], autonomic failure [31–33] and during convalescence after a long period in bed with a severe illness [51]. Patients with Cushing's syndrome lack a cortisol rhythm, but also have abnormal circadian rhythms for electrolyte excretion [52]; abnormal rhythms for water and electrolyte excretion are also reported in patients who have been treated with corticosteroids in divided doses over the day [53].

Abnormal rhythms are sometimes the cause of clinical symptoms. Nocturnal enuresis is probably at least in some cases due to an abnormal circadian rhythm for urine flow. This in turn may be caused by the absence of a rise in ADH levels during the night [54]. Administration of vasopressin in the evening can cause the symptom to regress. In some patients other renal circadian rhythms can be abnormal too, both in amplitude and phase [55].

Circadian rhythms can also be demonstrated in the urinary excretion of abnormal substances (for instance tumour markers), provided that these substances are water-soluble and small enough to pass through the glomerular membrane and are not completely reabsorbed in the tubules [56,57].

In summary:

1. The phases of water, sodium and chloride rhythms are more often abnormal than the phase of the potassium rhythm in several clinical disorders.
2. The relative amplitudes of all renal rhythms tend to be lower in renal failure.
3. Pathological symptoms like marked proteinuria also have a circadian rhythm.
4. Abnormal renal rhythms could have implications for the renal elimination of drugs in some clinical disorders.

Possible causes of altered rhythms in clinical disorders
The usual explanation for the inverted circadian rhythms for urine flow and sodium excretion in oedematous disorders is that they result from an exaggerated response to a postural change. It is well recognized that lying down initiates diuretic and natriuretic reactions, but these are normally severely attenuated at night – that is the circadian influence outweighs these reflex effects. Patients with oedematous disorders retain water and sodium, especially during the day when they are in the upright position. This excess of fluid accumulates mainly in the interstitium of the lower part of the body. During the night, when the patient is supine, part of this excess will re-enter the circulation. Venous return to the heart will be larger than in health, and this (provided that the function of the 'cardiac pump' is not too impaired – in which case pulmonary oedema will develop) initiates a diuretic response that is large enough to over-ride the circadian antidiuresis. Excessive retention of water and sodium during the day with an abnormally large diuretic response during the night thus causes an inversion of the normal circadian rhythm. Similar changes might occur in convalescence after long bedrest and in patients with autonomic neuropathy. Strict recumbency around the clock restores the normal rhythms [58], but sitting in bed during the day with strict recumbency only during the night may maintain an abnormal rhythm in nephrotic patients [9].

The abnormalities of renal rhythms in severe renal failure probably have another explanation. Glomerular and tubular function in these patients are assumed to be so impaired that, even when 'circadian regulatory factors' are normal, the kidney is unable to generate a normal rhythm (though we accept that this begs the question as to how it does so in health).

In patients with glomerulopathies and normal GFR, the relative amplitude of the rhythm for urinary IgG excretion is much higher than for urinary albumin or transferrin excretion. IgG is a larger protein than albumin and serum concentrations show only minor variations over the day (the amplitude of these changes is less than 10% of the 24-h mean) in these patients. This means that the ratio (IgG clearance/albumin clearance), the selectivity index, also varies over the day. That is, urine with the lowest selectivity index – with the least amount of larger proteins – is produced during the night [9,10].

To explain the mechanism of the circadian rhythm for urinary protein excretion, and its increase in relative amplitude for larger proteins, is not easy. Although the passage of albumin and larger proteins through the glomerular membrane is increased in glomerulopathies, transfer is still very much restricted. We know that both GFR and the serum concentration of proteins have circadian rhythms with a low relative amplitude; it is very likely, therefore, that the filtered load of proteins will have a circadian rhythm too. An explanation for the higher relative amplitude of the protein rhythms in comparison with the GFR rhythm might be an additional day/night difference in this 'glomerular restriction'. The difference in relative amplitude between the albumin and IgG rhythms might also be caused by differences in glomerular restriction, although differences between the two proteins in tubular reabsorption cannot be excluded. The causes of circadian changes in 'glomerular restriction' are unknown but some mechanism based upon circadian variability in the size and/or charge selectivity of the 'barrier' to filtration provided by the glomerular basement membrane has to be postulated. Further studies in these areas are in progress now.

The circadian rhythms for urinary water and electrolyte excretion also have much higher relative amplitudes than the rhythms of GFR and of their filtered loads. In absolute quantities, the difference in filtered load between day and night is in excess of that required to account for the circadian difference in urinary excretion. By contrast, if the percentage reabsorption of the filtered load of a substance was the same during day and night, urinary excretion should fluctuate with the same relative amplitude as the filtered load. Therefore our hypothesis is that tubular reabsorptive mechanisms also have a circadian rhythm with a higher activity during the day than during the night but that the diurnal increase is (slightly) less than the increase in filtered load. In addition, there might be a small difference in phase in comparison with the GFR rhythm. The summation of the rhythms for filtered load and for one or more sites of tubular reabsorption or secretion would eventually determine the phase and amplitude of the rhythm for the urinary excretion rate of a substance [11]. Still unresolved is what regulates the circadian rhythms for GFR and tubular reabsorption. Clinical studies in healthy individuals in which one parameter is altered to see what happens to the circadian rhythms, as well as observations on renal rhythms in patients with certain well-known disorders, might help us to get more insight into this problem.

Hormones in urine

Recently, interest has been shown in the usefulness of hormone concentrations in urine in health and disease (see also Chapter 10). Radioimmunoassay was often a necessary prior development in order to be able to deal with the low concentrations involved. This is particularly the case for some molecules that are not filtered freely at the glomeruli; (for example, see the assay of melatonin [59]). Water-soluble metabolites are generally more concentrated in urine (having been filtered without restriction and then being less able to diffuse out of the tubule) and so might be expected to be more reliable. An example would be the assay of 6-hydroxymelatonin sulphate [60] (see Chapter 10). Three further examples of hormonal studies in urine are:

1. Bourguignon *et al.* [61] assayed gonadotropins in pubertal children. They were able to compare the rise on waking with the night-time sleep values at different stages of puberty.
2. Kathol and Gehris [62] assayed free cortisol in control subjects and others with a history of major depressive disorder. The recovered depressives showed a greater incidence of peaks in concentration (deviations from the mean) than did controls.
3. There are several claims that the circadian rhythms of urinary catecholamines are changed in some forms of depression (see Wehr and Goodwin [63]).

Other examples will be found during the course of this text. The point is that urine is not just a 'waste fluid'. Its study can give valuable information about the biochemistry and physiology of the body and the mechanisms by which the kidneys function and are controlled, information that can aid diagnosis and treatment.

References

1. Conroy, R.T.W.L. and Mills, J.N. *Human Circadian Rhythms*, Churchill, London (1970)
2. Minors, D.S., Mills, J.N. and Waterhouse, J.M. The circadian variations of the rates of excretion of urinary electrolytes and of deep body temperature. *Int. J. Chronobiol.*, **4**, 1–28 (1976)
3. Mills, J.N. Phase relations between components of human circadian rhythms. In *Chronobiology* (eds L.E. Scheving, F. Halberg and J.E. Pauly), Igaku Shoin, Tokyo, pp. 560–563 (1974)
4. Minors, D.S. and Waterhouse, J.M. Circadian rhythms of urinary excretion: the relationship between the amount excreted and the circadian changes. *J. Physiol.*, **327**, 39–51 (1982)
5. Blomhert, G., Gerbrandy, J.A., Molhuysen, J.A. and de Vries, L.A. Diuretic effect of isotonic saline solution compared with that of water. Influence of diurnal rhythm. *Lancet*, **ii**, 1011–1015 (1951)
6. Moore-Ede, M.C., Brennan, M.F. and Ball, M.R. Circadian variation of intercompartmental potassium fluxes in man. *J. Appl. Physiol.*, **38**, 163–170 (1975)
7. Mills, J.N. Human circadian rhythms. *Physiol. Rev.*, **46**, 128–171 (1966)
8. Mills, J.N. Transmission processes between clock and manifestations. In *Biological Aspects of Human Circadian Rhythms* (ed. J.N. Mills), Plenum, London, pp. 27–84 (1973)
9. Koopman, M.G., Krediet, R.T. and Arisz, L. Circadian rhythms and the kidney. A review. *Neth. J. Med.*, **28**, 416–423 (1985)
10. Koopman, M.G., Krediet, R.T., Koomen, G.C.M., de Moor, E.A.M. and Arisz, L. Circadian rhythm of proteinuria: Relationship with molecular weight (MW) of proteins and the influence of prostaglandin inhibition. *Contr. Nephrol.*, **68**, 114–120 (1988)
11. Koopman, M.G., Koomen, G.C.M., Krediet, R.T., De Moor, E.A.M., Hoek, F.J. and Arisz, L. Circadian rhythm in glomerular filtration rate in normal individuals. *Clin. Sci.*, **77**, 105–111 (1989)
12. Brenner, B.M., Baylis, C. and Deen, W.M. Transport of molecules across renal glomerular capillaries. *Physiol. Rev.*, **56**, 502–534 (1976)
13. Brod, J. and Fencl, V. Diurnal variations of systemic and renal hemodynamics in normal subjects and in hypertensive disease. *Cardiologia*, **31**, 494–497 (1957)
14. Smolensky, M.H., Tatar, S.E., Bergman, S.A., Losman, J.G., Barnard, C.N., Dasco, C.C. and Ktakt, I.A. Circadian rhythmic aspects of human cardiovascular function: a review by chronobiologic statistical methods. *Chronobiologia*, **3**, 337–371 (1976)
15. Delea, D.C. Chronobiology of blood pressure. *Nephron*, **23**, 91–97 (1979)
16. Baylis, C. and Blantz, R.C. Glomerular hemodynamics. *News Physiol. Sci.*, **1**, 86–89 (1986)

17. Gordon, R.D., Wolfe, L.K., Island, D.P. and Liddle, G.W. A diurnal rhythm in plasma renin activity in man. *J. Clin. Invest.*, **45**, 1587–1592 (1966)
18. Bowden, R.E., Ware, J.H., De Mets, D.L. and Keiser, H.R. Urinary excretion of immunoreactive prostaglandin E: a circadian rhythm and the effect of posture. *Prostaglandins*, **14**, 151–161 (1977)
19. Donckier, J., Anderson, J.V., Yeo, T. and Bloom, S.R. Diurnal rhythms in the plasma concentration of atrial natriuretic peptide. *Lancet*, **ii**, 710–711 (1986)
20. George, C.P.L., Messerli, F.H., Genest, J., Nowaczynski, W., Boucher, R., Kuchel, O. and Rojo-Ortega, M. Diurnal variations of plasma vasopressin in man. *J. Clin. Endocrinol. Metab.*, **41**, 332–338 (1975)
21. Lifschitz, M.D. Lack of a role for renal nerves in renal sodium reabsorption in conscious dogs. *Clin. Sci.*, **54**, 567–572 (1978)
22. Bello-Reuss, E., Colindres, R.E., Pastoriza-Munoz, E., Mueller, R.A. and Gottschalk, C.W. Effects of acute unilateral renal denervation in the rat. *J. Clin. Invest.*, **56**, 208–217 (1975)
23. Schneider, E., McLane-Vega, L., Hanson, R., Childers, J. and Gleason, S. Effect of chronic bilateral renal denervation on daily sodium excretion in the conscious dog. *Fed. Proc.*, **37**, 645 (1978)
24. Gordon, R.D., Peart, W.S. and Wilcox, C.S. Requirement of the adrenergic nervous system for conservation of sodium by the rabbit kidney. *J. Physiol.*, **293**, 24P (1979)
25. DiBona, G.F. and Sawin, L.L. Renal nerve activity in conscious rats during volume expansion and depletion. *Amer. J. Physiol.*, **248**, F15–23 (1985)
26. Katz, M.A. and Shear, L. Effects of renal nerves on renal hemodynamics; I. Direct stimulation and carotid occlusion. *Nephron*, **14**, 246–256 (1975)
27. Vander, A.J. Effect of catecholamines and the renal nerves on renin secretion in anaesthetized dogs. *Amer. J. Physiol.*, **209**, 659–662 (1965)
28. Berlyne, G.M., Mallick, N.P., Seedat, Y.K., Edwards, E.C., Harris, R. and Orr, W.M. Abnormal urinary rhythm after renal transplantation in man. *Lancet*, **ii**, 435–436 (1968)
29. Koene, R., Van Liebergen, F. and Wijdeveld, P. Normal diurnal rhythm in the excretion of water and electrolytes after renal transplantation. *Clin. Nephrol.*, **1**, 266–270 (1973)
30. Bell, G.M., Reid, W., Ewing, D.J., Cumming, A.D., Watson, M.L., Doig, A. and Clarke, B.F. Abnormal diurnal urinary sodium and water excretion in diabetic autonomic neuropathy. *Clin. Sci.*, **73**, 259–265 (1987)
31. Bradbury, S. and Eggleston, C. Postural hypotension: report of 3 cases. *Amer. heart J.*, **1**, 73–86 (1925)
32. Davidson, C.D., Smith, D.B. and Morgan, L.M. Diurnal pattern of water and electrolyte excretion and body weight in idiopathic orthostatic hypotension. The effect of three treatments. *Amer. J. Med.*, **61**, 709–715 (1976)
33. Minors, D.S. and Waterhouse, J.M. *Circadian Rhythms and the Human*, John Wright, Bristol (1981)
34. Richards, A.M., Tonolo, G., Fraser, R., Morton, J.J., Leckie, B.J., Ball, S.G. and Robertson, J.I.S. Diurnal changes in plasma atrial natriuretic peptide concentrations. *Clin. Sci.*, **73**, 489–495 (1987)
35. Williams, G.H., Cain, I.P., Dluhy, D.H. and Underwood, R.H. Studies on the control of plasma aldosterone concentration in normal man. Response to posture, acute and chronic volume depletion and sodium loading. *J. Clin. Invest.*, **51**, 1731–1742 (1972)
36. Armbruster, H., Vetter, W., Beckerhoff, R., Nussberger, J., Vetter, H. and Siegenthaler, W. Diurnal variations of plasma aldosterone in supine man: Relationship to plasma renin activity and plasma cortisol. *Acta Endocrinol.*, **80**, 95–103 (1975)
37. Mills, J.N. and Stanbury, S.W. A reciprocal relationship between K^+ and H^+ excretion in the diurnal excretory rhythm in man. *Clin. Sci. Mol. Med.*, **13**, 177–185 (1954)
38. Garland, H.O. Maternal adjustments to pregnancy. In *Variations in Human Physiology* (ed. R.M. Case), Manchester University Press, Manchester, pp. 1–19 (1985)
39. Houston, I.B. and Oetliker, O. Growth and development of the kidneys. In *Paediatrics*, 2nd edn (eds J.A. Davies and J. Dobbin), Heinemann, London, pp. 486–496 (1981)
40. Goldstein, A., Aronow, L. and Kalman, S.M. *Principles of Drug Action*, 2nd edn, John Wiley, London (1974)

41. Minors, D.S. and Waterhouse, J.M. Development of circadian rhythms in infancy. In *Paediatrics*, 2nd edn (eds J.A. Davies and J. Dobbing), Heinemann, London, pp. 980–997 (1981)
42. Gambertoglio, J.G. Effects of renal disease: altered pharmacokinetics. In *Pharmacological Basis for Drug Treatment* (eds L.Z. Benet, N. Massoud and J.G. Gambertoglio), Raven Press, New York, pp. 149–171 (1974)
43. Guite, H.F., Bliss, M.R., Mainwaring-Burton, R.W., Thomas, J.M. and Drury, P.L. Effects of posture on the circadian rhythm of urine flow and electrolyte excretion in elderly female patients. *Clin. Sci.*, **69**, Suppl. 12, 12P (1985)
44. Wesson, L.G. Diurnal circadian rhythms of electrolyte excretion and filtration rate in end stage renal disease. *Nephron*, **26**, 211–214 (1980)
45. Hillier, P., Knapp, M.S. and Cove-Smith, R. Circadian variation in urinary potassium excretion in chronic renal insufficiency. *Q. J. Med.*, **49**, 461–478 (1980)
46. Hishida, A., Kumagai, H., Sudo, M. and Nagase, M. Diurnal variation in urinary potassium excretion in chronic renal insufficiency. *Min. Elect. Metab.*, **7**, 20–27 (1982)
47. Koopman, M.G., Krediet, R.T., Zuyderhoudt, F.J.M., de Moor, E.A.M. and Arisz, L. A circadian rhythm of proteinuria in patients with a nephrotic syndrome. *Clin. Sci.*, **69**, 395–401 (1985)
48. Goldman, R. Studies on diurnal variation of water and electrolyte excretion: nocturnal diuresis of water and sodium in congestive cardiac failure and cirrhosis of the liver. *J. Clin. Invest.*, **30**, 1191–1199 (1951)
49. Jones, R.A., McDonald, G.O. and Last, J.H. Reversal of diurnal variation in renal function in cases of cirrhosis with ascites. *J. Clin. Invest.*, **31**, 326–334 (1952)
50. Baldwin, D.S., Sirota, J.H. and Villarreal, H. Diurnal variations of renal function in congestive heart failure. *Proc. Soc. Exp. Biol. Med.*, **74**, 578–581 (1950)
51. De Vries, L.S., Ten Holt, S.P., Van Daatselaar, J.J., Mulder, A. and Borst, J.C.G. Characteristic renal excretion patterns in response to physiological, pathological and pharmacological stimuli. *Clin. Chim. Acta*, **5**, 915–937 (1960)
52. Doe, R.P., Vennes, J.A. and Flink, E.B. Diurnal variation of 17-hydroxycorticosteroids, sodium, potassium, magnesium and creatinine in normal subjects and in cases of treated adrenal insufficiency and Cushing syndrome. *J. Clin. Endocrinol. Metab.*, **20**, 253–265 (1960)
53. Thomas, J.P., Coles, G.A. and El-Shaboury, A.H. Nocturia in patients on long term steroid therapy. *Clin. Sci.*, **38**, 415–425 (1970)
54. Norgaard, J.P., Petersen, E.B. and Djurhuus, J.C. Diurnal antidiuretic hormone levels in enuretics. *J. Urol.*, **134**, 1029–1031 (1985)
55. Lewis, H.E., Lobban, M.C. and Tredre, B.G. Daily rhythms of renal excretion in a child with nocturnal enuresis. *J. Physiol.*, **210**, 42–43P (1970)
56. Hrusheshky, W.J.M., Merdink, J. and Abdel-Monem, M.M. Circadian rhythmicity of polyamine urinary excretion. *Cancer Res.*, **43**, 3944–3947 (1983)
57. Tuckman, M., Robison, L.L., Maynard, R.C., Ramnarine, M.L. and Krivit, W. Assessment of the diurnal variations in urinary homovanillic and vanillylmandelic acid excretion for the diagnosis and follow-up of patients with neuroblastoma. *Clin. Biochem.*, **18**, 176–179 (1985)
58. Borst, J.C.G. and De Vries, L.A. The three types of 'natural' diuresis. *Lancet*, **ii**, 1–6 (1950)
59. Lang, V., Kornemark, M., Aubert, M.L., Paunier, L. and Sizonenko, P.C. Radioimmunological determination of urinary melatonin in humans: correlation with plasma levels and typical 24-hour rhythmicity. *J. Clin. Endocrinol. Metab.*, **53**, 645–650 (1981)
60. Arendt, J., Bojkowski, C., Franey, C., Wright, J. and Marks, V. Immunoassay of 6-hydroxymelatonin sulfate in human plasma and urine: abolition of the urinary 24-hour rhythm with atenolol. *J. Clin. Endocrinol. Metab.*, **60**, 1166–1173 (1985)
61. Bourguinon, J.P., Vanderschueren-Lodeweyckx, M., Reuter, A.M., Vrindts-Gevaert, Y., Gerard, A. and Franchimont, P. Radioimmunoassays of unextracted gonadotrophins in timed fractions of 24-hour urine: morning increase of gonadotrophin excretion, a circadian pattern in relation to puberty. *Horm. Res.*, **13**, 367–384 (1980)
62. Kathol, R.G. and Gehris, T. Peak amplitude and frequency of urinary free cortisol excretion in patients with a history of major depressive disorders. *Chronobiol. Int.*, **3**, 281–287
63. Wehr, T.A. and Goodwin, F.K. *Circadian Rhythms in Psychiatry*, Boxwood Press, California (1983)

Chapter 7

Clinical immunology and allergy

Francis Lévi, Alain Reinberg and Chantal Canon

Introduction

Immunity was first defined as the acquisition by an organism of specific defence
mechanisms, as a result of an infectious process. This concept has been extended
today. Immunological reactions involve both specific and non-specific responses of
an organism to an antigen. These reactions lead to the elimination of the antigenic
molecules and/or the cells that express them. Thus immunological processes
operate in several pathological states such as infectious, allergic, rheumatological
and malignant diseases. Clinical immunologists are concerned with the physiopathology and the diseases that affect lymphoid organs, just as cardiologists are
concerned with the physiopathology and the diseases that affect the heart [1,2].

Antigens include a broad variety of chemical substances (minerals, proteins,
drugs, autologous molecules, altered peptides etc.) from several origins (viruses,
bacteria, parasites, plants, animals, etc.). Antibodies, however, are molecules
synthesized by lymphocytes and plasmocytes as a specific response to an antigenic
stimulation. Since the defence processes of the organism are the topics of the
present chapter, both specific, i.e. truly immunological, and non-specific aspects,
such as inflammation, will be considered. Local symptoms (e.g. rubor, dolor, calor)
by which inflammation is clinically recognized also involve immunological
phenomena in which basophils, mast cells, antigens and antibodies as well as
humoral mediators such as histamine, bradykinin and arachidonic acid play an
important role. For instance, the excessive bronchial constriction responsible for
asthma is related to both allergic reactions and inflammatory processes [3].

Attempts to demonstrate *specific* antigens on human tumour cells have failed.
In several instances, however, quantitative differences in the amount of antigens
present at the cell surface have been found between cancerous and homologous
healthy tissue. Circadian and circannual rhythms, which characterize cellular
metabolism and division in healthy tissues but seldom in cancerous tissues [4], may
also modulate antigenic expression. If so, time may represent a critical factor for
the recognition of cancer cells by immune cells.

The transdisciplinary nature of both chronobiology and immunology has led us
to split this chapter into two sections. The first one will consider biological rhythms
in the immune net work and their implications for cancer aetiology and control.
The second one will deal with infectious and allergic diseases.

Biological rhythms in the immune network: implications for cancer aetiology and control

In this first section, we will review information indicating that immune defence mechanisms are organized along both a circadian and a circannual time scale in man. Following stimulation, the immune network organizes its response according to circaseptan (with a period, τ, $\simeq$ 7 days) [5] or other infradian (with $\tau > 28\,h$) time scales. Such rhythms are temporal features of the healthy immune network, just as macrophages, T and B lymphocytes constitute different cellular features of this system. The physiological rhythmicity of the immune network may be viewed as an index of good health, as is the case for some hormonal secretions, such as cortisol [6], LH [7] and prolactin [8] as well as body temperature [9]. Thus, a knowledge of the temporal organization of the immune network may be necessary to understand further its physiology, as well as its involvement in the aetiology and control of several diseases, including cancer. In this way we may also learn when the network is most receptive to instruction and control. Reproducible effects of 'immunomodulators' or other 'biological response modifiers' are not established at present, perhaps because time factors have been underestimated. This hypothesis is supported by the magnitude of circadian and circannual physiological changes in immune functions.

Circadian organization of the immune network

Dependence of the reactivity of the immune system on the circadian time of its exposure to an antigen

In a study designed by Cove Smith et al. [10], healthy subjects ($n=180$) were divided into seven groups and a purified protein derivative of tuberculin (PPD) was injected intradermally (Heaf test) at one of seven circadian times (01:00, 04:00, 07:00, 10:00, 13:00, 16:00, 19:00 or 22:00 h). In studies reported in this chapter human subjects were socially synchronized with diurnal activity (for example from $\simeq 07{:}00\,h$ to $\simeq 23{:}00\,h$) and nocturnal rest, unless otherwise mentioned. Therefore reference is made to local time rather than to the organism's biological time. The area of induration, as measured 48 h later, varied threefold as a function of the test time (Figure 7.1).

The response was maximal after tuberculin challenge at 07:00 h and minimal at 22:00 h. This was confirmed in subjects in whom the skin test was performed at these times, 6 weeks apart [10]. In another study, episodes of renal allograft rejection were also estimated to occur more commonly near 06:00 h in patients bearing a kidney transplant [11]. These results suggest that the cell-mediated immunity of man exhibits a physiological circadian rhythmicity with a large amplitude. Such findings are supported by results from several experiments on laboratory animals [12–16]. Many factors, however, are involved in the expression of immune reactivity *in vivo*.

Circadian rhythm in circulating immune cells
An insight into the temporal organization of the immune network may be gained from studies performed on circulating blood cells and their by-products. Most investigations performed on human beings have been carried out on circulating

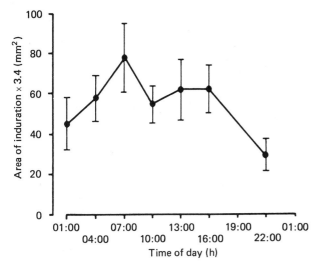

Figure 7.1 Circadian rhythm in skin reactivity to tuberculin (PPD). A total of 180 men and women were involved in this study. Areas (mm^2) of induration ($\times$ 3.4) were measured by two independent observers 48 h after the injection of PPD with the Heaf gun at various times. A measurable response was found in 122 subjects. The extent of this response varied as a function of time of antigenic challenge (After Cove-Smith *et al.* [10])

lymphocytes or monocytes–macrophages. These two cell types are closely involved in the development of an immune response. It is generally accepted that the monocyte–macrophage plays a key role in presenting the antigen to the lymphocytes. The numbers of circulating lymphocytes and monocytes vary predictably during the 24 h. The circadian rhythm in lymphocyte count is the more prominent. It was described as early as 1925 by Sabin *et al.* [17] and repeatedly confirmed [18,19]. In a study performed on 150 apparently healthy young and adult subjects sampled every 4 h for 24 h, a circadian rhythm in lymphocyte and monocyte count was documented by Haus *et al* [19]. Their group was comprised of 71 women and 79 men, age range 11–45 years. Figure 7.2 shows the temporal relationship of these two rhythms. The double amplitude (i.e. the difference between the peak and the trough of the rhythm) was 20% of ther 24-h-mean for monocytes and 35% for lymphocytes. The acrophase (peak time) was located near 20:00 h for monocytes and near 02:00 h for lymphocytes.

Lymphocytes are composed of several subtypes which exhibit different functions. These lymphocyte subtypes can now be identified with monoclonal antibodies directed specifically against surface membrane antigens.

Circadian rhythms in circulating lymphocyte subtypes
Whereas T lymphocytes are mainly involved in cell-mediated immunity, B lymphocytes are primarily responsible for humoral immunity. Both kinds of cells cooperate closely in the mounting of an immune response. For instance both T suppressor and B cells appear to be strongly involved in the production of immunoglobulin E (IgE) [20].

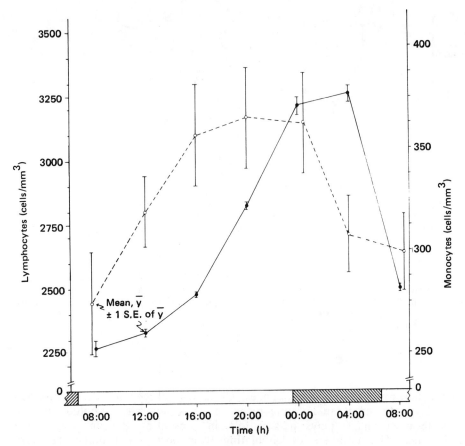

Figure 7.2 Circadian rhythm in the number of circulating lymphocytes (●) and monocytes (○) from peripheral blood; 150 apparently healthy young adult and adult subjects (71 women, 79 men) were studied six times over a 24-h span. The counting of formed elements was performed automatically. Two-hundred cell count differentials were done on Wright-stained smears (After Haus *et al.* [19])

A circadian rhythm in circulating T lymphocytes has been demonstrated with several complementary laboratory techniques. These include rosette formation with sheep erythrocytes and labelling with different monoclonal antibodies, Leu 4, OKT3, T28 [21–29]. Similar results were obtained in these studies even though the subjects differed in age, ethnic origin and sex. They were, moreover, performed in different seasons and according to different protocols (Table 7.1). In two studies, no night sample was obtained [22,27]. In another two studies, only four samples were obtained in 24 h [19,27]. In one study, each subject was sampled only once per day, with the sampling periods 1 week apart on the same day of the week. This was done in order to avoid a possible sequencing effect of repeated blood withdrawals within 24 h [19]. In yet another study, T cell count was determined directly on whole blood rather than on a suspension of isolated mononuclear cells [27]. These discrepancies may explain some of the differences in raw values. For these reasons, a further study was performed in five healthy young men. Blood

Table 7.1 Circadian rhythmicity of circulating lymphocyte subsets in man

Reference	Subjects			Samples		Month of study	Subsets investigated			
	No.	Sex	Age (years)	No.	Time (h)		T	Mature B	T helper	T suppressor cytotoxic
Abo et al. [35]*	4	M	26–32	6	8,12,16,20,0,4	April	En-RFC[a]	Anti-SIg	–	–
Bertouch et al. [22]**	9	M	24–49	6	6,9,12,15,18,21	?	T28	FMC1	OKT4	OKT8
Haus et al. [19]*	7	M	21–46	4	6,12,18,0	?	En-RFC	Anti-SIg	–	–
	8	F								
Lévi et al. [24]*	5	M	24–39	7	8,12,16,20,0,4,(8)	April, Nov.	OKT3	Anti-SIg	OKT4	OKT8
Miyakawi et al. [27][b]**	8	M	24–34	4	7,12,17,22	May	OKT3 OKT11	OKB2	OKT4	OKT8
Ritchie et al. [23]**	9	M	45–48	8	8,11,14,17,20,23,2.5	March	Leu 4	–	Leu 3a	Leu 2a Leu 2b
	1	F								
Lévi et al. [29]	5	M	25–35	33	8,12,16,20,0,4(8)	Jan., March, June, Aug., Nov.	OKT3	–	OKT4	OKT8

A summary of materials and methods used in different investigations. Labelled cells were counted under a microscope (*) or by flow cytometry (**).
[a]Laboratory technique used to characterize a given subset. En-RFC: rosette-forming cells. Anti-SIg: monoclonal antibody against immunoglobulins of different classes (IgG. IgA and IgM). All other symbols represent different monoclonal antibodies.
[b]Lymphocyte subsets were assessed on whole blood rather than on isolated mononuclear cells.

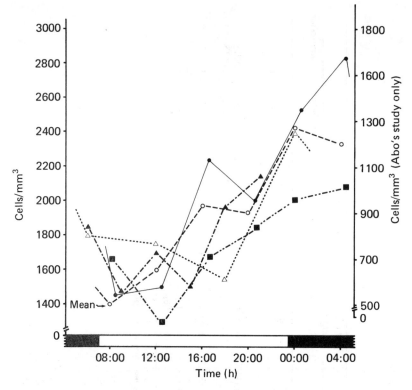

Figure 7.3 Circadian rhythm in number of circulating T cells from human peripheral blood. Summarized results from five different investigations (materials and methods given in Table 7.1). ○, RFC$^+$, Abo *et al.* [35]; ▲, T$_{28}^+$, Bertouch *et al.* [22]; △, RFC$^+$, Haus *et al.* [19]; ●, OKT3$^+$, Lévi *et al.* [26]; ■, OKT3$^+$, Lévi *et al.* [29]

was sampled every 4 h for 24 h each month for 5 months (January, March, June, August and November). The average circadian rhythm in circulating T lymphocyte subsets was thus determined across several circannual stages [29]. Figure 7.3 indicates that the circulating T lymphocyte count doubled between 08:00 h (trough time) and midnight or 04:30 h (peak times) in all these studies.

A circadian rhythm in circulating T helper lymphocytes has been demonstrated with two different monoclonal antibodies, Leu 3a and OKT4 [22–29]. The peak in circulating T helper cells occurred near 02:00 h in all studies: the number of these cells almost doubled in the course of 24 h (Figure 7.4). Thus the amount of all T and T helper cells that circulate in peripheral blood varies rhythmically along the circadian scale. Their respective numbers reach a peak in the middle of the night (rest) and a trough near wake-up time. The consistency of results obtained by different investigators argues for only minor interindividual differences in these rhythms. This may not be the case for suppressor-cytotoxic lymphocytes as well as for the helper/suppressor ratio.

Circadian variations in circulating T-suppressor-cytotoxic lymphocytes were found by Ritchie *et al.* [23] and ourselves [24]. T-suppressor-cytotoxic cells were respectively assessed with Leu 2b and OKT8 monoclonal antibodies and exhibited

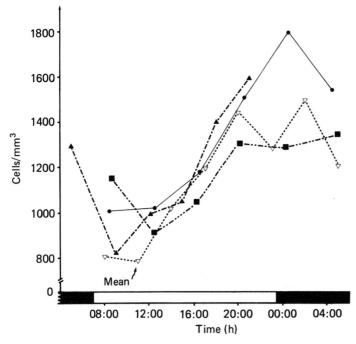

Figure 7.4 Circadian rhythm in number of circulating T helper cells from human peripheral blood. Summarized results from different investigations (materials and methods given in Table 7.1). ▲, OKT4+, Bertouch *et al.* [22]; ●, OKT4+, Lévi *et al.* [26]; ■, OKT4+, Lévi *et al.* [29]; ▽, Leu 3a+, Ritchie *et al.* [23]

Table 7.2 Circadian rhythmicity in circulating T-suppressor-cytotoxic lymphocytes

Reference	τ (h)	P^a	Mesor^b (cells/mm³)	Double amplitude^c (% mesor)	Acrophase^d (h)
Ritchie *et al.* [23]	24	<0.05	430	47	21:56
Lévi *et al.* [24]	24	0.003	570	67	20:30
Lévi *et al.* [29]	24	0.31	515	–	–
	12	<0.0001	515	36	08:30 and 20:30

From a cosinor analysis with a period τ = 24 or 12 h.
[a]*P* value of an F test of the rejection of the null-amplitude hypothesis.
[b]24-h mean.
[c]Difference between maximum and minimum of the rhythm.
[d]Time of estimated maximum.

similar rhythm characteristics (Table 7.2). However, subsequent investigations by ourselves [25,28,29] as well as studies by others [22,27] failed to demonstrate such a 24-h rhythm. Rather, a 12-h rhythm was statistically validated in five subjects in whom circadian studies were performed in 5 different months. Interindividual differences in peak and trough times may account for such observations and obliterate a 24-h rhythm as a group phenomenon.

The T helper/T suppressor-cytotoxic ratio seems to behave similarly. Whereas no circadian variation has been demonstrated at group level by most investigators

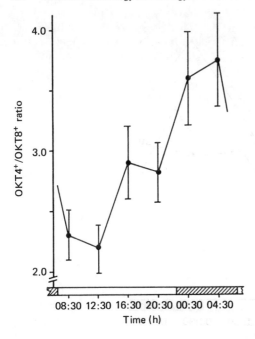

Figure 7.5 Circadian variation in helper/suppressor ratio from human peripheral blood of five healthy men studied in January, March, June, August and November. (After Lévi *et al.* [29])

[22,23,27] we found a large-amplitude circadian rhythm in the OKT4/OKT8$^+$ ratio from two subjects [24] and confirmed these results in a subsequent study (Figure 7.5) [29]. Bertouch *et al.* [22] have also pointed out that the lack of any group circadian variation in this ratio might result from interindividual differences, since the ratio doubled reproducibly during the test span in two of their subjects. In a subsequent study, we have also documented a statistically significant circadian rhythm in this ratio in three subjects but with different rhythm characteristics: the circadian peak was located 8 h earlier than in the first study [28].

These results and others [29] suggest that the circadian rhythmicity in T cells and that in the T helper subset may be species-specific. In comparison, the circadian variability in T suppressor-cytotoxic cells and that in helper/suppressor ratio may constitute a temporal feature of the individual's immunity, as a result, for example, of the genetic background and/or previous immune challenges: these last two variables may also respond more rapidly to an uncontrolled stimulus. Whether or not the presence of such a rhythm is of importance in subsequent development of disease is not known at present. It is also possible that a circannual or other low-frequency rhythm modulates the circadian peak time or periodicity of these two variables, as suggested from our studies [28]. If so, the circadian rhythmicity of these two T cell subsets may be under distinct hormonal control, as suggested by non-chronobiological studies [30].

In order to investigate this hypothesis further, T cell subsets and plasma cortisol and testosterone were determined at six circadian stages in each of 5 months in five healthy young men [29]. Circadian rhythms were demonstrated for circulating total, T and T helper lymphocytes with maxima localized in the first half of the night and double amplitudes exceeding 25% of the 24-h mesor. A 12 h rather than a 24 h rhythm was found for circulating T-suppressor-cytotoxic lymphocytes, with 2A (double amplitude) equal to 36% of the 24-h mesor and acrophases (ϕ) localized near 08:30 and 20:30 h. Such a 12-h rhythm may reflect a true circahemidian rhythm in the circulating count of suppressor-cytotoxic lymphocytes. A 12-h rhythm was documented for both DNA and RNA synthesis in circulating total lymphocytes [31] (S. Sanchez de la Pena, W. Hrushesky and F. Lévi, unpublished). Both OKT4$^+$ and HNKl$^+$ lymphocytes from peripheral blood may also express the T8 antigen at their surface [32,33]. The 12-h rhythmicity observed in OKT8$^+$ mononuclear cells may thus indicate that the T8 antigen is expressed predominantly at 08:30 h in a given subpopulation, and at 20:30 h in another. Double-labelling studies will be necessary to answer such questions.

The T helper suppressor-cytotoxic ratio exhibited a circadian rhythm with a pronounced double amplitude averaging 50% of the mesor and the acrophase localized at 01:00 h. This finding is consistent with our preliminary report in two subjects [24]. A circadian rhythm and an associated 12-h harmonic were documented in the present study for plasma total and free cortisol and testosterone concentrations, with characteristics similar to those reported earlier. No statistically significant correlation was found between plasma cortisol (either free or total) or testosterone and any of the five immunological variables investigated even though 162 pairs of data were used for testing each correlation. Because hormones often need a lag time to exert their metabolic effects, lag times of 4 and 8 h between plasma hormones and lymphocyte-related variables were also considered. Again no correlation was found between these two sets of variables. This suggests that adrenal cortex or testicular rhythmic secretions play only minor roles, if any, in the circadian organization of circulating total, T3, T4 or T8 lymphocytes and that of the T4/T8 ratio [28,29]. Other rhythmic controls need to be explored among the many potential contributing factors.

It is evident that a coincidence in time between peak and trough values of two variables does not necessarily imply any correlation or a fortiori any causal relationship (as was suspected for T lymphocytes and plasma cortisol (15,23,27,34,35]).

It is important to note that these findings relate to a physiological time structure, and that qualitatively different chronopharmacological effects may result from the exogenous administration of higher doses of these hormones for therapeutic purposes.

Mature B lymphocytes can be characterized by surface immunoglobulins (Ig) and identified by a monoclonal antibody directed against these Ig (SIg$^+$ lymphocytes). The number of circulating SIg$^+$ is reported to exhibit a circadian rhythm in healthy subjects [21,25,26]. Similar rhythm characteristics were found in two studies [24,34] (Figure 7.6) where the circadian acrophase was located near 20:00 h. This time is close to that of maximal skin reactivity to either house dust or penicillin in specifically sensitized patients [36,37]. B cells take part in this reaction. In one study, however, the acrophase of circulating B lymphocytes was located at 04:50 h [19]. This study involved four rather than six time points, and each sampling time differed from the next by 1 week. Such discrepancies may be accounted for by different laboratory techniques, study designs, and/or other infradian bioperiodicities. Thus passive adsorption of immunoglobulins on to lymphocytes and/or monocytes was minimized in our study [26] by preincubating mononuclear cells with 5% fetal calf serum. The consistent results obtained in two studies performed with a similar design [21,26,34] suggest that repeated sampling

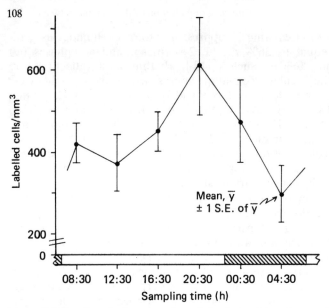

Figure 7.6 Circadian rhythm in number of circulating B lymphocytes (SIg^+). Seven circadian profiles in five apparently healthy subjects. (After Lévi *et al.* [26])

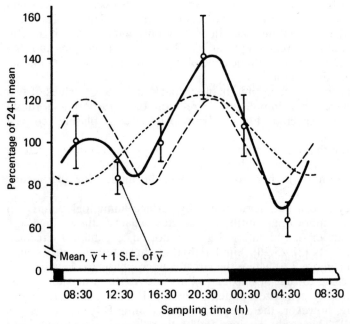

Figure 7.7 Circadian and circahemidian ($\tau \simeq 12\,h$) rhythms in circulating B lymphocytes. Seven circadian profiles in five apparently healthy subjects. Reconstruction of the rhythm's waveform according to Fourier's transform technique. Because of statistically significant interindividual differences in 24-h means, data from each individual were expressed as percentages of this subject's 24-h mean. Cosinor analysis revealed that both a 24-h rhythm and a 12-h rhythm component were statistically significant ($P<0.05$). The algebraic sum of these two periodic components represents a good approximation of the data (mean + 1 S.E.M. also plotted). – – –, 24-h component; ——, 12-h component. (After Lévi *et al.* [26])

along the 24-h scale had little effect. On the other hand, the circadian rhythm in circulating T lymphocytes was similar in all three studies (see above). A circahemidian rhythmic component with a period of 12 h was also found in our investigation which might account for these differences in circulating B lymphocytes. Thus circulating SIg$^+$ lymphocytes exhibited a composite pattern of two rhythms, which was reconstructed according to Fourier's transform technique (Figure 7.7). In addition, other infradian rhythms, circaseptan or circannual, may also influence the circadian rhythmicity of B lymphocytes, as discussed below.

Other circulating lymphocyte subsets have also been investigated with monoclonal antibodies. These include activated T and B subsets (anti-HLA-DR or OKIA) [23,26], light-chain-bearing B lymphocytes (anti-κ and anti-λ) [26], and pre-B lymphocytes (bearing at their surface the common associated lymphocytic leukaemia antigen, CALLA, assessed with both J5 and VILA1 monoclonal antibodies) [25,26]. For all these subtypes, a circadian and/or a circahemidian rhythm was found. The results are summarized in Table 7.3.

Table 7.3 Circadian variations in other lymphocyte (L) subsets from human peripheral blood

τ^a (h)	L subset	P^b	Double amplitude^c (% mesor)	Acrophase^d (h)
24	κ$^+$	0.17	–	–
	λ$^+$	0.06	54	20:40
	IA$^+$	0.82	–	–
	J5$^+$	<0.001	186	01:50
12	κ$^+$	0.04	54	21:05
	λ$^+$	0.22	–	–
	IA$^+$	0.04	44	23:50
	J5$^+$	0.01	116	14:50

Results are from cosinor analysis of data expressed as percentages of individual 24-h mean. Seven circadian profiles obtained in five healthy male subjects, sampled every 4 h for 24 h.
[a]Period.
[b]P value of an F test of the null-amplitude hypothesis.
[c]Difference between maximum and minimum of fitted cosine function.
[d]Time of maximum in fitted cosine function.

Since rhythm characteristics (including the dominant period) differ according to the cell type considered, a common regulation of the circadian rhythm in all circulating lymphocyte subsets is excluded. The mechanisms of these circadian variations may involve cell division in the thymus, lymph nodes and spleen: these are known to exhibit a circadian rhythm in various animal species [4,19,38,39]. Other mechanisms yet to be explored from a circadian point of view include cell trapping in the bone marrow, circulation from blood to lymph and back from lymph to blood and/or destruction by endogenous substances. For obvious reasons, such rhythms have not been documented in man.

Circadian rhythms in the metabolic activities of immune cells

The metabolic activity of circulating leucocytes has been found to vary predictably in the course of 24 h, as shown for RNA content (S. Sanchez de la Pena, W. Hrushesky and F. Lévi, unpublished) [40–42] and for several enzymic activities

Table 7.4 Circadian variations in metabolism of circulating lymphocytes in man (summarized results)

Reference	Subjects		Sampling		Variable measured	Period (h)	Time (s) of peak (h)
	No.	Sex	Interval (h)	Span (h)			
Carter et al. [31]	5	M	2	24	DNA synthesis	12	10 and 23
Heitbrock et al. [44]	8	?	6	48	RNA polymerase B activity	24	24
Hrusheshky, Sanchez and Levi (unpublished)	6	M	4	24	Total RNA content	12	6 and 18
Ramot et al. [43]	4	?	4	24	Glucose-6-phosphate dehydrogenase activity	24	16
					6-Phosphodehydrogenase activity	24	20
					Lactate dehydrogenase activity	24	16
					Hexokinase activity	12	12 and 20
					Glutamate–oxaloacetate transaminase activity	24	20
					All	24	16

Table 7.5 Circadian variation in in vitro transformability of human lymphocytes from peripheral blood (summarized results)

Reference	Subjects		Sampling interval[a] (h)	Kind of transformation	Technique	Time(s) of peak (h)
	No.	Sex				
Tavadia et al. [46]	6	M	4	PHA-induced	Isolated lymphocytes (72 h)	8
Eskola et al. [45]	6	M	6	Spontaneous	Whole blood (66 h)	8 and 20
				PHA-induced	Whole blood (66 h)	20
				Con A-induced	Whole blood (66 h)	20
				PPD-induced	Whole blood (66 h)	02
Carter et al. [31]	5	M	2	Spontaneous	Isolated lymphocytes (8 h)	10 and 22
Haus et al. [19]	9	M	4	PHA-induced	Isolated lymphocytes (48 h)	12
	8	F	6	PWM-induced		12
	9	?	1 week apart	PHA-induced	Isolated lymphocytes (48 h)	6

[a]Over a 24-h span.

[43,44]. Circulating lymphocytes are thus also affected by a rhythmic metabolism (Table 7.4). A circahemidian rhythm, with a period of 12 h stood out clearly for DNA synthesis, total RNA content and hexokinase activity. Figure 7.8 depicts the temporal relationships of such rhythms.

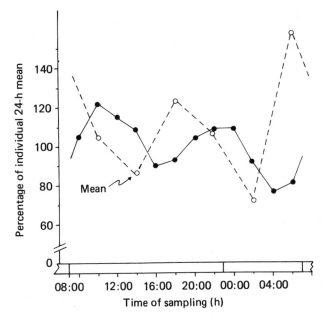

Figure 7.8 Circahemidian rhythms ($\tau \simeq 12\,h$) in the metabolic activities of circulating lymphocytes from peripheral blood. Tentative summary of circadian variations in DNA synthesis (●) (from Carter *et al.* [31]) and total RNA content (○) (Sanchez de la Pena, Hrushesky and Lévi, unpublished)

Other enzymic activities exhibited a rhythm with a period of 24 h rather than 12 h. These spontaneous circadian variations in the metabolism of circulating lymphocytes may account for those that characterize some of their functions.

Circadian rhythms in lymphocyte transformability
Once the immune system is stimulated, lymphocytes proliferate. This step is essential for cell-mediated immunity to operate properly. It can be explored by lymphocyte transformation tests. Lymphocyte transformation can occur either spontaneously or after exposure to an antigen or to mitogens, such as phyto-haemagglutinin (PHA), concanavalin A (Con A), purified protein derivative of tuberculin (PPD) or pokeweed mitogen (PWM). With all these agents, the transformation of peripheral lymphocytes exhibits a marked circadian rhythmicity (Table 7.5).

Spontaneous lymphocyte transformation
This follows a circahemidian (with $\tau = 12\,h$) rather than a circadian rhythm. Thus two peaks were found in 24 h, in two separate studies using different methodology [31,45]. In both studies, the peak–trough difference exceeded 40% of the 24-h mean, and the peaks were located at both 08:00 and 20:00 h.

Stimulated lymphocyte transformation with PHA, Con A, PPD and PWM or
streptokinase–streptodornase (SKSD)
This follows a unimodal circadian pattern [19,45,47]. In two studies, the circadian
maximum in PHA transformation occurred in the morning (08:00–10:00 h) and the
nadir in the late evening (18:00–00:00 h). These studies were performed on isolated
lymphocytes [19,46]. In the other study, the reverse was observed: the peak in
PHA transformation was located at 20:00 h and the nadir at 08:00 h [45]. Similar
results were also observed by these authors for Con A- and PPD-stimulated
transformation. This investigation was performed on whole blood. Differences in
methods and/or in seasons of study most likely account for these discrepancies in
stimulated lymphocyte transformation. In another circadian study conducted in
elderly subjects, Haus *et al.* [19] measured DNA formation by flow cytometry in
72-h PHA cultures using whole blood. They also found a nocturnal peak of the
number of cells in S phase. In the method using whole blood, both serum factors
and adjacent cells which affect the response are present [48–50]. Most likely, this
method mimics *in vivo* conditions better than conventional methods using purified
lymphocytes.

Natural killer (NK) cell activity and cells responsible for antibody-dependent cytotoxicity (ADCC) also exhibit circadian rhythms in man

In six healthy subjects, blood was sampled every 4 h for 24 h. Isolated mononuclear
cells were assayed against ^{51}Cr-labelled K562 chronic myelogenous leukaemia cells,
used as targets. A circadian rhythm in the NK activity of human blood was found,
with a large double amplitude (144% of the mesor) and a maximal activity

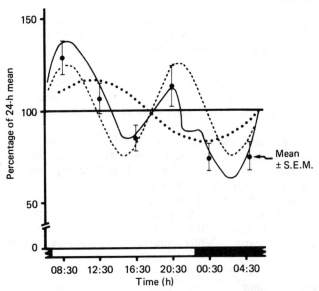

Figure 7.9 Circadian rhythm and circahemidian ($\tau \simeq 12$ h) component in circulating HNK1^{+}
lymphocytes. Reconstruction of the rhythm's waveform according to Fourier's transform technique.
Data are expressed as percentages of each individual's 24 h mesor. Cosinor analysis revealed statistically
significant rhythms with $\tau \simeq 24$ h and $\tau \simeq 12$ h ($P<0.001$) ······, 24-h component. -----, 12-h component.
(After Lévi *et al.*, [29])

Table 7.6 Circadian rhythm in different killer cell activities of circulating human mononuclear cells

Reference	No. of subjects	Method	Double amplitude[a] (% mesor)[b]	Acrophase[c] (h)
Williams et al. [51]	6	^{51}Cr-labelled K562 CML cells	140	11:00
Abo et al. [35]	4	^{51}Cr-labelled SRBC (ADCC)	70	13:00
Ritchie et al. [23]	10	HNK1 monoclonal ab	50	11:15
Lévi et al. [52]	5 (25 circadian profiles)	HNK1 monoclonal ab	35	11:30

A statistically significant circadian rhythm ($P<0.01$) was found in each study. All investigations involved six or more blood samples (every 4 h for 24 h).
[a]Difference between maximum and minimum in fitted cosine function.
[b]24-h mean.
[c]Time of maximum in fitted cosine function.

occurring near 11:00 h [51]. A similar circadian rhythm was also observed for the killing activity of human mononuclear cells in the ADCC system [35], both for the percentage of circulating killer cells (bearing receptors for the Fc fragment of IgG), and for the circulating number of lymphocytes labelled with HNK1 (Leu 7) monoclonal antibodies [23,52] (Table 7.6). A 12-h rhythmic component was also statistically validated. The reconstructed curve of circulating HNK1$^+$ lymphocyte count is shown in Figure 7.9 [52]. These results agree with those recently obtained by Gatti *et al.* [53] in seven healthy young men from whom blood was obtained every 4 h for 24 h in order to assess NK cell activity of separated mononuclear cells against K562 cells. Maximal activity was observed near 04:30 h. The circadian rhythm in NK cell activity seems to be inverted in nocturnally active rodents compared with diurnally active human beings: the NK activity of spleen cells of rats demonstrated a circadian rhythm with a maximum located in the early activity phase [54]. Thus processes that may lead to an immediate destruction of cancer cells vary in the course of 24 h, and reach their maximum around awakening.

Circadian rhythms in circulating immunoglobulins and complement

A circadian rhythm in circulating immunoglobulins of various classes and in fragment C3 of complement has been documented in man [55–58]. For IgA, IgG and IgM in mostly male subjects, and for C3 in female subjects, the double amplitude of the rhythm was 10–15% of the 24-h mean. For all these variables, the acrophase was located in the early afternoon. A circadian rhythm in total IgE has also been demonstrated in asthmatic children but not in healthy ones [59]. The peak time occurred during the night.

Circannual organization of the immune network

A circannual rhythm in the 24-h mesor of circulating leucocytes was demonstrated by Reinberg *et al.* [55] with the highest values occurring in early December, i.e. very close to the maximum found for total lymphocytes in our study [52]. No circannual rhythm in the morning values of total leucocytes or lymphocytes has been found by others [19,60]. In a recent study, large seasonal variations in morning total leucocyte count were found in young men, but not in men older than 40 years [61]. This indicates that age needs to be considered when evaluating the time structure of the immune system.

Rhythms over the course of a year have been documented for circulating B, T and NK lymphocyte subsets, for an enzymic activity of cultured lymphocytes and for the plasma concentrations of immunoglobulins in healthy subjects.

Circannual rhythm in B-cell immunity: Circulating SIg$^+$ lymphocytes exhibited a marked seasonal variation in five apparently healthy male subjects sampled at 08:30 h in both January and June (F. Lévi and C. Canon, unpublished results). The percentage of cells was twice as high in June as in January (Figure 7.10). These data agree with those obtained in eight Japanese subjects sampled between 09:00 and 10:00 h both in winter and summer [21]. In investigations of circannual rhythms, it is essential to specify the circadian sampling time and the sleep/activity patterns of the subjects in order to avoid so-called bioaliasing. This information was not provided in two other studies in which different results were reported [60,62]. The overall higher percentages of circulating B-cells found in the Japanese

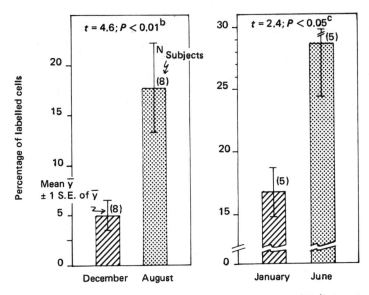

Figure 7.10 Circannual variation in circulating B lymphocytes (SIg$^+$) from human peripheral blood. The same male subjects were sampled between 08:30 and 10:00 h in winter and summer. Summarized results of our own data (unpublished)[c] and data from Abo *et al.* [21][b]

subjects [21], as compared to ours (of Caucasian origin) (C. Canon and F. Lévi, unpublished) may be accounted for by minor differences in the laboratory techniques used to characterize these cells.

Geographic, genetic and sex-related differences may all be of importance since the circannual rhythmicity of several hormones is reported to differ between Japanese, American and Italian women [8,63]. The most important factors appear to be genetic origin and/or the quality of food. Differences in circannual rhythms between female populations may relate to the variable incidence of several diseases, including breast cancer, T-cell lymphoma, etc., between Japanese and Caucasian populations.

The circannual rhythmicity of plasma immunoglobulins also exhibits a maximum in summer or in autumn and a minimum in winter. This has been shown for IgA, IgG and IgM [19,55,64,65]. A longitudinal study of rubella antibody titres in a young woman who had contracted German measles revealed reproducible peaks and troughs, in May and November, respectively, for 7 consecutive years. In November, titres were so low as to indicate lack of immunity against rubella, despite a history to the contrary [66]. Thus circulating immunoglobulins appear to reach their maximum near that in circulating B lymphocytes. This temporal relationship might tentatively be explained by an increased stimulation of B cells to proliferate and differentiate into plasma cells in summer. These plasma cells, mostly located in the lymph nodes, would then produce increased amounts of immunoglobulins in this season. Stimulation of B cells often results from the balanced activity of T helper and T suppressor cells, whose ratio seems to be higher in summer than in winter (as discussed subsequently). The catabolism of immunoglobulins may also be faster in winter than in summer. In view of the above we propose, as a testable hypothesis, the existence of a physiological winter depression in B-cell-mediated immunity.

A circannual rhythm in T-cell-mediated immunity was suggested by our preliminary findings in three apparently healthy donors. Whereas the number of circulating B cells in the morning reached its maximum in summer, that of T cells (OKT3[+]) appeared to have a peak in spring and a trough in winter [28]. In addition we have found an increase in the helper/suppressor ratio in both spring and summer as compared to winter (Figure 7.11). T-cell-mediated immunity was also lowest in

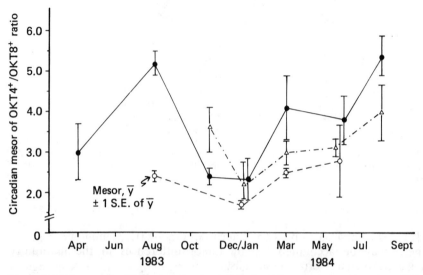

Figure 7.11 Circannual variation in helper/suppressor ratio from peripheral blood. Preliminary results from three apparently healthy men (aged 24–32) sampled every 4 h for 24 h in different seasons. (After Lévi *et al.* [52])

winter and highest in spring or summer in dogs and guinea-pigs, as well as in ground squirrels kept at a constant environmental temperature [67–70]. A study of circulating lymphocyte subsets was performed in January, March, June, August and November in five healthy young men [52]. The circadian mesor exhibited a circannual rhythm for total, T, T suppressor-cytotoxic and natural killer HNK1[+] (gauging NK cells) lymphocytes with maxima respectively estimated in November, March, December and October (Figure 7.12). A 6-month rhythm was documented for T helper lymphocytes, with estimated maxima occurring in both April and October. The double amplitudes of such circannual or circahemiannual rhythms ranged between 15 and 25% of the circannual mesor and were smaller than the corresponding circadian or circahemidian ones except for the HNK1[+] cells. The intraindividual reproducibility of these circannual rhythms was shown in the three subjects studied up to three times during the previous year. The results also support the view that pan-T, T helper, T suppressor-cytotoxic and HNK1[+] lymphocytes vary rhythmically in the course of the year. A similar circannual rhythmicity was also found for the T helper/T suppressor-cytotoxic ratio in a single individual followed for 2 years. This was not found at the group level. Interindividual differences may be found with regard to the circannual rhythmicity in this ratio.

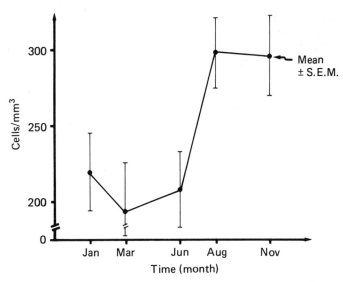

Figure 7.12 Circannual rhythm in 24-h mesor of circulating HNK1$^+$ mononuclear cells in five healthy young men

The arylhydrocarbon hydroxylase (AHH) activity of human lymphocytes was also found to vary with a circannual rhythmicity [71]. This microsomal oxidase was measured in cultured human lymphocytes from 977 donors over a span of 2.5 years. The highest induced AHH activity was observed during late summer, and the lowest one in winter. The peak–trough difference was 10-fold. This finding supports the hypothesis that the metabolic activity of immune cells is high in summer compared with winter. In the same study, the mitotic index of lymphocytes was highest in winter. An independent study reported similar findings [72]. Thus, both B- and T-cell-mediated immunities seem to be organized along the circannual time scale, with T-cell-amplified immunity predominating in spring and/or early autumn and B-cell immunity in summer. In winter, both kinds of immune defences appear to be depressed. This may be related to an increased number of circulating T suppressor-cytotoxic cells in this season. Among 22 environmental factors studied as possible causes of such a seasonal variation in human immunity, none was selected as a predictor [73]. It is possible that there exists a truly endogenous circannual organization of the immune network.

In the above study [52] two other circadian rhythm characteristics were affected by the season. The circadian double amplitude of total, T and T helper lymphocytes varied between 0 (no rhythm) in March and up to 46–60% of the mesor in November and January. A circadian rhythm of the T helper/T suppressor-cytotoxic ratio was not detected either in January or in March, but it was validated in the other seasons with 2As equal to 67% of the 24-h mesor in both June and August. Thus apparent discrepancies in the literature with regard to the presence or absence of a physiological circadian rhythm in T-lymphocyte-related variables [22–24,26–29] may be accounted for by a circannual modulation of circadian rhythmicity. In addition, the acrophases of the statistically validated circadian or circahemidian rhythms remained similar throughout the year. Such a seasonal modulation of the group circadian time structure is not an isolated case in man.

In healthy men, the circadian rhythm of plasma lutropin was absent in the first half of the year in two independent studies [74,75] and the circadian acrophase in plasma testosterone occurred 6 h later in summer than in winter [76]. These results represent data pooled from several individuals. The lack of a circadian rhythm at a group level may result from interindividual desynchronization, for example individual circadian rhythms may exhibit period lengths differing from precisely 24 h. This phenomenon might be more likely to occur at specific times of the year. Supporting this assumption, the endogenous so-called free-running circadian period of body temperature was shorter in March–April than in July–August in healthy human beings kept under temporal isolation [77]. In longitudinal studies carried out in Paris in June, oral temperature exhibited a period that differed from 24 h with statistical significance in two of five apparently healthy men, even though these subjects followed the usual social routine [78].

Circaseptan organization of the immune network

In 1938, Ask-Upmark [79] considered whether periods in the neighbourhood of 7 days (circaseptan rhythms) for numerous variables constituted a 'biological week'. Reimann [80] later grouped several cyclic diseases under the name of periodic diseases. Their most striking feature was the recurrence of symptoms at intervals of 7 days or integral multiples of 7 days in most cases. Hildebrandt [81] further emphasized the reactive nature of circaseptan rhythms, relative to an initial abrupt disturbance.

The circaseptan domain is part of the spectrum of biological rhythms which characterize living organisms. This bioperiodicity has been found in numerous species including mushrooms (Jerebzoff, personal communication), insects, rodents and man [5]. The circaseptan bioperiodicity is not just a part of the temporal structure of living organisms [82]: it has critical implications for human health maintenance and therapeutic intervention, with particular reference to defence mechanisms, cytokinetics and transplantation. Only these aspects will be discussed in the present chapter.

Dionigi et al. [83] have reported data in six healthy volunteers sampled between 08:30 and 09:30 h on Mondays, Wednesdays and Fridays for spans of 50 days or more, which suggest circaseptan rhythms in lymphocyte transformability. Three subjects developed infections during the study. These infections occurred at times of a severe depression in PHA transformation. Despite a sampling frequency inappropriate to the assessment of a circaseptan rhythm, a statistically significant 7-day period was found for one of their subjects as indicated by a periodogram. Further analysis of their data indicated that a circaseptan periodicity in PHA lymphoblastic transformation may be found in healthy subjects [5].

In patients who undergo kidney transplantation, rejection bouts may occur despite therapy. They may be transient and resolve. Sometimes they are irreversible and the graft needs to be removed. The incidence of rejection bouts in these patients is also characterized by a prominent circaseptan bioperiodicity. We have examined original data or published summaries of four series of patients from three geographic locations in whom a kidney transplant was performed [84,85]. Rejection criteria were similar in all series. Figure 7.13 indicates that the incidence of rejection episodes exhibited a 7-day cycle in each series. In patients treated with corticosteroid therapy and azathioprine, most rejection bouts occurred

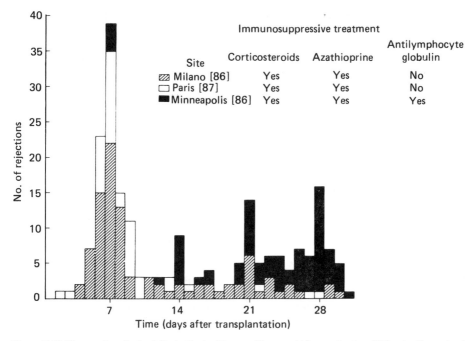

Figure 7.13 Circaseptan rhythmicity in the incidence of human kidney rejection (212 rejection episodes in a total of 579 kidney transplants). Similar timing of circaseptan bioperiodicity in the incidence of human kidney rejection in hospitals from three different geographic locations. 'Preventive' therapy with corticosteroids and immunosuppressors (azathioprine and/or antilymphocyte globulin). Antilymphocyte globulin appears to delay and reduce the incidence of rejection episodes but does not change their timing. (After Lévi *et al.* [5] and De Vecchi *et al.* [84])

on the 7th day after transplantation but some also occurred at integral multiples of 7 days. The addition of systemic antilymphocyte globulin to this preventive treatment in Minneapolis did not alter the circaseptan bioperiodicity in incidence of rejections. It did, however, decrease and delay the incidence of rejection episodes. Most of them now occurred on days 21 or 28 (1 or 2 weeks after cessation of antilymphocyte globulin on day 14). The circaseptan bioperiodicity in rejections and the effects of antilymphocyte globulin have recently been confirmed in another similar series of 157 kidney transplant recipients [86]. This type of rejection occurred despite 'preventive' corticosteroid therapy, was observed in all groups, did not respond to additional corticosteroid therapy and resolved spontaneously (even if corticosteroid therapy was decreased after its onset). It can be considered as an 'immunological characteristic'.

A circaseptan rhythm in the incidence of allograft rejection, a result of a host-versus-graft reaction, was also observed for kidney, heart and pancreatic transplants in rats [87,88] and for parabiotic animals [89]. Neither in rodent investigations nor in human ones was this rhythm synchronized by the societal 7-day week. Instead it was related to the day of transplantation.

Animal studies have suggested that the introduction of an antigen into an organism results in an immune response which is temporally organized along a circaseptan scale [5,90]. In man, a circaseptan rhythm in anti-Rh titre was observed in six of ten subjects immunized by pregnancy or transfusion [91].

A circaseptan bioperiodicity of T and B cell number has also been found in guinea-pigs, after antigenic induction of chronic relapsing allergic encephalomyelitis [92,93]. This experimental disease constitutes a model for the study of multiple sclerosis. One animal was sampled on 28 occasions during a total observation span of 387 days. Despite this relatively small number of observations, peripheral T and B cell numbers were shown to exhibit a statistically significant circaseptan bioperiodicity. The circaseptan acrophase in circulating T cell number preceded that in B cell number by 3 days. Three out of four symptomatic exacerbations occurred at integral multiples of 7 days, when the number of T lymphocytes was low.

Non-immunological inflammatory processes have also been shown to exhibit a circaseptan periodicity [94]. The extent of swelling following maxillofacial surgery varied according to a 7-day rhythm in 51 patients. Maximal swelling occurred on the 1st, 7th, 14th and 22nd post-operative day.

Both T and B 'arms' of the immune network seem to exhibit a circaseptan bioperiodicity in their response to an antigenic challenge. Such an antigen-promoted circaseptan bioperiodicity has been considered in the mathematical modelling of immunity [95]. Since inflammatory processes also appear to be organized along a 7-day time scale, it is likely that such periodicity indeed characterizes the time domain of host defences against attack.

Biological rhythms in infectious and allergic diseases

Circadian and circannual changes in infectious diseases

To epidemiologists, the clustering of illnesses in time suggests causality due to specific environmental factors [96]. To chronobiologists, the same phenomenon may infer a contribution of endogenous biological rhythms. With regard to human infectious diseases, no research has yet been conducted in order specifically to evaluate bioperiodicity in pathogen virulence, transmission etc. In addition, circadian rhythms have been documented in unicellular eukaryote species but not in prokaryote bacteria [97]. In consequence this part of the chapter will focus on biological rhythms in immunological and inflammatory processes.

Circadian rhythms in infectious diseases

Early experiments in rodents revealed 24-h rhythms in the response of animals to bacterial endotoxins (e.g. *Escherichia coli*) and other infectious agents [98–100]. Hejl [101] in studies involving 2044 persons reported that the onset of fever resulting from bacterial infection occurred predominantly in the morning between 05:00 and 12:00 h while that resulting from viral infection predominated during the late afternoon and evening, between 15:00 and 22:00 h. Circadian rhythms in infectious diseases are compatible with circadian changes in both immunological [26,102] and inflammatory processes [103]. Moreover, 12-h rhythms in certain aspects of these processes may account for peak time differences observed between bacterial and viral infections.

Circannual rhythms in infectious diseases

An earlier review by Smolensky *et al.* [96] found the morbidity and the mortality from infectious diseases (mainly upper respiratory infections including the common cold, influenza and pneumonia) was greatest in winter and least in summer in both the northern and southern hemispheres, in children as well as in adults. This circannual staging differs from that of infectious diseases that primarily affect children (e.g., mumps, chicken pox, rubella and rubeola). The latter are most frequent in spring. As emphasized by Smolensky [96] the crowding of children in school does not fully account for the timing of infectious diseases in this age group [104]. Annual peak incidence does not fit with the annual schedule of school attendance, which would predict a peak in the autumn. Undoubtedly, seasonal changes in environmental conditions conducive to the virulence and spread of infectious agents are critical. However, since annual rhythms characterize human immune functions [26,27,55,59,66–68], the aetiology of the seasonality of infection is likely to be multifactorial and involve both exogenous (e.g. environmental) and endogenous (e.g. immunological) cyclic phenomena. Connections between predictable-in-time changes in immune functions and those of either inflammation or endocrine function (e.g. adrenocortical secretion) will now be considered.

Circadian and circannual changes in inflammation. Role of corticosteroids

Inflammation is clinically recognized by the development of local redness, swelling, pain and heat (rubor, dolor, calor). The inciting agent can be physical (radiant, mechanical), chemical (toxic substances, pollutants, drugs) or biological (viral or bacterial infections or antigens). In sensitized patients, histamine is released from mast cells of peripheral tissues (e.g. skin, airways, etc.) as a result of the antigen–antibody reaction. Local reactions (e.g. itching, erythema and wheal) result from the intradermal (i.d.) injection of either histamine, a histamine liberator or antigens in sensitized patients. These are related to neural stimulation, as well as to changes in both vascular diameter and permeability, with transfer of fluids and oedema. A large-amplitude circadian rhythm in erythema and wheal resulting from i.d. injection of either histamine or various antigens (in patients with specific allergies) has been demonstrated by Reinberg *et al.* [36,105], Lee *et al.* [37] and Smolensky *et al.* [106]. Peaks occurred around 23:00 h and troughs around 11:00 h (Figure 7.14). These times fit well with the nocturnal peak of bronchial reactivity to histamine when this agent is inhaled in aerosol form [107,108].

Labrecque *et al.* [109] were first to show circadian variations in the oedema and the symptoms of inflammation produced by carraggenin (carr) into the hind paw of rats. The rate of formation of oedema was fastest (e.g. 2.5 h) when the phlogistic agent was injected at the end of the activity span compared to the end of the rest span (e.g. 4 h). Annual changes with a peak in May also characterized this phenomenon in the rat.

Three possible mechanisms underlying the time-dependent variation of carr-induced oedema and inflammation have been proposed by Labrecque and Belanger [109,110]. The first takes into account the circadian rhythm of corticosteroid secretion. These authors have shown that adrenalectomy abolishes

122

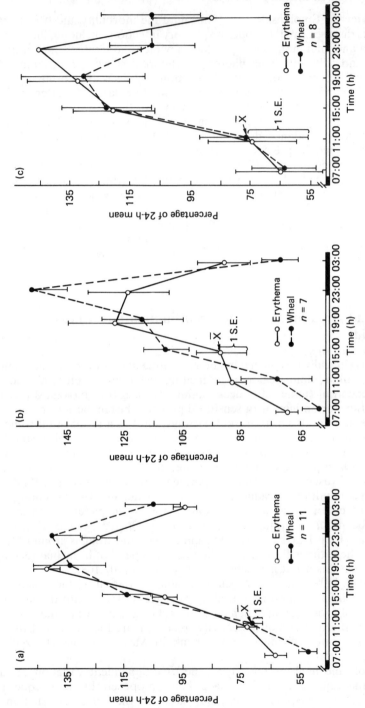

Figure 7.14 Cutaneous reaction to histamine (a), house dust (b) and grass pollen (c) extracts has a circadian rhythm. Highest sensitivity occurs between 19:00 and 23:00h; lowest sensitivity occurs at 07:00h. During the period of greatest reactivity, response to histamine is at least twice the lowest level. Light and shaded portions of the abscissa correspond to times of activity and rest respectively for the sample. (From Reinberg *et al.* [105] and Smolensky *et al.* [106] with permission)

the circadian variation in the rate of formation of carr-induced oedema. It can be restored by injections of a corticosteroid to adrenalectomized rats with dosing times calculated to mimic the hormonal rhythm.

Pertinent also are the findings of Bureau *et al.* [111] demonstrating a circadian rhythm in the BCG-induced migration of polymorphonuclear leucocytes in intact mice and its obliteration in adrenalectomized mice. These data strongly suggest that the corticosterone circadian rhythm helps to regulate that of the BCG-induced granulocyte migration in mice.

The second possible explanation considers that the tissue sensitivity (chronesthesy) to inflammatory agents may vary with hours of the day and days of the year, as shown by Labrecque *et al.* [110]. This idea is supported by data showing a strong correlation between the time course of exudation of protein-bound Evan's Blue and the rate of formation of oedema [110]. In addition, the susceptibility of vascular tissue to equally-spaced-in-time doses of either bradykinin or prostaglandin E2 or arachidonic acid exhibits a circadian rhythm [110].

The third possible explanation is that circadian and circannual changes in inflammatory reactions relate to changes in number and functions of white blood cells: for example, the uptake of carr by macrophages is necessary to obtain the inflammatory effect of this agent. These three possible mechanisms could well be complementary in their effects.

With regard to corticosteroids, their major pharmacological property is to prevent or suppress the development of inflammation. They have long been recognized as suppressors of histamine- and bradykinin-induced vasodilation. Inflammation is, of course, associated with allergic reactions which are frequently involved in diseases such as asthma, eczema, urticaria, etc. At the molecular level, corticosteroids are believed to control the rate of protein synthesis. The many types of cells present in an inflamed airway contribute to the inflammatory response as effector cells and regulatory cells. Their release of mediators, proteinases and reactive oxygen species can be down-regulated by corticosteroids [112]. This phenomenon helps to reduce macrophage, neutrophil and eosinophil effects and functions. The activities of corticosteroids are rather complex and not fully characterized; moreover the time structure is almost never taken into account at this molecular level of interpretation.

Predictable-in-time changes in allergic reactions

There is no doubt that the occurrence of asthma at night depends upon many synchronized circadian rhythms [113–116] (see also Chapter 5). Both nocturnal exacerbation of dyspnoea and minimum bronchial patency coincide in time with the nadirs of corticosteroid secretion [113, 115–117], catecholamine secretion [115,116], threshold of bronchial susceptibility to inhaled acetylcholine [114] and inhaled histamine [107,108]. These aspects are discussed by P. Barnes in Chapter 5 of this book.

In fact we are dealing here with physiological rhythms, including that of the vagal tone of airways which can be demonstrated in both healthy subjects and asthmatics. The critical difference is precisely the hyper-reactivity of airways in sensitized patients. De Vries *et al.* [107] and Tammeling *et al.* [108] initially demonstrated that the nocturnal distress of asthma, bronchitis and emphysema is dependent on

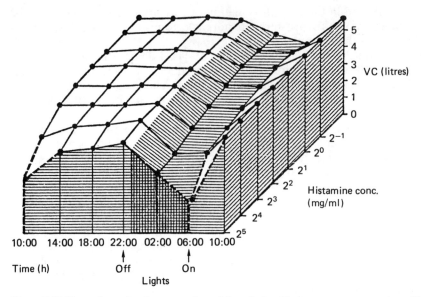

VC (litres)

Histamine conc.
(mg/ml)

10:00   14:00 18:00 22:00   02:00 06:00 10:00

Time (h)   Off   On

Lights

Figure 7.15 Three-dimensional presentation of the relationship between concentration of inhaled histamine to the absolute value of the vital capacity (VC) at various times of the day in a patient with slight symptoms of obstructive lung disease. At two time points (10:00 and 06:00 h) the highest histamine concentration was not administered. (After De Vries *et al.* [107] and Tammeling *et al.* [108])

the circadian rhythmicity of hyper-reactivity in airways (Figure 7.15). Patients with asthma and other chronic obstructive pulmonary diseases, when challenged by the inhalation of histamine in aerosol at different times of day and night, exhibit very large variations in the threshold dose required to produce a 15% loss of bronchial patency. In diurnally active patients, the airways are much more hyper-reactive when challenged at 00:00 and 04:00 h than at 12:00 and 16:00 h.

Investigations by Reinberg *et al.* [114] using aerosols of acetylcholine confirmed the large-amplitude circadian rhythm of airway hyper-reactivity in asthmatic patients (Figure 7.16). Last but not least Gervais *et al.* [118] have also demonstrated changes in bronchial patency [both forced expiratory volume per 1 s (FEV 1) and peak expiratory flow (PEF)] as a function of the timing of airway stimulation with house dust extract in house-dust-sensitive asthmatic patients. Tests, using a fixed dose of house dust, were conducted at 08:00, 15:00, 19:00 and 23:00 h on different days while patients were housed in an allergen-shielded area. A challenge at 15:00 and 19:00 h resulted in minimal effects on bronchial patency (Figure 7.17). At 08:00 h there was a 15% fall in patency while at 23:00 h the most severe bronchoconstriction (22% fall) occurred. This was associated with rales and wheezing lasting for several hours in some patients. These findings indicate that timing of exposure to offending agents may be just as important as the degree of exposure. The circadian rhythm of cutaneous and airway reactivity to antigens and other agents has important implications in the interpretation of skin tests and results from bronchial challenge.

The hyper-reactivity of airways in allergic patients does not only include response to specific antigens (e.g. house dust extracts) and mediators (histamine,

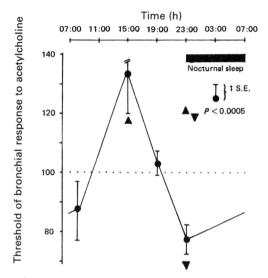

Figure 7.16 Eight healthy adults – smokers or exsmokers (four women, 28–47 years of age, and four men, 24–48 years of age) – were synchronized with light (07:00–23:00 h) and dark (23:00–07:00 h). Serial determinations of the bronchial response to acetylcholine (ACh) were made at fixed hours (08:00, 15:00, 19:00 and 23:00 h) as one test per day on five different days, each separated by an interval of about 1 week. The order of the tests was randomized among the subjects. The ACh test at 15:00 or at 08:00 h was done twice. Each measurement session began with three determinations of 1-s forced expiratory volume (FEV1). By successive assays the smallest quantity of ACh via aerosol inhalation (particle size ∼ 1 nm) was determined which provoked a 15–20% decrease in the FEV1 recorded at the beginning of each session. The lowest threshold occurred at 23:00 h and the highest at 15:00 h. (The variation between test times is shown as relative values from the group mean for all tests.) (From Reinberg *et al.* [114] with permission)

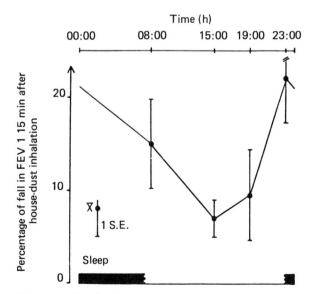

Figure 7.17 Circadian changes in the airways' susceptibility to house dust in diurnally active house-dust-sensitive asthmatic patients. The pre- to post-test difference in the FEV1 at 15:00 h was relatively minor compared to that at 23:00 h. Reproduced from Gervais *et al.* [118] with permission

acetylcholine) but also to non-specific agents such as toxicants (smoke, etc.) resulting from pollution. In patients removed from a polluted environment (e.g. shielded rooms, sojourn in areas of high and low air pollution, etc.) circadian changes in bronchial patency persist but the 24-h mean increases progressively and may reach a level that is above the threshold for asthma [115, 117]. Pertinent to this discussion is the observation that in certain occupational settings non-immediate and recurrent nocturnal asthmatic reactions may follow a single daytime exposure to allergens [119–121]. According to Taylor *et al.* [121] workers suffering from recurrent nocturnal asthmatic reactions may only complain of minor symptoms and may exhibit almost normal airway patency during the daytime (Figure 7.18). Despite the fact that antigen exposure occurs during the diurnal working span, dyspnoea mostly occurs at night, and may recur for several consecutive nights.

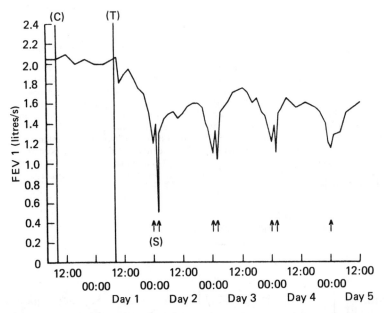

Figure 7.18 Temporal variation in airway patency of one presumably diurnally active asthmatic patient following a single pulmonary challenge on the test day (numbered 1) with an antigen to which hypersensitivity had previously developed (budgerigar serum) through occupational exposure. Although the FEV1 was close to normal during the day it was extremely low during the night, giving rise to severe episodes of dyspnoea over several consecutive nights. C, control; T, test hour on day one; S, inhaled puffs of a sympathoagonist. Reproduced from Taylor *et al.* [121] with permission

Circadian changes in effectiveness of vaccinations

Predictable changes in the effectiveness of vaccination are the consequence of the circadian time structure of immune networks. The effectiveness of vaccination with live attenuated Venezuelian equine encephalomyelitis virus can be gauged by the number of specific fluorescent antibody particles. Forty healthy young men were vaccinated at 08:00 h or at 20:00 h. Some 75% of the subjects immunized at 08:00 h demonstrated specific intracellular fluorescing particles by day 2 post vaccination, as compared to 15% of those vaccinated at 20:00 h [122]. Two studies have documented serum antibody levels as a function of the daily time when vaccination was performed.

In a preliminary study, 125 volunteers, aged 16–77 years, received 0.5 ml of Connaught influenza vaccine in summer between 08:30 and 17:00 h. Circulating specific antibody concentrations were determined 21–30 days later. This period corresponds to their maximum rise following vaccination. For A/Philippines and A/Chile, a circadian variation was statistically validated with the highest response corresponding to early afternoon. Vaccination near noon was also associated with increased arm soreness but no significant differences were found with other side effects (including fever) (Langlois et al. [123]). In 500 subjects receiving hepatitis B vaccine, serum antibodies were determined 4–8 weeks after the third vaccine injection. Highest antibody concentrations (anti-HBS) were associated with early afternoon administration. This vaccination time also yielded more pain and swelling (Pöllmann et al. [124]). Taken together these results suggest that the immunopharmacological effect of vaccination against viral diseases may be optimized by administering the vaccine near the middle of the active span (near the nadir of circulating total, pan-T and T-helper lymphocytes, which also corresponds to the nadir of circulating T-suppressor-cytotoxic lymphocytes). A number of questions arise, however. Is the time course of antibody response similar, whatever the vaccination time? Are there large circadian variations in specific immunoglobulins following such vaccinations, and could these confuse the issue? These studies nevertheless demonstrate the clinical relevance of searching for an optimal time of day for vaccination. Furthermore, circannual changes also deserve thorough scrutiny, in order to improve the prevention of infectious diseases in children. A pertinent vaccination calendar is now actively requested by paediatricians [125].

Discussion

Periodic, and therefore predictable, variations characterize all the immunological variables investigated to date in laboratory animals and in man. Whereas circadian and circannual rhythms have well-known geophysical counterparts, other periodicities do not. This is the case for circahemidian rhythms (with a period $\simeq$ 12 h) and circaseptan rhythms ($\simeq$ 7 days). Circatrigintidian rhythms ($\simeq$ 30 days) in immunity have been little explored, and thus have not been mentioned. Such rhythms have, however, been documented for the immediate skin reactivity of sensitized women to several antigens and to histamine [106,107].

Many biological rhythms are endogenous and of genetic origin. External cycles (e.g. zeitgebers) are not required for their expression. They may, however, influence some parameters of these rhythms within certain limits.

We are only beginning to understand the rhythms that affect the human immune network in health. Nevertheless, a rather good agreement characterizes results from investigations performed with different experimental designs and laboratory techniques. Most immune variables investigated in man have shown very large amplitudes and similar acrophases in both circadian and circannual periodicity.

The hormonal regulation of such rhythms is likely to be complex since many hormones, such as cortisol, adrenaline, testosterone, growth hormone, lymphokines, etc., exert various actions on different targets of the immune network [126–128 and many others], and themselves exhibit both circadian and circannual variations [8,129,130].

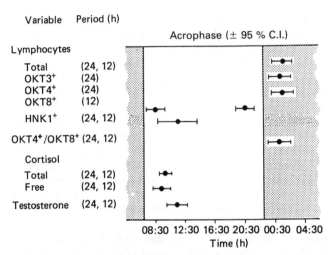

Figure 7.19 Acrophase chart of circulating total lymphocytes, T and HNK1+ subsets and plasma cortisol and testosterone in five diurnally active healthy men (24–36 years). Data from all five study months (January, March, June, August, November, 1984) were pooled. The periods detected for each variable are indicated. Black dots indicate the location in time of the acrophase and the horizontal line its 95% confidence interval. When a 24-h rhythm was detected, the circadian acrophase is the only one shown. When a 12-h rhythm was detected alone (no 24-h rhythm), as was the case for T suppressor-cytotoxic cells, two acrophases are shown in the 24-h scale. The level of statistical significance of these circadian or circahemidian rhythms was $P<0.001$

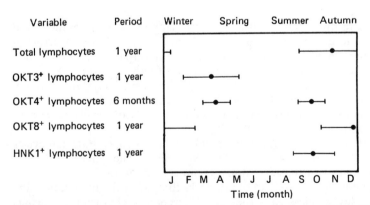

Figure 7.20 Seasonal time structure of circulating total lymphocytes and T and HNK1+ subtypes in five healthy young men (aged 24–36 years), as represented by an acrophase chart. The maximum (acrophase, ϕ) is shown with its 95% confidence limits, as yielded by cosinor analysis, for a period τ $\equiv$ 1 year or 6 months

At present, the effects of such hormones on circulating immune cells have been documented at only one circadian stage. For example exogenous corticosteroids given at 08:00 h resulted in a profound decrease in circulating lymphocytes (mostly T cells and monocytes, which was maximal 4–6 h after administration, at the time of their spontaneous nadir [126]). A glucocorticoid-induced redistribution of these cells in other compartments of the body was suggested. Other studies performed in rodents and in man have indicated a role for corticosteroids in the regulation of immune rhythms [15,34,131]. Nothing is known, however, about the effects that exogenous corticosteroids exert upon the immune network if they are given at other times of the day. In asthmatic patients, morning dosing of exogenous corticosteroids was found to be more effective in increasing bronchial patency than evening dosing [132]. Thus chronopharmacological investigations of hormonal actions upon immunity appear mandatory.

T-cell-mediated immunity was found to be more efficient at night and in spring or summer in healthy subjects (Figures 7.19 and 7.20). The relationship of such immune rhythms to the aetiology and development of infectious, allergic and malignant diseases is suggested by some sparse data [133,134].

The circadian rhythmicity in the metabolic activity of lymphocytes appeared to differ between healthy subjects (Figure 7.8) and women with advanced ovarian tumours [42], and a chronopathology of immune functions may characterize some illnesses. Thus, the circadian rhythmicity in the activity of several enzymes from circulating lymphocytes was found to differ between healthy subjects and patients with chronic lymphocytic leukaemia (CLL) [41,43]. A similar observation was made with circulating lymphocyte subsets in CLL patients [134]. The documentation of large-amplitude circadian, circaseptan and circannual rhythms in human immunity suggests a further evaluation of the role of these rhythms in the development of several acute or chronic diseases, including infections, rheumatological processes, allergy and cancers. The demonstration that a change in the timing of immunomodulators may result in a favourable or an unfavourable effect upon the growth of a transplantable tumour in rats also emphasizes the need for further studies in chronoimmunopharmacology [102,135].

References

1. Holborow, E.J. and Reeves, W.G. *Immunology in Medicine,* Academic Press, London (1977)
2. Paul, W.E. *Fundamental Immunology*, Raven Press, New York (1984)
3. Charpin, J. *Allergologie*, 2nd edn, Flammarion Medecine Science, Paris (1987)
4. Scheving, L.E., Pauly, J.E., Tsai, T.H. and Scheving, L.A. Chronobiology of cell proliferation. Implications for cancer chronotherapy. In *Biological Rhythms and Medicine; Cellular, Metabolic, Physiopathologic and Pharmacologic Aspects* (eds A. Reinberg and M. Smolensky), Springer Verlag, New York, pp. 79–130 (1983)
5. Lévi, F. and Halberg, F. Circaseptan (about 7-days) bioperiodicity – spontaneous and reactive – and the search for pacemakers. *La Ricerca Clin. Lab.*, **12**, 323–370 (1981)
6. Ceresa, F., Angeli, A., Bocuzzi, G. and Molino, G. Once a day stimulated and basal ACTH secretion phases in man; their response to corticoid inhibition. *J. Clin. Endocrinol. Metab.*, **29**, 1074–1079 (1969)
7. Zumoff, B., Freeman, R., Coupey, S., Saenger, P., Markowitz, M. and Kream, J. Chronobiologic abnormality in luteinizing hormone secretion in teenage girls with the polykystic-ovary syndrome. *N. Engl. J. Med.*, **309**, 1206–1209 (1983)
8. Halberg, F., Cornelissen, G., Sothern, R. *et al.* International geographic studies of oncologic interest on chronobiologic variables. *Neoplasms – Comparative Pathology of Growth in Animals, Plants and Man* (ed. H. Kaiser), Williams & Wilkins, Baltimore, pp. 563–595 (1981)

9. Reinberg, A. and Smolensky, M. Chronobiology and thermoregulation. *Pharmacol. Ther.*, **22**, 425–464 (1983)
10. Cove-Smith, M.S., Kabler, P.A., Pownall, R. and Knapp, M.S. Circadian variation in an immune response in man. *Brit. Med. J.*, **ii**, 253 (1978)
11. Knapps, M.S., Cove-Smith, M.S., Dugdale, R., MacKenzie, N. and Pownall, R. Possible effect of time on renal allograft rejection. *Brit. Med. J.*, **i**, 75–77 (1979)
12. Fernandes, G., Halberg, F., Yunis, E.J. and Good, R.A. The circadian rhythmic plaque-forming cell response of spleens from mice immunized with SRBC. *J. Immunol.*, **117**, 962–966 (1976)
13. Pownall, R., Kabler, P.A. and Ķnapp, M.S. The time of day of antigen encounter influences the magnitude of the immune response. *Clin. Exp. Immunol.*, **36**, 347–354 (1979)
14. Ratte, J., Halberg, F., Kuhl, J.F.W. and Najarian, J.S. Circadian variation in the rejection of rat kidney allografts. *Surgery*, **73**, 102–108 (1973)
15. Knapp, M.S. and Pownall, R. Biological rhythms in cell-mediated immunity: findings from rats and man, and their potential clinical relevance. In *Recent Advances in the Chronobiology of Allergy and Immunology* (eds M. Smolensky, E. Reinberg and J.P. McGovern), Pergamon Press, Oxford, pp. 323–331 (1980)
16. Hayashi, O. and Kikuchi, M. The effect of the light–dark cycle on humoral and cell-mediated immune responses of mice. *Chronobiologia*, **9**, 291–300 (1982)
17. Sabin, F.R., Cunningham, R.S., Doan, C.A. and Kindwall, J.A. The normal rhythm of the blood cells. *Bull. Johns Hopkins Hosp.*, **37**, 14–67 (1925)
18. Bartter, F.C., Delea, C.S. and Halberg, F. A map of blood and urinary changes related to circadian variations in adrenal cortical function in normal subjects. *Ann. NY Acad. Sci.*, **98**, 969–983 (1962)
19. Haus, E., Lakatua, D.J., Swoyer, J. and Sackett-Lundeen, L. Chronobiology in hematology and immunology. *Amer. J. Anat.*, **168**, 467–517 (1983)
20. Feldman, M. Les cellules qui suppriment l'immunité. *La Recherche*, **17**, 692–695 (1986)
21. Abo, T. and Kumagai, K. Studies on surface immunoglobulin on human B lymphocytes. *Clin. Exp. Immunol.*, **33**, 441–452 (1978)
22. Bertouch, J.V., Roberts-Thomson, P.J. and Bradley, J. Diurnal variation of lymphocyte subsets identified by monoclonal antibodies. *Brit. Med. J.*, **286**, 1171–1172 (1983)
23. Ritchie, W.S., Oswald, I., Micklem, H.S., Boyd, J.E., Elton, R.A., Jazwinska, E. and James, K. Circadian variation of lymphocyte subpopulations: a study with monoclonal antibodies. *Brit. Med. J.*, **286**, 1773–1775 (1983)
24. Lévi, F., Canon, C., Blum, J.P., Reinberg, A. and Mathé, G. Large-amplitude circadian rhythm in helper: suppressor ratio of peripheral blood lymphocytes. *Lancet*, **ii**, 462–463 (1983)
25. Canon, C., Lévi, F., Reinberg, A. and Mathé, G. Circulating CALLA positive lymphocytes (L) exhibit a circadian rhythm in Man. *Leukemia Res.*, **9**, 1539–1546 (1985)
26. Lévi, F., Canon, C., Blum, J.P., Mechkouri, M., Reinberg, A. and Mathé, G. Circadian and/or circahemidian rhythms in nine lymphocyte-related variables from peripheral blood of healthy subjects. *J. Immunol.*, **134**, 217–225 (1985)
27. Miyakawi, T., Taga, K., Nagaoki, T., Seki, H., Suzuki, Y. and Tahiguchi, N. Circadian changes of T lymphocytes subsets in human peripheral blood. *Clin. Exp. Immunol.*, **55**, 618–622 (1984)
28. Canon, C., Lévi, F., Touitou, Y., Sulon, J., Demey-Ponsard, E., Reinberg, A. and Mathé, G. Variations circadiennes et saisonnièires du rapport inducteur: suppresseur (OKT4$^+$:OKT$^+$) dans le sang veineux de l'homme adulte sain. *C.R. Acad. Sci. Paris (III)*, **302**, 519–524 (1986)
29. Lévi, F., Canon, C., Touitou, Y., Sulon, J., Demey-Ponsard, R., Mechkouri, M., Mowrowicz, I., Touboul, J.P., Reinberg, A. and Mathé, G. Circadian rhythms in circulating T lymphocyte subsets, plasma total and free cortisol and testosterone in healthy men. *Clin. Exp. Immunol.*, **71**, 320–335 (1988)
30. Cohen, J.H., Danel, L., Cordier, G., Saez, S. and Revillard, J.P. Sex steroids receptors in peripheral T cells: absence of androgen receptors and restriction of estrogen receptors to OKT8-positive cells. *J. Immunol.*, **131**, 2767–2771 (1983)
31. Carter, J.B., Barr, G.D., Levin, A.S., Byers, V.S., Ponce, B. and Fudenberg, H. Standardization of tissue culture conditions for spontaneous thymidine-2 ^{14}C incorporation by unstimulated normal human peripheral lymphocytes: circadian rhythm of DNA synthesis. *J. Allergy Clin. Immunol.*, **56**, 191–205 (1975)

32. Porwit-Kaiazek, A., Amar, P., Skiazek, T. and Biberfeld, P. Leu 7$^+$ (HNK-1$^+$) cells. II Characterization of blood Leu 7$^+$ cells with respect to immunophenotype and cell density. *Scand. J. Immunol.*, **18**, 495–499 (1983)

33. Lanier, L., Engleman, E., Gatenby, P., Badcock, G., Werner, N. and Herzenberg, L. Correlation of functional properties of human lymphoid cell subsets in surface marker phenotypes using multiparameter analysis and flow cytometry. *Immunol. Rev.*, **74**, 143–160 (1983)

34. Abo, T., Kawate, T., Hinuma, S., Itoh, K., Abo, W., Sato, J. and Kumagai, K. The circadian periodicities of lymphocyte subpopulations and the role of corticosteroid in human beings and mice. In *Recent Advances in the Chronobiology of Allergy and Immunology* (eds M. Smolensky, A. Reinberg and J.P. McGovern), Pergamon Press, Oxford, pp. 301–316 (1980)

35. Abo, T., Kawate, K., Itoh, K. and Kumagai, K. Studies on the bioperiodicity of the immune response. I. Circadian rhythms of human T, B and K cell traffic in the peripheral blood. *J. Immunol.*, **126**, 1360–1363 (1981)

36. Reinberg, A., Zagula-Mally, Z., Ghata, J. and Halberg, F. Circadian reactivity rhythm of human skin to house dust, penicillin and histamine. *J. Allergy Clin. Immunol.*, **44**, 292–306 (1969)

37. Lee, R.E., Smolensky, M.H., Leach, C. and McGovern, J.P. Circadian rhythms in the cutaneous sensitivity to histamine and selected antigens including phase relationships to urinary cortisol excretion. *Amer. Allergy,* **38**, 231–236 (1977)

38. Laguchev, S.S. and Pivarova, A.I. Diurnal changes in the mitotic index and number of DNA synthesizing cells in the lymph nodes. *Dokl. Akad. Nauk. SSR,* **179**, 493–495 (1968)

39. Kirk, H. Mitotic activity and cell degeneration in the mouse thymus over a period of 24 hours. *Z. Zellforsch.*, **129**, 188–195 (1972)

40. Kohler, W.C., Karacan, I. and Renert, O.M. Circadian variation of RNA in human leucocytes. *Nature*, **238**, 94–96 (1972)

41. Hrushesky, W., Sanchez, S., Lévi, F., Brown, H., Halberg, F., Haus, E., Sothern, R. and Kennedy, B.J. Total RNA content of cancer patient's mononuclear cells demonstrate marked circadian rhythmicity. *Blood*, **54**, 596 (1979)

42. Hrushesky, W. The clinical application of chronobiology to oncology. *Amer. J. Anat.*, **168**, 519–542 (1983)

43. Ramot, B., Brok-Simoni, F., Chiveidman, E. and Ashkenazi, Y.E. Blood leucocyte enzymes. III. Diurnal rhythm of activity in isolated lymphocytes of normal subjects and chronic lymphatic leukemia patients. *Brit. J. Haematol.*, **34**, 79–85 (1976)

44. Heitbrock, H.W., Mertelsmann, R. and Garbrecht, M. Circadian rhythm of RNA polymerase B activity in human peripheral blood lymphocytes. *Int. J. Chronobiol.*, **3**, 255–261 (1976)

45. Eskola, J., Frey, H., Molnar, G. and Soppi, E. Biological rhythm of cell-mediated immunity in man. *Clin. Exp. Immunol.*, **26**, 253–257 (1976)

46. Tavadia, H.B., Fleming, K.A., Hume, P.D. and Simpson, H.W. Circadian rhythmicity of plasma cortisol and PHA-induced lymphocyte transformation. *Clin. Exp. Immunol.*, **22**, 190–193 (1972)

47. Kaplan, M.S., Byers, V.S., Levin, A.S., German, D.F., Fudenberg, H.H. and Lecam, L.N. Circadian rhythm of stimulated blastogenesis. A 24 hour cycle in the mixed leucocyte culture reaction and with SKDS stimulation. *J. Allergy Clin. Immunol.*, **58**, 180–193 (1976)

48. Hedfors, E., Holm, G. and Petterson, D. Activation of human peripheral blood lymphocytes by concanavalin A: dependence of monocytes. *Clin. Exp. Immunol.*, **22**, 223–229 (1975)

49. Heilman, D.H., Gambrill, M.R. and Leichner, J.P. The effect of hydrocortisone on the incorporation of tritiated thymidine by human blood lymphocytes cultured with phytohaemagglutinin and pokeweed mitogen. *Clin. Exp. Immunol.*, **15**, 203–210 (1973)

50. Rosenstreich, D.I., Farrar, J.J. and Dougherty, S. Absolute macrophage dependency of T lymphocyte activation by mitogens. *J. Immunol.*, **116**, 131–137 (1976)

51. Williams, R., Kraus, L.J., Dubey, D.P., Yunis, E.J. and Halberg, F. Circadian bioperiodicity in natural killer cell activity of human blood. *Chronobiologia*, **6**, 172 (1980)

52. Lévi, F., Canon, C., Touitou, Y., Reinberg, A. and Mathé, G. Seasonal modulation of the circadian time structure of circulating T and natural killer lymphocyte subsets from healthy subjects. *J. Clin. Invest.*, **81**, 407–413 (1988)

53. Gatti, G., Cavallo, R., Sartori, M.L., Carignola, R., Delponte, D., Salvadori, A. and Angeli, A. Circadian variations of interferon-induced enhancement of human natural killer (NK) cell activity. *Cancer Det. Prev.*, **12**, 431–438 (1988)

54. Fernandes, G., Carandente, F., Halberg, E., Halberg, F. and Good, R.A. Circadian rhythm in activity of lymphocytic natural killer cells from spleens of Fischer rats. *J. Immunol.*, **123**, 662–628 (1979)

55. Reinberg, A., Schuller, E., Delasnerie, N., Clench, J. and Helary, M. Rythmes circadiens et circannuels des leucocytes, protéines totales, immunoglobulines A, G et M; Etude chez 9 adultes jeunes et sains. *Nouv. Press Med.*, **6**, 3819–3823 (1977)
56. Halberg, F., Duffert, D. and von Mayersbach, H. Circadian rhythm in serum immunoglobulins of clinically healthy young men. *Chronobiologia*, **4**, 114 (1977)
57. Pallansch, M., Kim, Y., Halberg, E. *et al.* Circadian rhythm in several components of the complement cascade in healthy women. *Chronobiologia*, **6**, 139–140 (1979)
58. Kim, Y., Pallansch, M., Carandente, F., Reissman, G., Halberg, E. and Halberg, F. Circadian and circannual aspects of the complement cascade. New and old differing in specificity. *Chronobiologia*, **7**, 189–204 (1980)
59. Gaultier, C., De Montis, G., Reinberg, A. and Motohashi, Y. Circadian rhythm of serum total immunoglobulin E (IgE) in asthmatic children. *Biomed. Pharmacother.*, **41**, 186–188 (1987)
60. Bratescu, A. and Teodorescu, M. Circannual variation in the B cell/T cell ratio in normal human peripheral blood. *J. Allergy Clin. Immunol.*, **68**, 273–280 (1981)
61. Gidlow, D.A., Church, J.P. and Clayton, B.E. Haematological and biochemical parameters in an industrial workforce. *Ann. Clin. Biochem.*, **20**, 341–348 (1983)
62. MacMurray, J.P., Barker, J.P., Armstrong, J.D., Bozzetti, L.P. and Kuhn, I.N. Circannual changes in immune function. *Life Sci.*, **32**, 2363–2370 (1983)
63. Haus, E., Lakatua, D.J., Halberg, F. *et al.* Chronobiological studies of plasma prolactin in women in Kyushu, Japan and Minnesota, USA. *J. Clin. Endocrinol. Metab.*, **51**, 632–640 (1980)
64. Lyngbye, J. and Kroll, J. Quantitative immunoelectrophoresis of proteins in serum from a normal population: season-, age-, and sex-related variations. *Clin. Chem. (NY)*, **17**, 495–500 (1971)
65. Deleanu, M., Lupsaia, S. and Neumann, E. Seasonal fluctuations of some serum globulins in blood donors. *J. Interdiscipl. Cycle Res.*, **8**, 243–245 (1977)
66. Rosenblatt, L.S., Shifrine, M., Hetherington, N.W., Paglieroni, T. and McKenzie, R. A circannual rhythm in rubella antibody titers. *J. Interdiscipl. Cycle Res.*, **13**, 81–88 (1982)
67. Shifrine, M., Taylor, N.J., Rosenblatt, L.S. and Wilson, F.D. Seasonal variation in cell-mediated immunity of clinically normal dogs. *Exp. Hematol.*, **8**, 318–326 (1980)
68. Shifrine, M., Rosenblatt, L.S., Taylor, N., Hetherington, N.W., Matthews, V.J. and Wilson, F.D. Seasonal variations in lectin-induced lymphocyte transformation in Beagle dogs. *J. Interdiscipl. Cycle Res.*, **11**, 219–231 (1980)
69. Godfrey, H.P. Seasonal variation of induction of contact sensitivity and of lymph node T lymphocytes in guinea pigs. *Int. Arch. Allergy Appl. Immunol.*, **49**, 411–414 (1975)
70. Sidky, Y.A., Hayward, J.S. and Ruth, R.F. Seasonal variations of the immune response of ground squirrels kept at 22–24°C. *Canad. J. Physiol. Pharmacol.*, **50**, 203–206 (1972)
71. Paigen, B.E., Ward, E., Reilly, A., Houten, L., Gurtoo, H., Minowada, J., Steenland, K., Harens, M.B. and Sartori, P. Seasonal variation of arylhydrocarbon hydroxylase activity in human lymphocytes. *Cancer Res.*, **41**, 2757–2761 (1981)
72. Sinha, A., Linscombe, A., Gollapudi, B., Jersey, G. and Flake, R. Cytogenic variability of lymphocytes from phenotypically normal men. Influence of smoking, age, season and sample storage. *J. Toxicol. Environ. Health*, **17**, 325–345 (1986)
73. Shifrine, M., Garsd, A. and Rosenblatt, L.S. Seasonal variation in immunity of humans. *J. Interdiscipl. Cycle Res.*, **13**, 157–165 (1982)
74. Reinberg., A., Lagoguey, M., Cesselin, F., Touitou, Y., Legrand, J.C., Delasalle, A., Antreassian, J. and Lagoguey, A. Circadian and circannual rhythms in plasma hormones and other variables of five healthy young human males. *Acta Endocrinol.*, **88**, 417–425 (1978)
75. Touitou, Y., Lagoguey, M., Bogdan, M., Reinberg, A. and Beck, H. Seasonal rhythms of plasma gonadotropins: their persistence in elderly men and women. *J. Endocrinol.*, **96**, 15–22 (1983)
76. Reinberg, A., Lagoguey, M., Chauffournier, J.M. and Cesselin, F. Circannual and circadian rhythms in plasma testosterone in five healthy young Parisian males. *Acta Endocrinol.*, **80**, 732–741 (1975)
77. Wirz-Justice, A., Wever, R. and Aschoff, J. Seasonality in free-running circadian rhythms in man. *Naturwissenschaften*, **71**, 316–322 (1984)
78. Reinberg, A., Lévi, F., Bicakova-Rocher, A., Blum, J.P., Ouechni, M.M. and Nicolai, A. Biologic time-related changes in antihistamine and other effects of chronic administration of mequitazine in healthy adults. *Annu. Rev. Chronopharmacol.*, **1**, 61–64 (1984)
79. Ask-Upmark, E.V. On periodic fever. *Acta Soc. Med. Suec.*, **64**, 5–25 (1938)
80. Reiman, H.A. *Periodic Diseases*, Davis, Philadelphia (1963)
81. Hildebrandt, G. Physiologische Gesichtspunkte zur Rehabilitation. *Z. Phys. Med.*, **1**, 373–381 (1970)

82. Halberg, F., Engeli, M., Hamburger, C. and Hillman, D. Spectral resolution of low-frequency small-amplitude rhythms in excreted 17-ketosteroids; probable androgen-induced circaseptan desynchronization. *Acta Endocrinol. (kbh)* (suppl. 103), **5**, 54 (1965)

83. Dionigi, R., Zonta, A., Albertario, F., Galeazzi, R. and Bellinzona, G. Cyclic variation in the response of lymphocytes to phytohemagglutinin in healthy individuals. *Transplantation*, **16**, 550–559 (1973)

84. De Vecchi, A., Carandente, F., Fryd, D.S., Halberg, F., Sutherland, D.E., Howard, R.J., Simmons, R.L. and Najarian, J.S. Circaseptan (about 7 days) rhythms in human kidney allograft rejection in different geographic locations. *Adv. Biosci.*, **19**, 193–202 (1979)

85. Kreis, H., Lacombe, M., Noel, L.H., Descamps, J.M., Chailley, J. and Crosnier, J. Kidney-graft rejection: has there been the need for steroids to be reevaluated? *Lancet*, **ii**, 1169–1172 (1978)

86. Besarab, A., Wesson, L., Jarrell, B. and Burke, J.F. Effects of delayed graft function and ALG on the circaseptan (about 7 days) rhythm of human renal allograft rejection. *Transplantation*, **35**, 562–566 (1983)

87. Ratte, J., Halberg, F., Kuhl, J.F.W. and Najarian, J.S. Circadian and circaseptan variations in rat kidney allograft rejection. In *Chronobiology in Allergy and Immunology* (eds J. McGovern, A. Reinberg and M. Smolensky), C.C. Thomas, Springfield, IL, pp. 250–257 (1977)

88. Kawahara, K., Lévi, F., Halberg, F., Rynasiewicz, J. and Sutherland, D. Circaseptan bioperiodicity in rat allograft rejection. In *Toward Chronopharmacology* (eds R. Takahashi, F. Halberg and C.A. Walkers), Pergamon Press, New York, pp. 273–280 (1982)

89. Cornelius, E.A., Yunis, E.J. and Martinez, C. Parabiosis intoxication: clinical, hematologic and serologic features. *Transplantation*, **5**, 112–134 (1967)

90. Stimpfling, J.H. and Richardson, A. Periodic variations of the hemagglutinin response of mice following immunization against sheep red blood cells and alloantigens. *Transplantation*, **5**, 1496–1503 (1967)

91. Rubinstein, P. Cyclic variations in anti-RH titer detected by automatic quantitative hemagglutination. *Vox Sang*, **23**, 508–522 (1972)

92. Raine, C.S., Traugott, V. and Stone, S.H. Suppression of chronic allergic encephalomyelitis: relevance to multiple sclerosis. *Science*, **201**, 445–448 (1978)

93. Lévi, F., Halberg, F., Nesbit, M., Haus, E. and Lévine, H. Chronooncology. In *Neoplasms – Comparative Pathology of Growth in Animals, Plants and Man* (ed. H.E. Kaiser), Williams & Wilkins, Baltimore, pp. 267–316 (1981)

94. Pöllmann, L. and Hildebrandt, G. Long-term control of swelling after maxillo-facial surgery: a study of circaseptan reactive periodicity. *Int. J. Chronobiol.*, **8**, 105–114 (1982)

95. Grossman, Z., Asofsky, R. and De Lisi, C. The dynamics and antibody secreting cell production: regulation of growth and oscillations in the response of T-independent antigens. *J. Theor. Biol.*, **84**, 49–61 (1980)

96. Smolensky, M.H., Halberg, F. and Sargent, F. Chronobiology of the life sequence. In *Advances in Climatic Physiology* (eds S. Itoh, K. Ogata and H. Yohimura), Igaku Shoin, Tokyo, pp. 281–318 (1972)

97. Edmunds, L.N. (ed.). *Cell Cycle Clocks*, Marcel Dekker, New York (1984)

98. Halberg, F., Johnson, E.A., Brown, B.I.V. and Bittner, J.J. Susceptibility rhythm to *E. coli* endotoxin and bioassay. *Proc. Soc. Exp. Biol. Med.*, **103**, 142–144 (1960)

99. Feigin, R.D., San Joaquin, V.H., Haymond, M.W. and Wyatt, R.G. Daily periodicity of susceptibility of mice to pneumococcal infection. *Nature*, **224**, 379–380 (1969)

100. Wongwiwat, M., Sukapanit, S., Triyanond, C. and Sawyer, W.D. Circadian rhythm of the resistance of mice to acute pneumococcal infection. *Infect. Immun.*, **5**, 442–448 (1972)

101. Hejl, Z. Daily, lunar, yearly and menstrual cycles and bacterial or viral infections in man. *J. Interdiscipl. Cycle Res.*, **8**, 250–253 (1977)

102. Lévi, F., Halberg, F., Chihara, G. and Byram, J. Chronoimmunomodulation: circadian, circaseptan and circannual aspects of immunopotentiation or suppression with lentinan. In *Toward Chronopharmacology* (eds R. Takahashi, F. Halberg and C.A. Walker), Pergamon Press, Oxford, pp. 289–311 (1982)

103. Bureau, J.P., Coupé, M., Labrecque, G. and Vago, P. Chronobiologie de l'inflammation. *Path. Biol.*, **35**, 942–950 (1987)

104. Lilienfeld, A.M. and Lilienfeld, D.E. *Foundations of Epidemiology*, Oxford University Press, Oxford (1980)

105. Reinberg, A., Sidi, E. and Ghata, J. Circadian rhythms of human skin to histamine or allergen and the adrenal cycle. *J. Allergy Clin. Immunol.*, **36**, 279–283 (1965)

106. Smolensky, M.H., Reinberg, A., Lee, R. and McGovern, J.P. Secondary rhythms related to

hormonal changes in the menstrual cycle: special reference to allergology. In *Biorhythms and Human Reproduction* (eds M. Ferrin, R.L. Vande Wiele and F. Halberg), John Wiley & Sons, London, pp. 287–306 (1974)

107. De Vries, K., Goei, J.T., Booy-Noord, H. and Orie, N.G. Changes during 24 hours in the lung function and histamine hyperreactivity of the bronchial tree in asthmatic and bronchitis patients. *Int. Arch. Allergy,* **20**, 93–101 (1962)

108. Tammeling, G.J., De Vries, K. and Kruyt, E.W. The circadian pattern of the bronchial reactivity to histamine in healthy subjects and in patients with obstructive lung diseases. In *Chronobiology in Allergy and Immunology* (eds M.H. Smolensky, A. Reinberg and J. McGovern), C.C. Thomas, Springfield, IL, pp. 139–150 (1977)

109. Labrecque, G., Doré, F., Lapierre, A., Perusse, F. and Belanger, P.M. Variation in the carrageenin induced edema in the action and the plasma levels of indomethacin. In *Chronopharmacology* (eds A. Reinberg and F. Halberg), Pergamon Press, Oxford, pp. 231–238 (1979)

110. Labrecque, G. and Belanger, P. The chronopharmacology of the inflammatory process. *Annu. Rev. Chronopharmacol.,* **2**, 291–325 (1986)

111. Bureau, J.P., Coupé, M. and Labrecque, G. Chronopharmacological study of the effect of corticosterone on BCG induced granulocyte migration in normal and in adrenalectomized mice. *Annu. Rev. Chronopharmacol.,* **3**, 309–312 (1986)

112. Greening, A.P. Asthma: mechanism of action of corticosteroids. Fokus-Atemwegserkrankungen heute. *Fifth International Kongress Therapie der Atemwegserkrankungen,* Springer Verlag, Berlin, pp. 28–34 (1986)

113. Reinberg, A., Ghata, J. and Sidi, E. Nocturnal asthma attacks; their relationship to the circadian adrenal cycle. *J. Allergy Clin. Immunol.,* **34**, 323–330 (1963)

114. Reinberg, A., Gervais, P., Morin, M. and Abulker, C. Rythme circadien humain du seuil de la réponse bronchique à l'acétylcholine. *Comptes-Rendus Acad. Sci. (Paris),* **272**, 1879–1881 (1971)

115. Reinberg, A., Gervais, P. and Ghata, J. In *Chronobiology in Allergy and Immunology* (eds J.P. McGovern, M. Smolensky and A. Reinberg), C.C. Thomas, Springfield, IL (1977)

116. Barnes, P., Fitzgerald, G., Brown, M. and Dollery, C. Nocturnal asthma and changes in circulating epinephrine histamine and cortisol. *N. Engl. J. Med.,* **303**, 263–267 (1980)

117. Reinberg, A. and Smolensky, M. Biological rhythms and medicine. *Cellular, Metabolic, Physiopathologic and Pharmacologic Aspects,* Springer Verlag, New York, p. 305 (1983)

118. Gervais, P., Reinberg, A., Gervais, C., Smolensky, M.H. and DeFrance, O. Twenty-four hour rhythm in the bronchial hyperreactivity to house dust in asthmatics. *J. Allergy Clin. Immunol.,* **59**, 207–213 (1977)

119. Smolensky, M.H. Chronobiology and epidemiology. *Pathol. Biol.,* **35**, 991–1004 (1987)

120. Pepys, J. Clinical and therapeutic significance of patterns of allergic reactions of the lungs to extrinsic agents. *Amer. Rev. Resp. Dis.,* **116**, 573–587 (1977)

121. Taylor, A.N., Davies, R.J., Hendrick, D.J. and Pepys, J. Recurrent nocturnal asthmatic reactions to bronchial provocation tests. *Clin. Allergy,* 213–219 (1979)

122. Feigin, R. Metabolic changes in infectious diseases. *Clin. Ped.,* **9**, 84–93 (1970)

123. Langlois, P.H.N., White, R.F. and Gklezen, W.P. Diurnal variation in human response to influenza vaccination? A pilot study of 125 volunteers. *Annu. Rev. Chronopharmacol.,* **3**, 1213 (1986)

124. Pöllmann, L. and Pöllmann, B. Circadian variations of the efficiency of hepatitis B vaccination. *Annu. Rev. Chronopharmacol.,* **5**, 45–48 (1988)

125. Reinberg, A., Lévi, F. and Smolensky, M. Chronobiologie et pathologie infectieuse. *Médecine et Maladies Infectieuses,* **17**, 348–350 (1987)

126. Fauci, A.S. and and Dale, D.C. The effect of *in vivo* hydrocortisone on subpopulations of human lymphocytes. *J. Clin. Invest.,* **53**, 240–246 (1974)

127. Yu, D.T.Y. and Clements, P.J. Human lymphocyte subpopulations: effect of epinephrine. *Clin. Exp. Immunol.,* **25**, 472–479 (1976)

128. Bhakri, H.L., Jones, H., pettingale, K.W. and Dee, D.E.H. Circadian variation of lymphocyte subpopulations. *Brit. Med. J.,* **287**, 562 (1983)

129. Reinberg, A., Lagoguey, M., Cesselin, F., Touitou, Y., Legrand, J.C., Delasnerie, A., Antreassian, I. and Lagoguey, A. Circadian and circannual rhythms in plasma hormones and other variables of five healthy young human males. *Acta Endocrinol.,* **88**, 417–427 (1978)

130. Touitou, Y., Suton, J., Bogdan, A. *et al.* Adrenal circadian system in young and elderly human subjects: a comparative study. *J. Endocrinol.,* **83**, 201–210 (1982)

131. Kawate, T., Abo, T., Hinnma, S. and Kumagai, K. Studies on the bioperiodicity of the immune response. II. Covariations of murine T and B cells and a role of corticosteroid. *J. Immunol.,* **126**, 1364–1367 (1981)

132. Reinberg, A., Gervais, P., Chaussade, M., Fraboulet, G. and Duburque, B. Circadian changes in effectiveness of corticosteroids in eight patients with allergic asthma. *J. Allergy Clin. Immunol.*, **71**, 425–433 (1983)
133. Cohen, P. The influence on survival of season of onset of childhood acute lymphoblastic leukemia (ALL). *Annu. Rev. Chronopharmacol.*, **3**, 217 (1986)
134. Canon, C., Lévi, F., Bennaceur, M., Touboul, J.P., Pati, A., Reinberg, A. and Mathé, G. Alterations of circadian rhythms in lymphocyte subpopulations of patients with hematologic malignancies. *Proc. 12th Annu. Meet. Eur. Soc. Med. Oncol.*, Nice, Nov. 28–30, 1986. *Cancer Chemother. Pharmacol.*, **18** (suppl. 1), 58 (abstr.) (1986)
135. Tsai, T.H., Burns, E.R. and Scheving, E. Circadian influence on the immunization of mice with live bacillus Calmette-Guérin (BCG) and subsequent challenge with Ehrlich ascites carcinoma. *Chronobiologia*, **6**, 187–201 (1979)

Chapter 8

Circadian rhythms of plasma amino acids, brain neurotransmitters and behaviour

Peter Leathwood

Introduction

In several recent popular books [1,2] and scientific publications [3,4] strong claims have been made suggesting that the macronutrient content of meals can influence mood, aid in adaptation to jet lag and influence behaviour. The mechanism proposed is that the proportions of protein and carbohydrate in a meal influence plasma amino acid levels, changing the availability to the brain of the amino acids that are precursors for serotonin (5-hydroxytryptamine, (5-HT)) and the catecholamines, directly influencing synthesis, release and function of these neurotransmitters. A corollary of this idea is that the circadian rhythms of biogenic amines and plasma amino acids might depend upon, or be modulated by, diet. If true, these ideas would have major theoretical and practical importance in understanding control and manipulation of neurotransmitter function and behaviour in chronobiology.

For these reasons the editors of this book decided to include a chapter reviewing some of these ideas. The topic is difficult to cover coherently, first because the chains of (proposed) causality are so long and complex (i.e. from changes in food intake, via changes in plasma amino acids, changes in brain levels of precursors, changes in neurotransmitter synthesis, storage, release and function to changes in mood and behaviour); second because at almost every link in the chain, current understanding is incomplete; and third because the measures used are often crude and sometimes of doubtful relevance to the mechanism under consideration (e.g. using measures of neurotransmitter levels to estimate rates of synthesis or turnover). In spite of these reservations, it is well worth summarizing the main experimental results and examining how the whole picture fits together. As the reader will see, this chapter provides a splendid illustration of the observation that what currently passes as the 'scientific approach' to phenomena is very useful for dissecting a problem into smaller and smaller pieces, but it is often less useful in putting the pieces together again.

The first section will consider in some detail the potential role of circadian and food-induced changes in plasma amino acids on precursor availability in the synthesis and function of serotonin, showing how, under carefully chosen and rather limited circumstances, current results are compatible with the idea that dietary manipulation of tryptophan availability can influence serotoninergic function, but that there is little or no serious evidence to support the hypothesis that consumption of different foods can, via the same mechanism, influence serotoninergic function or behaviour.

The second section will deal more briefly with the idea that influencing precursor availability can affect catecholaminergic function, behaviour and mood. It is now well established that L-dopa (L-dihydroxyphenylalanine) can increase striatal dopamine synthesis and restore motor control in patients with Parkinson's disease. The idea that tyrosine availability might, in any practical circumstances, also influence central catecholamine synthesis and function is still extremely speculative, while suggestions that meal composition might, by influencing precursor availability, have similar effects, are still in the realm of wishful thinking since there is really no supporting evidence for this idea.

Serotonin (5-HT)

Figure 8.1 illustrates the sequence of events by which diet is supposed to influence serotoninergic function. In parallel are noted some of the questions that need to be addressed. The section will begin with an examination of the quantitative relationships at each step and then, in the light of this analysis, examine the plausibility of suggestions that tryptophan alone, diet, or circadian amino acid patterns might, via changes in central tryptophan availability, influence serotoninergic function.

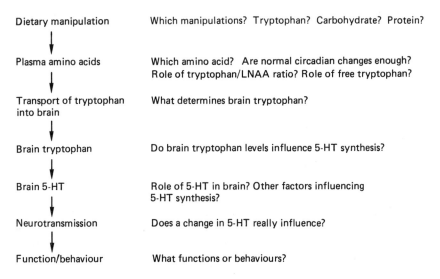

Figure 8.1 Sequence of events linking dietary manipulation to serotonergic function and some of the questions that need to be addressed in analysing suggestions that any particular dietary manipulation really does operate via this pathway to change behaviour

Brain tryptophan and 5-HT synthesis

5-HT in the brain is synthesized from the essential amino acid, tryptophan. The rate-limiting step is the hydroxylation of tryptophan to 5-hydroxytryptophan by the enzyme tryptophan 5-monooxygenase. A variety of factors, including firing frequency of the neurone, time of day and concentration of tryptophan, can influence the rate of this reaction [5,6]. The enzyme is usually about half-saturated *in vivo* (this means that in some circumstances, the rate of delivery of tryptophan to the brain may be the rate-limiting step in 5-HT synthesis), so changes in brain concentrations of tryptophan can influence the rate of 5-HT synthesis and thus levels of 5-HT and/or 5-hydroxyindoleacetic acid (5-HIAA), the metabolite produced by oxidative deamination of 5-HT. In the rat, doubling brain tryptophan from say 15 to 30 μM usually, but not always [6,7], leads to an increase of about 10–15% in 5-HT or 5-HT+5-HIAA. This is within the normal range of circadian

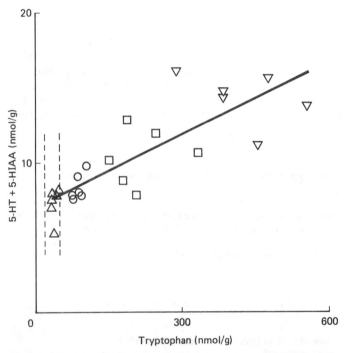

Figure 8.2 Relationship, in cynomolgus monkeys, between brain (striatal) tryptophan and the sum of 5-HT and 5-HIAA in brain stem. Brain tryptophan levels were manipulated by oral administration of tryptophan 1 h before. The treatments were as follows: △, controls; ○, tryptophan, 20 mg/kg; □, 90 mg/kg; ▽, 400 mg/kg. The dashed lines indicate the range of control values for tryptophan ± 2 standard deviations. The slope of this plot suggests that very large increases in tryptophan are needed to obtain a reliable change in brain 5-HT + 5-HIAA, with a 5-fold increase in tryptophan leading to a 25% rise in 5-HT + 5-HIAA. (Note: it was not possible to measure tryptophan and 5-HT in both regions.) (Drawn from data in Leathwood and Fernstrom [14])

variations in brain tryptophan [8–10]. Smaller changes (see Figure 8.2) do not seem to influence brain 5-HT or 5-HIAA reliably [11,12]. In primates and man, increases in brain tryptophan can also lead to increases in 5-HIAA in brain or cerebrospinal fluid [13,14], but it seems that, at least in primates, much larger increases in tryptophan are needed to get reliable changes in 5-HT (Figure 8.2).

Control of brain tryptophan levels

Tryptophan is carried into the brain by the large neutral amino acid (LNAA) transport system of the blood–brain barrier, and must compete with valine, leucine, isoleucine, phenylalanine, tyrosine and methionine for access to the carrier binding site [15]. Increasing plasma tryptophan concentration while keeping the other LNAAs constant will increase the rate of tryptophan transport into the brain. Similarly, raising (or lowering) levels of the other LNAAs while maintaining plasma tryptophan constant will also change the rate of transport. When it varies over a large range, the tryptophan/LNAA ratio is in many circumstances a fairly good predictor of brain tryptophan; within the normal range it is not [6,7,12,16] (see also Figure 8.3). Thus, as several groups have shown, in rats, a 3-fold rise in

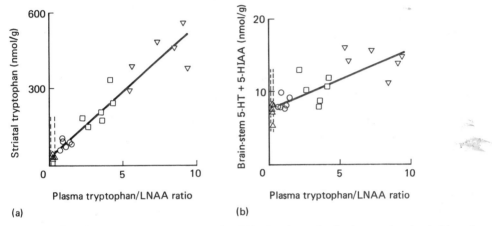

(a)   (b)

Figure 8.3 Correlations between plasma tryotphan/LNAA ratios and striatal tryptophan levels (a), and brainstem 5-HT + 5-HIAA levels (b). These results suggest that a large increase in the ratio reliably raises brain 5-HT; within the normal range (dashed lines) it does not. (Drawn from data in Leathwood and Fernstrom [14]). Symbols as for Figure 8.2

the ratio (e.g. from 0.1 to 0.3) will produce an 80–100% rise in brain tryptophan and a 10–15% increase in 5-HT and/or 5-HIAA. (As Figure 8.3 shows, a similar relationship may exist in primates, since a 4-fold increase in the plasma tryptophan/ LNAA ratio increased brain-stem 5-HT + 5-HIAA by about 10%, although interanimal variability was high.) With larger changes, the shifts in brain tryptophan and 5-HT are more reliable. With changes of less than 2-fold, most researchers have been unable to find any consistent effects of plasma tryptophan/ LNAA ratios on brain tryptophan or 5-HT. Since, to measure brain tryptophan and 5-HT, one must kill the experimental animal, it is not yet possible to know if, in individual animals, small changes in the plasma tryptophan/LNAA ratio (±50%) really influence 5-HT levels or rates of synthesis. Studies with simultaneous measures of plasma amino acids and intracerebral voltammetry or dialysis should soon be able to tell if such small changes in the ratio (within the circadian range) influence 5-HT and 5-HIAA release. Current evidence from these techniques suggests that only very large changes in brain tryptophan, accompanied by marked increases in serotoninergic activity, actually lead to detectable increases in 5-HT release [17,18]. Recent evidence suggests that the activity of the brain uptake system for LNAA is increased by β-adrenergic agonists [19] so that factors such as exercise, arousal or stress might also increase availability of tryptophan to the brain independently of changes in the plasma tryptophan/LNAA ratio.

Tryptophan in plasma binds reversibly to albumin, and estimates of dialysable tryptophan suggest that only 15–20% is 'free'. It is often thought that transport into the brain should depend more on 'free' than on 'total' tryptophan in plasma. However, as Pardridge [15] has pointed out, interactions that are valid *in vitro* do not necessarily hold *in vivo*, so during passage through the brain capillaries when the carrier is also competing for tryptophan, 70–80% of plasma tryptophan is effectively 'free' and available for transport into the brain, and albumin binding normally plays only a minor role in determining brain tryptophan levels. Our own results comparing the ability of free tryptophan, total tryptophan, [free tryptophan]/LNAA and [total tryptophan]/LNAA to predict brain tryptophan levels tend to confirm this conclusion [20].

On the other hand, situations such as prolonged starvation, stress or sustained exercise, which produce major increases in plasma free tryptophan also increase brain tryptophan. This has been interpreted as evidence that plasma free tryptophan is an important determinant of brain tryptophan. The results of Ericksson and Carlsson with β-adrenergic agonists suggest that the increase in brain tryptophan may equally be due to a non-specific increase in transport of all LNAAs into the brain. Since researchers have rarely measured brain levels of the other LNAAs, this possibility cannot be ruled out.

Diet and plasma tryptophan/LNAA ratios

In rats, consumption of large amounts (200–400 mg/kg or more) of tryptophan in the absence of LNAA can produce sharp increases in plasma tryptophan/LNAA ratios (and plasma tryptophan), enough to increase brain tryptophan and 5-HT [7]. Smaller amounts (50–100 mg/kg) increase brain tryptophan but do not always change 5-HT or 5-HIAA (e.g. [21]). Primates show a similar pattern [14].

Combining tryptophan with a carbohydrate load, which tends to lower plasma levels of all the LNAA [22], accentuates the increase in the ratio. In quantitative terms, in man, 400 mg of tryptophan combined with a small carbohydrate load increases the plasma tryptophan/LNAA ratio 3-fold [23]. If the transport characteristics of the blood–brain barrier are similar in rats and man, and they seem to be [24], this should be enough to produce a small increase in brain 5-HT synthesis.

If, however, tryptophan is consumed with a protein-rich meal (when levels of all LNAAs rise) its effects on the tryptophan/LNAA ratio should be dampened [6]. For clinical use, it is often recommended that dose levels of about 2 g of tryptophan be taken with a meal [25]. As Table 8.1 shows, according to its composition, the meal could accentuate, attenuate or not influence the availability of tryptophan to the brain and hence its potential effects on 5-HT synthesis. This could, at least in part, explain the inconsistent results from clinical studies using tryptophan [25].

As Fernstrom and Wurtman [7,26] have shown, under some conditions, meal composition can also influence brain 5-HT synthesis. If rats are starved overnight and then fed carbohydrate, the increase in muscle glucose metabolism accelerates muscle uptake of the branched chain amino acids leucine, valine and isoleucine, so lowering their levels in plasma. Since plasma tryptophan usually remains quite stable, the tryptophan/LNAA ratio rises, and at 2 h after feeding begins, can

Table 8.1 Estimated changes in plasma tryptophan, plasma total LNAAs, brain tryptophan and brain 5-HT+5-HIAA after consumption of 2 g of tryptophan with different midday meals in man

Variable	Protein content of meal (g)			References
	50	25	0	
Plasma tryptophan 2 h after meal (mM)	80	60	40	Values taken from Fernstrom et al. [40]
Plasma LNAA 2 h after meal (mM)	1140	630	270	Values taken from Fernstrom et al. [40]
Increase in plasma tryptophan 2 h after 2 g of tryptophan (mM)	150	150	150	Extrapolated from Eccleston et al. [78]
Tryptophan/LNAA ratio	0.2	0.33	0.77	
Expected change in brain tryptophan	+30%	+100%	+230%	Extrapolated from Fernstrom & Wurtman [7]
Expected change in brain 5-HT + 5-HIAA	+7%	+14%	+50%	Extrapolated from Fernstrom & Wurtman [7]

The estimated changes in plasma tryptophan after consumption of 2 g of tryptophan are extrapolated from Eccleston et al. [78]. Estimated values for plasma tryptophan and LNAA after different meals from Fernstrom et al. [40]. Their 'expected' effects on brain tryptophan and 5-HT are extrapolated from the values of Fernstrom and Wurtman [7]. The last publication was chosen because it is the most frequently cited as evidence for the quantitative effects of manipulating plasma tryptophan/LNAA ratios on brain 5-HT synthesis. As can be seen, according to the predictions of the hypothesis, the same 2 g dose of tryptophan might be expected to increase brain 5-HT availability by anything from 7 to 50% according to the composition of concurrently eaten food.

increase from a baseline level of 0.1 to about 0.3 [26]. As can be seen from the above discussion, this might be expected to increase brain tryptophan and brain 5-HT and/or 5-HIAA. Some researchers (e.g. [27]) have suggested that a high-protein meal fed to rats starved overnight might (by increasing LNAA levels more than those of tryptophan) lower the tryptophan/LNAA ratio and hence decrease brain tryptophan and 5-HT levels. The experimental evidence available does not support this hypothesis since protein meals under these circumstances decrease neither the plasma tryptophan/LNAA ratio nor brain tryptophan or 5-HT [6,7,28] (see also [29] for a detailed review). Several reviews state that protein meals lower brain tryptophan and 5-HT, either citing paper by Fernstrom and Wurtman [7] which concludes '... however, when even larger elevations of plasma tryptophan are produced by the ingestion of protein-containing diets, brain tryptophan and serotonin do not change.', or without giving any evidence at all (e.g. [32]). One study did report decreased brain tryptophan after feeding fasted rats a protein-rich meal, but found no increase in brain tryptophan after the protein-free meal, suggesting an unusual control group [33].

To what extent do these results with carbohydrate fed to overnight-starved animals generalize to free-feeding rats? Will any carbohydrate meal increase brain 5-HT? A surprising number of scientists appear to assume this is so (see [6] for some examples). The vast majority of published experimental results suggest that it is not. In free-feeding rats or in rats fasted for short periods and then allowed to eat carbohydrate, either the plasma tryptophan/LNAA ratio simply does not change or the shifts are so small that brain tryptophan and 5-HT are unaffected [8,11,12,34,35].

Protein-containing meals taken after a short fast or by free-feeding rats do not change the ratio [11] (P.D. Leathwood and L. Arimanana, unpublished work; see Table 8.2). Curiously, Li and Anderson [10] reported what appears to be a small increase in the ratio and in brain 5-HT, but no change in brain tryptophan in rats eating protein-rich meals following a short fast. In free-feeding animals given a choice of high- and low-protein diets, or fixed levels of protein, no robust

Table 8.2 Lack of effect of protein-free and protein-rich meals on brain 5-HT synthesis in free-feeding rats

Parameter	Protein content of meal (%)			
	0	55 (casein)	73 (casein)	55 (beef)
Meal size (g)	3.6 ± 0.6	3.8 ± 0.7	4.0 ± 0.4	4.2 ± 0.4
Plasma				
Tryptophan (μmol/l)	80 ± 6	170 ± 7	211 ± 13	197 ± 11
Tryptophan/LNAA	0.13 ± 0.01	0.12 ± 0.02	0.11 ± 0.03	0.14 ± 0.06
Brain				
Tryptophan (nmol/g)	15 ± 1	15 ± 1	14 ± 2	15 ± 2
5-HT (nmol/g)	2.0 ± 0.05	1.7 ± 0.05	1.9 ± 1.0	1.8 ± 1.1
5-HIAA (nmol/g)	1.1 ± 0.04	0.8 ± 0.04	0.9 ± 0.04	0.9 ± 0.04

The animals were killed 2 h later and plasma amino acids and brain tryptophan, 5-HT and 5-HIAA were measured. There were small but statistically significant differences in the plasma tryptophan/LNAA ratio ($F = 4.3$; df = 3, 28; $P<0.025$), but the highest value was after beef protein. brain tryptophan and 5-HT levels were unchanged after the different treatments. In contrast, brain 5-HIAA levels were significantly lower after protein-containing meals as compared to carbohydrate. Thus, there may be a difference in brain 5-HT turnover after eating meals of different composition, but the difference does not seem to be driven by changes in plasma tryptophan/ LNAA ratio of brain tryptophan levels.

systematic relationships among dietary carbohydrate/protein intake, plasma tryptophan/LNAA ratios, brain tryptophan or 5-HT metabolism have emerged (see Fernstrom [29] and Leathwood [36], for detailed reviews, and Li and Anderson [10] for a contrary view). In man, carbohydrate-rich protein-free 'meals' eaten at lunchtime or in the evening have no significant effect on the plasma tryptophan/LNAA ratio [23,37] (see also Figure 8.4).

In the morning, after an overnight fast, a carbohydrate meal may increase the ratio by 10–20% [38,39]. After a mixed meal containing 20–25 g of protein, the ratio remains stable [23,40]; if taken in the morning it may fall by 10–20% [23].

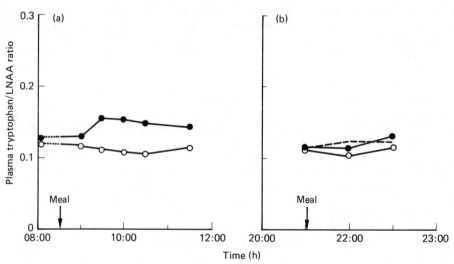

Figure 8.4 Changes in plasma tryptophan/LNAA ratios in healthy young men after breakfast (a) or evening (b) meals supply 500 kcal and containing 93 g of carbohydrate and 1.6 g of protein (●), 73 g of carbohydrate and 21.6 g of protein (○). In the evening, neither the protein nor the carbohydrate meals influenced plasma tryptophan/LNAA ratios. In the morning, the carbohydrate-rich meal produced a small but significant increase in the ratio; replacing 20 g of carbohydrate with protein led to a small decrease in the ratio. (Redrawn from [23] and [38])

With a 'meal' consisting of 75 g or more of protein (e.g. 300 g of turkey breast) the ratio may fall by nearly 20% over the next 3 h [37]. As shown above, in rats and monkeys, change of this order would not influence brain tryptophan or 5-HT, but one cannot be absolutely sure that the same holds for some individual animals (or men).

Neurotransmission

The reader will already have noticed that many of the published studies of effects of tryptophan administration on brain 5-HT metabolism describe changes in 5-HT and/or 5-HIAA levels. In fact, increases in brain tryptophan are often accompanied by increases in 5-HIAA but no change in 5-HT, and it is possible that the extra 5-HT may be metabolized intracellularly to 5-HIAA without ever entering the 'functional' pool. Attempts to resolve this question have, so far, produced equivocal results. In isolated synaptosomes, increasing tryptophan in the medium increases 5-HT synthesis, but the 5-HT is metabolized to 5-HIAA without being released. If the synaptosomes are depolarized, 5-HT release is increased [41]. In rats given tryptophan (100 mg/kg i.p.), hypothalamic 5-HIAA levels rise. Giving a 5-HT reuptake blocker (fluoxetine) decreases 5-HIAA levels by 10–40%, suggesting that most of the 5-HT is metabolized to 5-HIAA without being released. If, however, the rats are subjected to supramaximal electrical stimulation in the Raphé nuclei, giving tryptophan does increase 5-HT release [17,42]. It remains to be seen whether small increases in 5-HT availability during periods of high (but physiological) firing rates also lead to increased 5-HT release.

A second possible adaptation to changed intraneuronal 5-HT levels is that firing rates may change. This certainly occurs after major increases in 5-HT, but with small variations (±12%), firing rates did not adapt [43], so changes in neurotransmission could have occurred. Thus, in summary, although 5-HIAA may increase, it is usually impossible to know what proportion (if any) comes from the functional pool. The results of Lookingland [17,42], however, do suggest that tryptophan increases the 'releasable' pool of 5-HT so that when the neurones are activated, more of the neurotransmitter can be released.

The role of 5-HT in the brain

The vast majority of central serotoninergic neurones are found in the Raphé nuclei. From there, fine slowly conducting fibres spread throughout the brain making multiple and often ill-defined connections with other neurones. Both electrical stimulation of serotoninergic neurones in the Raphé nuclei and application of small amounts of 5-HT depress firing rates or reactivity in a wide range of central neurones [44]. These observations have led to speculation that 5-HT sometimes acts as a neuromodulator having broad, tonic 'down-regulatory' effects, in contrast to the global 'up-regulatory' action of noradrenergic systems (see Jouvet [45] and Koella [44] for review). This speculation is to some extent supported by an analysis of the effects of 5-HT on behaviour. Increasing 5-HT release or activity by drug treatments, electrical stimulation of the Raphé nuclei, or intraventricular delivery of small amounts of 5-HT tends to decrease arousal and facilitate sleep onset [44]. Similar treatments have been reported to down-regulate other systems, for example, decreasing pain sensitivity, sexual behaviour, aggression and food intake [6]. Lowering 5-HT by pharmacological means or by Raphé lesions often leads to sustained arousal and insomnia [45]. Although these global effects are quite reliable and have been incorporated into theories of arousal, vigilance, sleep and satiety, too little is known about the details of 5-HT function and too many inconsistent or contradictory results have been reported for these ideas to be taken as more than a guide towards some useful target behaviours to examine after treatments thought to influence 5-HT release.

Behavioural effects of tryptophan

Taking into account the predictions (and limitations) of the hypothesis as outlined above, the behavioural effects of tryptophan administration are surprisingly consistent with the idea that it is acting via a small increase in 5-HT availability. In man, large doses of tryptophan (3 g or more) often lead to decreased arousal, sleepiness and even mild euphoria [46]. In searching for the smallest effective dose, we found that 0.5 g, combined with a carbohydrate load, produced fatigue or lethargy and decreased sleep latency in a significant proportion of test subjects, although some subjects noted no effect at all [47,48].

The apparently inconsistent effects on sleep latency should not really be surprising. 5-HT is not a central depressant like most pharmacological sedatives. From what is understood about its mode of action, it could only be expected to facilitate sleep onset [45]. Good sleepers rarely notice the effects of tryptophan (probably because they fall asleep easily anyway), nor do people with severe insomnia (perhaps because their problems are beyond the reach of a weak sleep facilitator). In a carefully chosen target population of people with mild insomnia and problems getting to sleep, as little as 1 g of tryptophan reliably increases sleepiness (P.D. Leathwood and F. Chauffard, unpublished work). With less than 0.5 g of tryptophan, behavioural effects are no longer observed [46,48]. This is entirely consistent with the above analysis, since changes in the plasma tryptophan/LNAA ratio should be too small to influence brain tryptophan.

Decreasing the plasma tryptophan/LNAA ratio to less than 0.02 (by consumption of 100 g of mixed amino acids minus tryptophan) can induce a lowering of mood and increased nervousness [25]. This might be linked to decreased cerebral availability of tryptophan for 5-HT synthesis. Nobody has yet reported on the effects of this type of treatment on sleepiness or sleep onset.

Behavioural effects of foods and meals

As outlined above, in some circumstances carbohydrate can increase brain 5-HT (although in the particular model used–the rat starved overnight–no behavioural sequelae have been recorded). In man, however, carbohydrate either has no effect on the plasma tryptophan/LNAA ratio or increases it only by 10–20%. This would at best produce a 0–2% increase in 5-HT. On the other hand, one can never be sure that in some individuals or in some crucial brain region, functionally significant changes in 5-HT availability do not occur. It is, therefore, worth examining the behavioural effects of these dietary manipulations to see if they produce changes coherent with modulation of serotoninergic function.

In one double-blind experiment a carbohydrate breakfast had no effect at all on mood or sleepiness scores [47]. Volunteers ate a 400 kcal meal on four occasions; with it they took a pill containing 500 mg of tyrosine, 500 mg of tryptophan, 100 mg of caffeine or a placebo. The carbohydrate intake could be expected to increase the plasma tryptophan/LNAA ratio by 10–20% in the placebo group; the addition of 500 mg of tyrosine should have been enough to prevent the increase. Mood and sleepiness ratings were practically identical after the two treatments. In contrast, if 500 mg of tryptophan was taken with the meal (a treatment that should about triple the plasma tryptophan/LNAA ratio), a significant proportion of volunteers reported feeling more sleepy. With 100 mg of caffeine most reported feeling more wide awake.

Studies comparing the effects of protein and carbohydrate 'meals' on mood and performance have produced almost entirely negative results. (This is quite surprising in that such studies are rarely double-blind, and people's expectations as to the effects of meat, sweets or bread could be expected to influence their responses.) Spring *et al.* [3] compared the effects of 75 g of carbohydrate (as sherbert) or 75 g of protein (as cold turkey). There was no significant main effect of meal composition, but a (non-predicted) significant meal × sex interaction emerged: women rated themselves as slightly more sleepy after carbohydrate as compared to protein, men as slightly less sleepy. In contrast, women reported feeling a little less calm after carbohydrate, men a little more calm, again with no significant main effect. Reaction times were not significantly affected by diet. The only clear-cut result was that the group of older people receiving carbohydrate at lunchtime produced more omission errors in a dichotic listening test during the afternoon. (In this test the subject wears stereo earphones and is presented with two simultaneous messages, one to each ear, and is asked to attend to one message and ignore the other. Subjects repeat each word of the message while listening to the next word. Errors in 'shadowing' the target message are used as a measure of distractability.) Since this was a between-groups difference which only appeared at one time point, its interpretation is unclear. In a second study [37], comparing a starch 'meal' (a special pita bread) with a protein 'meal' (cold turkey), the pretest scores for vigour and sleepiness ratings were different and this difference was maintained during the next 2 h. Performance in a simple auditory reaction time test was slower 1.75 h after eating carbohydrate, and digit symbol substitution was slightly less efficient at 3.5 h. No pretest measures were made. Again, this type of result should be interpreted very conservatively. It is interesting to note that, although the authors of these two studies took great care to underline the inconclusiveness of their results, these studies have been cited as evidence that subjects feel 'less alert after eating carbohydrate than after protein'.

The only clear-cut positive results are in what appears to be the opposite direction to that predicted by the 'serotoninergic' hypothesis. In an elegantly designed double-blind cross-over study, glucose (20 g taken every 30 min) significantly increased vigilance and decreased errors in a driving simulator [49]. In other double blind studies [50] (K. Mercurio, personal communication), high-protein meals were shown to be more satiating than high-carbohydrate meals. (According to the hypothesis, protein meals are supposed to lower 5-HT availability, and decreased serotoninergic activity is supposed, if anything, to decrease satiation.)

In summary, results so far really offer no support at all for the hypothesis that, in normal living, carbohydrate meals increase and protein meals decrease precursor availability for brain 5-HT synthesis and, via this mechanism, have an effect on serotoninergic activity or behaviour. An additional point is worth mentioning here. Although researchers discuss the effects of 'carbohydrate meals' and 'protein meals' as if these occur in normal eating, a whole meal consisting entirely of one macronutrient is an artificial construct and would rarely occur in normal eating.

Even a 'coffee and a Danish pastry' contains enough protein [51] to ensure that the plasma tryptophan/LNAA ratio would not change, and 300 g of turkey breast (without bread) is a fairly unusual meal.

Diet and circadian rhythms of 5-HT metabolism

Several research groups have suggested that circadian changes in brain 5-HT may be secondary to diurnal cycles in feeding and to the influence of feeding on plasma amino acids (e.g. [52]). Subsequent measures of circadian variations in 5-HT levels (and/or its metabolite 5-HIAA), its release and turnover, or in firing frequency of serotoninergic neurones have produced such inconsistent and contradictory results that any hypothesis aimed at explaining them is still bound to be speculative. In rats, brain 5-HT levels tend to peak in the light period (usually near the end), and are lowest in the dark period [8,9,53,54] (see also Figure 8.5), although some

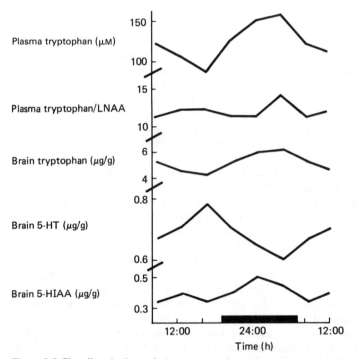

Figure 8.5 Circadian rhythms of plasma tryptophan, plasma tryptophan/LNAA ratios and brain tryptophan, 5-HT and 5-HIAA in male rats eating a 30% casein diet. Each point represents the mean of six animals. On analysis of variance, all measures except the plasma tryptophan/LNAA ratios showed significant circadian rhythms. The bar indicates the dark period. (Redrawn from [8])

researchers have reported either no significant rhythm [10,16] or even the opposite pattern [55,56].

If one includes measures of 5-HIAA, the situation becomes more complex, because its circadian pattern in the rat, with some exceptions [9], usually exhibits a peak during the dark period [8,10,44,53], suggesting perhaps that 5-HT release is higher during arousal, leading to a rise in 5-HIAA and a fall in 5-HT (Figure

8.5). This interpretation fits well with observations that: (i) an increase in serotoninergic activity is often accompanied by a fall in 5-HT and a rise in 5-HIAA [57]; (ii) 5-HT release, as estimated by *in vivo* voltammetry or dialysis, is higher during arousal than in sleep ([45,58], S. Leibowitz, personal communication); and (iii) firing rates of serotoninergic neurones seem to be highest during arousal, slightly lower during slow-wave sleep and much lower during paradoxical sleep [45]. In fact, the observed circadian rhythms of firing rates of serotoninergic neurones [44] may simply be a function of a state of arousal because, at different times of day, in conscious animals, serotoninergic neurones have similar firing rates [59].

These observations pose a paradox. On one hand, 5-HT seems to function as a 'down regulator', decreasing firing rates and sensitivity of target neurones and generally decreasing vigilance and behavioural reactivity. On the other hand, circadian studies suggest that firing rates of serotoninergic neurones and release of 5-HT are probably highest during arousal. Jouvet and Koella have suggested different explanations which may in fact be complementary. Jouvet [45] observed that in animals rendered insomniac by drugs or Raphé lesions, re-establishing 5-HT availability did not immediately lead to sleep onset. Instead, a consistent delay of about 45 min preceded sleep. He suggested that, in addition to its neurotransmitter role, 5-HT might act as a neurohormone whose release leads to formation of a stable sleep-inducing substance which needs to accumulate to a critical level before sleep onset can be facilitated. Koella [44] suggested that, during the waking stage, as (adrenergic-generated) arousal approaches an optimum level, serotoninergic tone begins to increase, thus preventing over-arousal and setting off the next cycle of sleep. As these two suggestions show, there are sufficient uncertainties to sustain a great deal of imaginative theorizing in this domain.

The level of brain tryptophan is consistently found to be increased during the arousal/eating phase of the 24 h [8–10,54–56], although Fernstrom [16] reported no change. The amplitude of the circadian change is usually reported as about 20% (range ± 6–40%) of the mean value. Thus the pattern of brain tryptophan tends to correlate with estimates of 5-HT release (and tryptophan intake–see next paragraph). There is no clear evidence to show whether or not these changes in tryptophan availability to any extent drive the circadian changes in 5-HT release.

It is equally difficult to identify the factors controlling the circadian changes in brain tryptophan. Several studies have followed plasma tryptophan, plasma tryptophan/LNAA ratios and brain tryptophan. One found a significant and similar correlation between both these plasma measures and brain tryptophan [10], but discussed only the tryptophan/LNAA:brain tryptophan relationship (if anything, plasma tryptophan seemed to correlate better with brain tryptophan). A second noted a significant positive correlation between plasma tryptophan and brain tryptophan but not between the ratio and brain tryptophan [8], and a third found no correlations at all [60]. These results offer little or no support for the idea that plasma tryptophan/LNAA ratios drive brain tryptophan levels. This is not surprising since experimental manipulations of plasma tryptophan/LNAA ratios within the normal circadian range (0.08–0.2) have generally been found to have little or no influence on brain tryptophan. What is perhaps surprising is the tenacity of the idea that they do. In circadian studies, plasma total and free tryptophan tend to correlate rather well with brain tryptophan. But again, this is not evidence of a causal relationship. Thus, Morgan and Yndo [56] found that changes in the eating cycle (by giving rats food in the light phase) shifted the circadian peak of plasma total tryptophan from the dark phase into the light phase, leading only to a small shift in the pattern of brain tryptophan. In addition, Fernstrom *et al.* [60] found that lowering plasma tryptophan (by feeding a 12% protein diet) did not influence brain tryptophan levels. Thus overall, neither plasma total tryptophan (nor free tryptophan) nor plasma tryptophan/LNAA ratios emerge as really convincing predictors of brain tryptophan. A possible explanation for this pattern of results is that during arousal there may be a general enhancement of LNAA transport across the blood–brain barrier. This phenomenon has already been demonstrated with β-adrenergic drugs [19] and stress [57] but it remains to be seen if transport capacity really exhibits a circadian variation.

Diet and circadian changes in plasma amino acids

The earliest studies of circadian variation in plasma amino acids in man showed that plasma total amino acids are relatively stable, tending to be higher in the daytime than at night. While these global changes were relatively independent of food intake, levels of the large neutral amino acids did seem to be influenced by timing of meals [61,62]. More recent studies have shown that plasma levels of these amino acids are also influenced by the protein content of the diet and of each meal. Fernstrom *et al.* [40] showed that in young men fed a protein-free diet for 5 days, morning levels of LNAA were slightly lower than if they were given 75 g of protein per day, and fell by 30–50% during the daytime. With 150 g/day, morning levels were 10–20% higher and rose by 50–80% during the day. With 75 g of protein, levels remained constant during the day and rose 10–30% in the evening. With the protein-free diet, the plasma tryptophan/LNAA ratio rose (from 0.12 to 0.16) during the day; with 75 g of protein it remained stable at around 0.1, and with 150 g it was lower and stable at about 0.08 (see Figure 8.6).

Extrapolating from the animal studies, one would not expect changes of this order to influence brain tryptophan or 5-HT metabolism. Although as there have

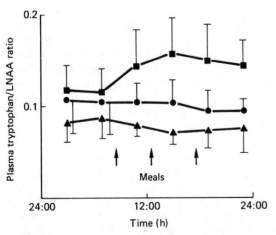

Figure 8.6 Circadian changes in plasma tryptophan/LNAA ratios in healthy young men consuming diets containing 0 (■), 75 (●) or 150 (▲) g of egg protein per day. Each point represents the mean (± S.D.) of two determinations on seven subjects. Blood samples were collected on the 4th and 5th days of feeding the diets. (Redrawn from ref. [40])

been no studies on the biochemical or behavioural effects of 'clamping' the ratio at different levels in the range 0.07–0.16, one cannot be sure there will be no effect. It should also be remembered that eating a protein-free diet for 5 days would be an unusual occurrence in the lives of most people, so that normal variation could be smaller than seen in Fernstrom's study.

Fernstrom and his colleagues [60] have also examined the effects on circadian changes in plasma LNAA, brain tryptophan, 5-HT and 5-HIAA of feeding rats 12, 24 and 40% protein diets. Plasma LNAA showed significant diurnal variations at all protein levels (peaking in the dark period), with increasing dietary protein producing higher overall levels and greater amplitudes for each LNAA. Plasma tryptophan was lower at all times of day with 12% protein but there was no fall in brain tryptophan. The plasma tryptophan/LNAA ratio showed no overall significant change with time of day, but was influenced by dietary protein (it was slightly lower with the highest level). There was also a significant diet × time interaction, with 12% and 24% protein producing a peak in plasma tryptophan/LNAA at the end of the night, while animals eating 40% protein showed a peak at the end of the light period. Overall, brain tryptophan was uninfluenced by dietary protein level: there were circadian changes, different across proteins but they bore no evident relationship to plasma tryptophan or tryptophan/LNAA [60].

Diet and circadian changes in mood and behaviour

As can be seen from the above analysis, the biochemical predictions of the model have not stood up well to dissection and reconstruction. Because one can never be absolutely sure that, within individuals, diet cannot influence 5-HT function, it is interesting to check to what extent observed circadian mood patterns or behaviours fit with the predictions of the model.

One prediction is that mood might link with macronutrient selection [2]. This hypothesis has been directly tested in the context of circadian rhythms of food selection and mood in man [63]. The researcher commented as follows: 'Diets rich in carbohydrate should increase plasma tryptophan and in turn increase brain serotonin levels resulting in lethargy and somnolence. In fact the opposite was found, with subjects ingesting diets higher in carbohydrate reporting higher energy levels. This finding might have occurred because normal subjects were used'. It is interesting to note that the author (1) accepts the serotoninergic hypothesis (in spite of the contrary evidence already published), (2) reports an observation that apparently contradicts the predictions, and (3) introduces an 'explanation' of the contradiction without calling into question the hypothesis.

A second idea is that the proportions of protein and carbohydrate in a meal influence brain 5-HT synthesis and that, in turn, 5-HT availability influences macronutrient selection, thus driving circadian rhythms of protein/carbohydrate selection. Although circadian changes in protein and carbohydrate selection have been reported in rats [64,65] (Figure 8.7), the patterns show no evident relationship to 5-HT metabolism [12] (see also Figure 8.5), and one cannot be sure that the rats were actually selecting particular macronutrients (as opposed to exhibiting circadian changes in taste or texture preference).

Consumption of carbohydrate or protein meals by free feeding animals had no effect on brain tryptophan [6]. In addition, in the one study that compared effects of fixed proportions of protein (30% protein diet) with dietary selection (from 0

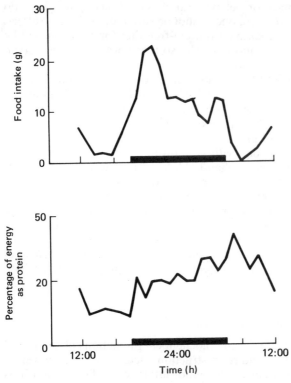

Figure 8.7 Circadian rhythms of food intake and protein energy selection in young adult male rats. Male rats (250 g) were offered a choice of 0% and 60% protein diets over 9 days. Diet pellets (75 mg) were obtained by lever press. Within 3 days the selection patterns were stable and the results for the next 6 days were used for analysis. Each point represents the mean of 12 rats. The bar indicates the dark period. (Redrawn from ref. [65])

or 60% protein) on plasma amino acids and brain 5-HT metabolism [8], the changes seen (a tendency for higher levels of brain 5-HT following the peak of protein selection) were opposite to those predicted by the model. Thus, the idea that protein/carbohydrate selection is controlled by a serotoninergic feedback mechanism is contradicted by current evidence (see Fernstrom [29] for a detailed review).

The last idea that will be considered here is that dietary manipulation of neurotransmitters can help overcome jet lag. Two recent books [1,2] give almost identical recommendations on how to counteract jet lag. The dietary aspects of their ideas seem to be based on the results of animal studies (see Graeber *et al.* [66] for a review). They suggest careful programming of social life and meal times to the new time zone (to aid resynchronizing) and restriction of caffeinated beverages to appropriate times in the circadian cycle (to maintain arousal in the daytime but not disrupt sleep at night). They both explain that a high-protein meal (meat, dairy products, beans) stimulates the adrenaline pathway giving 5 h worth of energy, while carbohydrate foods (pasta, salad, rich fruit desserts) give a surge of energy for up to an hour and then, by influencing the indoleamine pathway, help induce sleep. Taking these foods at appropriate times is supposed to help one adapt to the phase shift.

Even in the context of the diet/5-HT hypothesis, these nutritional recommendations are odd. If one ate a meal consisting of pasta, salad and fruit, it would probably contain 7–8% protein [51], enough to ensure that plasma tryptophan/ LNAA ratios did not change at all. A military adaptation of the dietary treatment recommended by Ehret has been tested on a small group of US military personnel [66]. The adaptation included taking 100 mg of dimenhydrinate in flight [at 22:20 h central european time (CET) (16:00 h US time)] and 'at 23:00 h CET the lights were turned off and everyone was instructed to sleep'. The only macronutrient manipulation was that the soldiers received a steak and a two-egg omelette for breakfast plus coffee at 14:30 h CET. The authors report that the experimental group were less fatigued than the controls but confidence in the results (or the state of arousal of those taking countermeasures) is somewhat diminished by the author's admission that six out of the 15 experimentals and one of the 15 controls had to be dropped from the analysis because they either lost their fatigue questionnaires or gave contradictory responses! This particular treatment did not seem to be very effective, but the military constraints and complexity of the design make it impossible to interpret. I could find no study that had attempted to test the effects of Ehret or Wurtman's dietary recommendations on jet lag.

There is, however, one well-designed study aimed precisely at testing the effects of dietary manipulation of 5-HT metabolism on jet lag. Spinweber [67] reported the effects of 2 g of tryptophan or a placebo, given to 51 US Navy Marines travelling from San Diego to Okinawa. The aim was, by using tryptophan as a short-acting sedative, to reduce the sleep-loss component of the jet lag syndrome. Tryptophan was administered in flight and 1 h before bedtime during the first 3

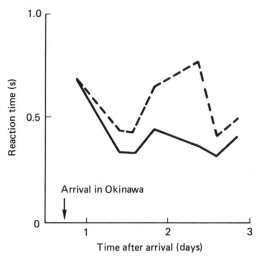

Figure 8.8 Performance in a four-choice reaction time test by US Marines after flying from California to Okinawa. The x axis shows days (marked at 00:00 h). The arrow indicates arrival time in Okinawa. Tryptophan (2 g) was taken in flight and at 22:00 h on the first 3 days after arrival. Subjects receiving tryptophan (——) had significantly faster reaction times at 21:00 h than subjects receiving placebo (–––) on the first day after arrival. (Redrawn from ref. [67])

days after arrival. Performance measures, taken morning, afternoon and evening for several days before and after travelling, included four-choice reaction time, digit-symbol substitution, word memory, and addition tests. Sleep recordings during the voyage were made on 12 of the volunteers. Tryptophan did not significantly increase in-flight sleep but it improved sleep on the first night in Okinawa ($274.5 \pm 9.9\,min$ vs $222.3 \pm 4.8\,min$ ($P=0.034$)). Sleep was not enhanced in the following 2 nights. Subjects receiving tryptophan reported feeling more alert on arrival, but both groups showed impaired reaction time performance. In contrast, the next evening and the following morning, the group receiving tryptophan showed normal reaction times while the group receiving placebo were still impaired (Figure 8.8).

Results for short-term word memory also showed improved performance with tryptophan. These results, although not spectacular, suggest that tryptophan might aid sleep onset and improve performance after travel through several time zones. The results of this study are extremely promising but, before this anti-jet lag strategy can be fully accepted, they need to be repeated with east and west travel, and perhaps combined with dietary manipulation (e.g. tryptophan could be taken with low-protein meals to diminish competition for transport across the blood–brain barrier, and caffeinated drinks could be taken in the morning as recommended by Ehret and Scanlon[1]).

Catecholamines

The first successful clinical application of a neurotransmitter precursor was the use of L-dihydroxyphenylalanine (L-dopa), a LNAA which is the direct precursor of dopamine, in the treatment of Parkinson's disease. In the mid 1950s, clinicians observed that patients treated with reserpine (used as an antihypertensive drug) often exhibited the symptoms of Parkinson's disease. Subsequent experiments on mice showed that reserpine produced a similar akinesia in these animals. In addition it lowered brain levels of the neurotransmitter dopamine. Treating the mice with dopa restored brain dopamine levels and abolished the akinesia [68]. These animal studies were quickly followed by observations that parkinsonian patients have marked deficits in striatal dopamine. The first clinical tests of L-dopa were not very successful, and it took nearly 10 years before it was established as the treatment of choice for Parkinson's disease. This success was an important stimulus for research into other potential neurotransmitter precursors.

Two points in this story are of particular interest to the present discussion. First, in the treatment of Parkinson's disease, L-dopa was often found to be more efficient in the morning. This was generally thought to be linked to circadian changes in dopamine function. In 1975, Mena and Cotzias [69] suggested an alternative explanation. They noted that even a single high-protein meal could exacerbate Parkinsonian symptoms and showed that L-dopa is more active and side effects are fewer if patients are maintained on a low but adequate protein diet. These effects are almost certainly due to competition between L-dopa and other LNAAs for transport across the blood–brain barrier [70]. Second, L-dopa often produces behavioural side effects ranging from a positive 'awakening' effect to psychosis. The increased alertness, vigour and well-being experienced by some patients could well be linked to concomitant increases in noradrenaline synthesis, while the serious psychotic symptoms seen in 10–15% of patients treated with L-dopa may well be triggered by excess dopamine in the limbic system.

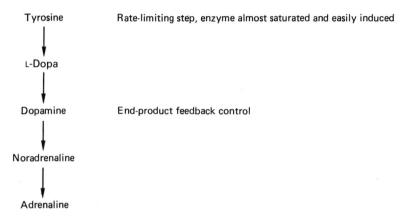

Figure 8.9 Steps in synthesis of dopamine, noradrenaline and adrenaline from the precursor amino acid, tyrosine. The rate-limiting step is the hydroxylation of tyrosine to dopa. Since the enzyme appears to be almost saturated, is easily induced and the rate of reaction is subject to end-product feedback control, it is not surprising that in most circumstances small changes in tyrosine availability seem to have no effect on catecholamine synthesis and release

Tyrosine as a precursor of catecholamines

The catecholamines, dopamine and noradrenaline, are synthesized from the amino acid, tyrosine (Figure 8.9). The rate-limiting step in this synthesis is the hydroxylation of tyrosine to L-dopa. The rate of this reaction is regulated by a variety of factors including: end-product inhibition, firing rate of the neurone, induction and activation of the enzyme, presynaptic receptors, cofactor and (under some situations) substrate availability [71]. It appears that, *in vivo*, with physiological levels of tyrosine, the enzyme is almost completely saturated [71], so that even very large increases in tyrosine availability are unlikely to increase catecholamine synthesis by more than 10–20%. This suggests that decreasing brain tyrosine might be an interesting experimental strategy in searching to establish if manipulation of precursor availability has any influence on dopamine and noradrenaline synthesis.

As Sved [71] has shown, increasing brain tyrosine in experimental animals consistently produces no change in the rate of catecholamine synthesis (of nine published studies using large doses of tyrosine, seven found no effect and two reported increases of 13 and 15%). Very recently, Ackworth *et al.* [30] observed that sustained increases in brain tyrosine produced by giving 200 mg of tyrosine per kg, i.p., produced an early transient rise in striatal and nucleus acumbens dopamine release, suggesting that sudden large increases in precursor availability may influence catecholamine synthesis but that end-product inhibition rapidly re-establishes control.

If animals are given a pretreatment that markedly increases catecholamine release (e.g. haloperidol, yohombine and perhaps stress) and are then injected with tyrosine, the rate of catecholamine synthesis can show an increase. The drug effects are robust but not all experimenters have been able to confirm an effect of stress [71]. The practical significance of these observations is difficult to assess because the doses of tyrosine needed are large (usually about 200 mg/kg) and the levels of stress are severe (e.g. unavoidable electric shocks for 1 h).

Effects of diet on brain tyrosine and catecholamines

With dietary manipulations the results seem fairly clear but interpretations are contradictory. Fernstrom and Faller [28], using overnight-starved rats, noted that, relative to fasted animals, 0% and 20% protein meals increased the tyrosine/LNAA ratio by about 60% and increased brain tyrosine by about 70%; a 40% protein diet at least doubled both the plasma tyrosine/LNAA ratio and brain tyrosine. Similarly, Gibson and Wurtman [72] observed that protein-free and 40% protein meals increased brain tyrosine by 50 and 130% respectively. They also noted that (in the presence of a decarboxylase inhibitor) these meals increased dopa levels by 75% and 62% respectively. Thus, in the absence of feedback inhibition, the protein-free meal led to a greater accumulation of dopa than did the high-protein meal. These results were at first interpreted to imply that dopamine synthesis was under precursor control and that perhaps a protein meal specifically increases catecholamine synthesis. However, as Sved and Fernstrom (unpublished observations reported in [71]) have shown, while protein-containing meals fed to rats starved overnight did indeed increase brain tyrosine levels and dopamine metabolites, rats given non-nutritive agar showed no change in brain tyrosine but levels of dopamine metabolites still increased, suggesting that eating *per se*, no matter what the meal composition, increases dopamine turnover (Figure 8.10), and that perhaps, by a mechanism yet to be defined, protein can potentiate this effect.

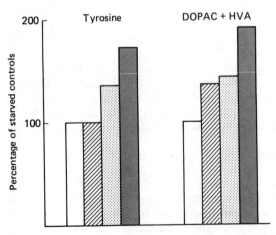

Figure 8.10 Dopamine metabolites in the striatum in rats (six per treatment) fasted overnight and then allowed access to different diets for 2 h. The non-nutritive diet did not change brain tyrosine but did increase dopamine metabolites, suggesting that the process of eating itself rather than precursor availability influenced brain dopamine metabolism. □, Starved; ▨, agar; ▨, carbohydrate; ▨, 40% protein; DOPAC, dihydroxyphenylacetic acid; HVA, homovanillic acid. (Drawn from data presented in ref. [71])

Furthermore, Johnson and Balachandran [73] have recently demonstrated that increasing protein intake tends to decrease sympathetic noradrenaline turnover, but these diet-induced changes are not mediated by tyrosine or altered by tyrosine supplementation. They also found no effect of the high-protein diet on brain tyrosine or noradrenaline turnover. In addition, tyrosine supplementation (which did increase brain tyrosine) was without effect on noradrenaline turnover.

In man, protein-rich diets, if anything, tend to lower plasma tyrosine/LNAA ratios [40], and so could not conceivably increase brain tyrosine levels or influence catecholamine synthesis, at least via this particular mechanism.

Returning to animal studies, in rats, chronic feeding of tyrosine-supplemented diets had no detectable effects on central catecholamine levels [74]. Feeding tyrosine for a few days increases brain tyrosine but does not seem to influence catecholamine turnover [73].

Functional effects of manipulating tyrosine availability

In animals, treatment with tyrosine can interact with some drug treatments in a manner suggesting that, with marked increases in catecholamine turnover, precursor availability can also influence catecholaminergic function. Again, results have been inconsistent. For example, L-valine (which might be expected to lower brain tyrosine levels) has been reported to attenuate behavioural and hypothermic responses to amphetamine [75] but others could not confirm the effect [76]. Tyrosine has also been reported to decrease blood pressure in spontaneously hypertensive rats, and to diminish reserpine-induced increases in plasma prolactin [71]. This could mean that tyrosine availability influences catecholamine turnover only if neurones are maximally activated.

Several research groups have examined the effects of tyrosine on mood and performance in normal human subjects. The results were negative [37,47]. Similarly, although preliminary tests of tyrosine in depressed patients were promising, larger scale studies were negative (A.J. Gelenberg, personal communication). Several review articles mention positive therapeutic effects of tyrosine in the early stages of Parkinson's disease, but the original article referred to [77] did not discuss this subject.

In summary, giving large doses of tyrosine might, in extreme (and still rather ill-defined) situations where catecholamine turnover is enormously increased, influence catecholamine synthesis. On the other hand, current experimental evidence gives no support at all to the idea that dietary manipulation of carbohydrate or protein levels can, via changes in precursor availability, influence catecholaminergic activity. It is therefore difficult to understand how reviewers and writers of popular books on control of mood by food [1,2] manage to conclude that high-protein meals will, by preferentially increasing (!) tyrosine availability, potentiate catecholaminergic function.

Conclusions

The discoveries that, in appropriate conditions, brain dopamine synthesis can be influenced by L-dopa administration and that brain 5-HT synthesis can be influenced by tryptophan, tryptophan/carbohydrate mixes or even by the carbohydrate in a meal led to a wealth of speculation, hypotheses and research on the potential functional and practical consequences. Some of the ideas led nowhere, but others, such as the use of L-dopa in the treatment of Parkinson's disease, are major scientific successes. A third group such as tryptophan to aid sleep (or even counter the effects of jeg lag) show some promise, while yet others remain to be explored. Unfortunately, the idea that the composition of meals will, via the mechanism outlined in Figure 8.1, influence circadian rhythms of brain 5-HT metabolism and behaviour seems to be one of those that did not lead very far.

References

1. Ehret, C.F. and Scanlon, L.W. *Overcoming Jet Lag*, Berkley, New York (1983)
2. Wurtman, J.J. *Managing your Mind and Mood through Food*, Rawson, New York (1986)
3. Spring, B.J., Maller, O., Wurtman, J.J., Digman, L. and Cozolino, L. Effects of protein and carbohydrate meals on mood and behaviour. *J. Psychiatr. Res.*, **17**, 155–167 (1983)
4. Wurtman, R.J. Nutrients affecting brain composition and behaviour. *Integr. Psychiatry*, **5**, 226–257 (1987)
5. Fernstrom, J.D. Role of precursor availability in the control of monoamine biosynthesis in the brain. *Physiol. Rev.*, **63**, 484–546 (1983)
6. Leathwood, P.D. Tryptophan availability and serotonin synthesis. *Proc. Nutr. Soc.*, **46**, 143–156 (1987)
7. Fernstrom, J.D. and Wurtman, R.J. Brain serotonin content: physiological regulation by plasma amino acids. *Science*, **178**, 414–416 (1972)
8. Blatter, F., Leathwood, P.D. and Ashley, D.V.M. Rats free to select protein and energy separately show decreased circadian rhythm of brain serotonin. *Annu. Rev. Chronopharmacol.*, **3**, 5–8 (1986)
9. Hillier, J.G. and Redfern, P.H. Twenty four hour rhythms in serum and brain indoleamine concentrations: Tryptophan-5-hydroxylase and monoamine oxidase activity in the rat. *Int. J. Chronobiol.*, **4**, 197–210 (1976)
10. Li, E.T.S. and Anderson, G.H. Self selected meal composition, circadian rhythms and meal responses in plasma and brain tryptophan and 5-hydroxytryptamine in rats. *J. Nutr.*, **112**, 2001–2010 (1982)
11. Ashley, D.V.M., Leathwood, P.D. and Moennoz, D. Carbohydrate meal increases brain 5-hydroxytryptamine in the adult rat only after prolonged fasting. In *Progress in Tryptophan and Serotonin Research* (eds H.G. Schlossberger, W. Kochen, B. Linzen and H. Steinhart), de Gruyter, Berlin, pp. 591–594 (1984)
12. Leathwood, P.D. and Ashley, D.V.M. Strategies of protein selection by weanling and adult rats. *Appetite*, **4**, 97–112 (1983)
13. Gillman, P.K., Bartlett, J.R., Bridges, P.K., Hunt, A., Patel, A.J., Kantermaneni, B.D. and Curzon, G. Indolic substances in plasma, cerebrospinal fluid, and frontal cortex of humans infused with saline or tryptophan. *J. Neurochem.*, **37**, 410–417 (1981)
14. Leathwood, P.D. and Fernstrom, J.D. Effects of oral tryptophan administration on serotonin and 5-hydroxyindoleacetic acid levels in monkey brain. *J. Neural Trans.* (in press) (1989)
15. Pardridge, W.M. Brain metabolism: a perspective from the blood–brain barrier. *Physiol. Rev.*, **63**, 1481–1535 (1983)
16. Fernstrom, J.D. Acute and chronic effects of protein and carbohydrate ingestion on brain tryptophan levels and serotonin synthesis. *Nutr. Rev.*, **44**, (suppl), 25–36 (1986)
17. Lookingland, K.J., Shannon, N.J. and Moore, K.E. Effects of tryptophan administration on synthesis, storage and metabolism of serotonin in the hypothalamus of normal and raphé stimulated rats. In *Amino Acid Availability and Brain Function in Health and Disease* (ed. G. Huether), Springer Verlag, Berlin, pp. 159–166 (1988)
18. Hutson, P.H., Sarna, G.S., Kantamaneni, B.D. and Curzon, G. Monitoring the effect of a tryptophan load on brain indole metabolism in freely moving rats by simultaneous cerebrospinal fluid sampling and brain dialysis. *J. Neurochem.*, **44**, 1266–1273 (1985)

19. Ericksson, T. and Carlsson, A. β-Adrenergic control of brain uptake of large neutral amino acids. *Life Sci.*, **42**, 1583–1589 (1983)
20. Leathwood, P.D. Neurotransmitter precursors and brain function. *Bibl. Nutr. Dieta.*, **38**, 54–71 (1986)
21. Arimanana, L., Ashley, D.V.M., Furniss, D. and Leathwood, P.D. Protein/carbohydrate selection in rats following administration of tryptophan, glucose, or a mixture of amino acids. In *Progress in Tryptophan and Serotonin Research* (eds H.G. Schlossberger, W. Kochen, B. Linzen and H. Steinhart), de Gruyter, Berlin, pp. 549–552 (1984)
22. Martin du Pan, R., Mauron, C., Glaeser, B. and Wurtman, R.J. Effects of various oral glucose doses on plasma neutral amino acid levels. *Metabolism*, **31**, 937–943 (1982)
23. Ashley, D.V.M., Barclay, D.V., Chauffard, F., Moennoz, D. and Leathwood, P.D. Plasma amino acid responses to evening meals of differing nutritional composition. *Amer. J. Clin. Nutr.*, **36**, 143–153 (1982)
24. Choi, T.B. and Partridge, W.M. Phenylalanine transport at the human blood–brain barrier. *J. Biol. Chem.*, **261**, 6536–6541 (1986)
25. Young, S.N. The clinical pharmacology of tryptophan. In *Nutrition and the Brain* (eds R.J. Wurtman and J.J. Wurtman), Raven, New York, Vol. 6, pp. 223–276 (1985)
26. Fernstrom, J.D. and Wurtman, R.J. Brain serotonin content: increase following ingestion of carbohydrate diet. *Science*, **174**, 1023–1025 (1971)
27. Wurtman, R.J. Ways that foods can affect the brain. *Nutr. Rev.*, **44**, (suppl), 2–6 (1986)
28. Fernstrom, J.D. and Faller, D.V. Neutral amino acids in the brain: Changes in response to food ingestion. *J. Neurochem.*, **30**, 1531–1538 (1978)
29. Fernstrom, J.D. Food-induced changes in brain serotonin synthesis: Is there a relationship to appetite for specific macronutrients? *Appetite*, **8**, 163–182 (1987)
30. Ackwoth, I.N., During, M.J. and Wurtman, R.J. Processes that couple amino acid availability to neurotransmitter synthesis and release. In *Amino Acid Availability and Brain Function in Health and Disease* (ed. G. Huether), Springer Verlag, Berlin, pp. 117–136 (1988)
31. Wurtman, R.J. and Wurtman, J.J. Nutritional control of central neurotransmitters. In *The Psychobiology of Anorexia Nervosa*. (eds K.M. Pirke and D. Ploog), Springer Verlag, Berlin, pp. 4–11 (1984)
32. Young, S.N. The clinical psychopharmacology of tryptophan. In *Nutrition and the Brain* (eds R.J. Wurtman and J.J. Wurtman), Raven, New York, Vol. 7, pp. 49–88 (1986)
33. Glaeser, B.S., Maher, T.J. and Wurtman, R.J. Changes in brain levels of acidic, basic, and neutral amino acids after consumption of single meals containing different proportions of protein. *J. Neurochem.*, **41**, 1016–1021 (1983)
34. Peters, J.C. and Harper, A.E. Protein and energy consumption, plasma amino acid ratios and brain neurotransmitter concentrations. *Physiol. Behav.*, **27**, 287–298 (1981)
35. Reeves, P.G. and O'Dell, B.L. Short term zinc deficiency in the rat and self selection of dietary protein. *J. Nutr.*, **111**, 375–383 (1981)
36. Leathwood, P.D. Dietary manipulation of serotonin and behaviour. In *Amino Acid Availability and Brain Function in Health and Disease* (ed. G. Huether), Springer Verlag, Berlin, pp. 309–324 (1988)
37. Leiberman, H.R., Spring, B.J. and Garfield, G.S. The behavioural effects of food constituents: strategies used in studies of amino acids, protein, carbohydrate and caffeine. *Nutr. Rev.*, **44** (suppl.), 61–70 (1986)
38. Ashley, D.V., Liardon, R. and Leathwood, P.D. Breakfast meal composition influences plasma tryptophan to large neutral amino acid ratios of healthy lean young men. *J. Neur. Trans.*, **63**, 271–283 (1985)
39. Schweiger, U., Warnoff, M., Pahl, J. and Pirke, K.M. Effects of carbohydrate and protein meals on large neutral amino acids, glucose and insulin plasma levels of anorectic patients. *Metabolism*, **35**, 938–943 (1986)
40. Fernstrom, J.D., Wurtman, R.J., Hammarstrom-Wiklund, B., Rand, W.M., Munro, H. and Davidson, C.S. Diurnal variations in plasma concentrations of tryptophan, tyrosine, and other large neutral amino acids: effect of dietary protein intake. *Amer. J. Clin. Nutr.*, **32**, 1912–1922 (1979)

41. Wolf, W.A. and Kuhn, D.M. Uptake and release of tryptophan and serotonin: an HPLC method to study flux of endogenous 5-hydroxyindoles through synaptosomes. *J. Neurochem.*, **46**, 61–67 (1986)
42. Lookingland, K.J., Shannon, N.J., Chapin, D.S. and Moore, K.E. Exogenous tryptophan increases synthesis, storage and intraneuronal metabolism of 5-hydroxytryptamine in the rat hypothalamus. *J. Neurochem.*, **47**, 205–212 (1986)
43. Trulson, M.E. Dietary tryptophan does not alter the function of brain serotonin neurons. *Life Sci.*, **37**, 1067–1072 (1985)
44. Koella, W.P. Serotonin and sleep. In *Sleep '84* (eds W.P. Koella, E. Rüther and H. Schulz), Fischer, Stuttgart, pp. 6–39 (1984)
45. Jouvet, M. Hypnogenic indoleamine-dependent factors and paradoxical sleep rebound. In *Sleep 1982 – 6th Eur. Congr. Sleep Res.* (ed. W.P. Koella), Karger, Basel, pp. 2–18 (1982)
46. Hartmann, E. and Greenwald, D. Tryptophan and human sleep: an analysis of 43 studies. In *Progress in Tryptophan and Serotonin Research* (eds H.G. Schlossberger, W. Kochen, B. Linzen and H. Steinhart), de Gruyter, Berlin, pp. 297–304 (1984)
47. Leathwood, P.D. and Pollet, P. Diet-induced mood changes in normal populations. *J. Psychiatr. Res.*, **17**, 147–154 (1983)
48. Leathwood, P.D. and Pollet, P. Tryptophan (500 mg) decreases subjectively perceived sleep latency and increases sleep depth in man. In *Progress in Tryptophan and Serotonin Research* (eds H.G. Schlossberger, W. Kochen, B. Linzen and H. Steinhart), de Gruyter, Berlin, pp. 311–314 (1984)
49. Keul, J., Huber, G., Lehman, M., Berg, A. and Jacob, E.-F. Einfluss von Dextrose auf Fahrleistung, Konzentrationsfähigkeit Kreislauf und Stoffwechsel im Kraftfahrzeug-Simulator (Doppelblind-Studie im cross-over design). *Akt. ErnährMed.*, **7**, 7–14 (1982)
50. Hill, A.J. and Blundell, J.E. Macronutrients and satiety: effects of a high protein or a high carbohydrate meal on subjective motivation to eat and food preferences. *Nutr. Behav.*, **3**, 133–144 (1986)
51. Paul, A.A. and Southgate, D.A.T. *The Composition of Foods*, Elsevier, Amsterdam (1978)
52. Perez-Cruet, J., Tagliamonte, A., Tagliamonte, P. and Gessa, G.L. Changes in brain serotonin metabolism associated with fasting and satiation in rats. *Life Sci.*, **11**, 31–39 (1972)
53. Hery, F., Rouer, E. and Glowinski, J. Daily variations in serotonin metabolism in the rat brain. *Brain Res.*, **43**, 445–465 (1972)
54. Sugden, D. Circadian change in rat pineal tryptophan content: lack of correlation with serum tryptophan. *J. Neurochem.*, **33**, 811–812 (1979)
55. Fernstrom, J.D., Madras, B.K., Munro, H.N. and Wurtman, R.J. Nutritional control of 5-hydroxytryptamine in the brain. In *Aromatic Amino Acids and the Brain – Ciba Foundation Symposium*, Elsevier, Amsterdam, pp. 153–165 (1974)
56. Morgan, W.W. and Yndo, C.A. Daily rhythms in tryptophan and serotonin content in mouse brain: The apparent independence of these parameters from daily changes in food intake and from plasma tryptophan content. *Life Sci.*, **12**, 395–408 (1973)
57. Dunn, A.J. Changes in plasma and brain tryptophan and brain serotonin and 5-hydroxyindoleacetic acid after footshock stress. *Life Sci.*, **42**, 1847–1853 (1988)
58. Cespuglio, R., Faradji, H., Gomez, M.E. and Jouvet, M. Single unit recordings in the nuclei Raphé dorsalis and magnus during the sleep waking cycle of semi-chronic prepared cats. *Neurosci. Lett.*, **24**, 133–138 (1981)
59. Trulson, M.E. and Jacobs, B.L. Raphé unit activity in freely moving cats: lack of diurnal variation. *Neurosci. Lett.*, **36**, 285–290 (1980)
60. Fernstrom, J.D., Fernstrom, M.H., Grubb, P.E. and Volk, E.A. Absence of chronic effects of dietary protein content on brain tryptophan concentration in rats. *J. Nutr.*, **115**, 1337–1344 (1985)
61. Feigin, R.D., Beisal, W.R. and Wannemacher, R.W. Rhythmicity of plasma amino acids and relation to dietary intake. *Amer. J. Clin. Nutr.*, **24**, 329–341 (1971)
62. Wurtman, R.J. Diurnal rhythms in mammalian protein metabolism. In *Mammalian Protein Metabolism* (ed. H. Munro), Academic Press, New York, Vol. 4, pp. 445–479 (1970)
63. De Castro, J.M. Macronutrient relationships with meal patterns and mood in the spontaneous feeding behaviour of humans. *Physiol. Behav.*, **39**, 561–569 (1987)

64. Johnson, D.J., Li, E.T.S., Coscina, D.V. and Anderson, G.H. Different diurnal rhythms of protein and non-protein energy intake by rats. *Physiol. Behav.*, **22**, 777–780 (1979)
65. Leathwood, P.D. and Arimanana, L. Circadian rhythms of food intake and protein selection in young and old rats. *Annu. Rev. Chronopharmacol.*, **1**, 255–258 (1984)
66. Graeber, R.C., Sing, H.C. and Cuthbert, B.N. The impact of transmeridian flight on deploying soldiers. In *Biological Rhythms, Sleep and Shiftwork* (eds L.C. Johnson, D.I. Tepas and W.P. Colquhoun), MTP Press, Lancaster, pp. 513–537 (1981)
67. Spinweber, C.L. *L-Tryptophan, Sleep and Performance*. Naval Health Research Center report no. 87-4, San Diego, California (1987)
68. Carlsson, A., Lindqvist, M. and Magnusson, T. 3,4-Dihydroxyphenylalanine and 5-hydroxytryptophan as reserpine antagonists. *Nature (London)*, **180**, 1200 (1958)
69. Mena, I. and Cotzias, G.C. Dietary protein content and the "on/off" phenomenon in Parkinson's disease. *New Engl. J. Med.*, **292**, 181–184 (1975)
70. Nutt, J.G., Woodward, W.R., Hammerstad, J.P., Carter, J.H. and Anderson, J.L. The "on-off" phenomenon in Parkinson's disease: relation to levodopa absorption and transport. *New Engl. J. Med.*, **310**, 483–488 (1984)
71. Sved, A.F. Precursor control of the function of monoaminergic neurons. In *Nutrition and the Brain* (eds R.J. Wurtman and J.J. Wurtman), Raven, New York, Vol. 6, pp. 223–276 (1983)
72. Gibson, C.J. and Wurtman, R.J. Physiological control of brain catechol synthesis by brain tyrosine concentration. *Biochem. Pharmacol.*, **26**, 1137–1142 (1977)
73. Johnson, J. and Balachandrian, J. Effects of dietary protein, energy and tyrosine on central and peripheral norepinephrine turnover in mice. J. Nutr., **117**, 2046–2053 (1987)
74. Thurmond, J.B., Kramarcy, N.R., Lasley, S.M. and Brown, J.W. Dietary amino acid precursors: effect on central monoamines, aggression and locomotor activity in the mouse. *Pharmacol. Biochem. Behav.*, **12**, 525–532 (1980)
75. Chiel, H.J. and Wurtman, R.J. Suppression of amphetamine-induced hypothermia by the neutral amino acid valine. *Psychopharmacol. Commun.*, **2**, 207–217 (1976)
76. Fernando, J.C. and Curzon, G. Behavioural responses to drugs releasing 5-hydroxytryptamine and catecholamines: effects of treatments altering precursor concentrations in brain. *Neuropharmacology*, **20**, 115–122 (1981)
77. Growdon, J.H., Melamed, E., Logue, M., Hefti, F. and Wurtman, R.J. Effects of oral L-tyrosine administration on CSF tyrosine and homovanillic acid levels in patients with Parkinson's disease. *Life Sci.*, **30**, 827–832 (1982)
78. Eccleston, D., Ashcroft, G.W., Crawford, T.B.B. *et al*. Effect of tryptophan administration on 5-HIAA in cerebrospinal fluid in man. *J. Neurol. Neurosurg. Psychiatr.*, **33**, 269–272 (1970)

Chapter 9

The relationship between biological rhythms and the affective disorders

Stuart Checkley

Introduction

Periodicity was one of the clinical features that first led to the distinction between the manic depressive and other psychoses [1]. This chapter will review clinical studies of the periodicity of manic depressive illness. It will describe the principal chronobiological hypotheses proposed to explain this periodicity. The clinical tests of these hypotheses will form the main part of the chapter which will describe studies of circadian rhythms of depressed patients under entrained and under free-running conditions. It will be seen that periodicity is a feature of some affective disorders ('manic depressive psychosis', 'bipolar affective disorder' and 'endogenous depression') but not of others ('depressive neurosis'). It is therefore necessary to begin by defining these different subcategories of the affective disorders.

Definitions

The affective disorders are those psychiatric disorders in which the primary disturbance is of affect or emotion. They include states of depression, mania, hypomania and anxiety. Anxiety states will not be discussed further as biological rhythms have not as yet been implicated in their pathogenesis.

Operational criteria for defining depression and mania are given in Tables 9.1 and 9.2. These are the official definitions approved by the American Psychiatric Association in their publication (DSM III) [97]. Most of the studies that will be reviewed in this chapter use either DSM III criteria or else the very similar Research Diagnostic Criteria (RDC) [2] from which DSM III was derived.

Depression as defined in DSM III is a large and heterogeneous entity which may affect 10% of the female population and 5% of the male population. For the purposes of biological studies it is appropriate to select more severe cases of depression in which biological symptoms such as anorexia, insomnia, retardation and fatigue are prominent: a wider range of biological abnormalities are more likely to be found in these types of depression than in the milder cases [3]. The DSM III category of major depression with melancholia (Table 9.2) describes this entity. In the RDC an almost identical condition is called endogenous depression. This latter term will be used as it is shorter. The entity is defined (Table 9.2) purely in terms of symptoms, regardless of whether or not these symptoms have been caused by exogenous factors.

Table 9.1 DSM III criteria for mania

Diagnostic criteria for a manic episode

A. One or more distinct periods with a predominantly elevated, expansive or irritable mood. The elevated or irritable mood must be a prominent part of the illness and relatively persistent, although it may alternate or intermingle with depressive mood.

B. Duration of at least one week (or any duration if hospitalization is necessary), during which, for most of the time, at least three of the following symptoms have persisted (four if the mood is only irritable) and have been present to a significant degree:
   (1) increase in activity (either socially, at work, or sexually) or physical restlessness
   (2) more talkative than usual or pressure to keep talking
   (3) flight of ideas or subjective experience that thoughts are racing
   (4) inflated self-esteem (grandiosity, which may be delusional)
   (5) decreased need for sleep
   (6) distractibility, i.e. attention is too easily drawn to unimportant or irrelevant external stimuli
   (7) excessive involvement in activities that have a high potential for painful consequences which is not recognized, e.g. buying sprees, sexual indiscretions, foolish business investments, reckless driving.

C. Neither of the following dominates the clinical picture when an affective syndrome is absent (i.e. symptoms in criteria A and B above):
   (1) preoccupation with a mood-incongruent delusion or hallucination (see definition below)
   (2) bizarre behaviour.

D. Not superimposed on either schizophrenia, schizophreniform disorder or a paranoid disorder.

E. Not due to any organic mental disorder, such as substance intoxication.
   (Note: A hypomanic episode is a pathological disturbance similar to, but not as severe as, a manic episode.)

Fifth-digit code numbers and criteria for subclassification of manic episode

6- In Remission. This fifth-digit category should be used when in the past the individual met the full criteria for a manic episode but now is essentially free of manic symptoms or has some signs of the disorder but does not meet the full criteria. The differentiation of this diagnosis from no mental disorder requires consideration of the period of time since the last episode, the number of previous episodes, and the need for continued evaluation or prophylactic treatment.

4- With Psychotic Features. This fifth-digit category should be used when there apparently is gross impairment in reality testing, as when there are delusions or hallucinations or grossly bizarre behaviour. When possible, whether the psychotic features are mood-incongruent should be specified. (The non-ICD-9-CM fifth-digit 7 may be used instead to indicate that the psychotic features are mood-incongruent; otherwise, mood-congruence may be assumed.)

   Mood-congruent Psychotic Features: Delusions or hallucinations whose content is entirely consistent with the themes of inflated worth, power, knowledge, identity, or special relationship to a deity or famous person; flight of ideas without apparent awareness by the individual that the speech is not understandable.

   Mood-incongruent Psychotic Features: Either (a) or (b):
   (a) Delusions or hallucinations whose content does not involve themes of either inflated worth, power, knowledge, identity or special relationship to a deity or famous person. Included are such symptoms as persecutory delusions, thought insertion and delusions of being controlled, whose content has no apparent relationship to any of the themes noted above.
   (b) Any of the following catatonic symptoms: stupor, mutism, negativism, posturing.

2- Without Psychotic Features. Meets the criteria for manic episode, but no psychotic features are present.

0- Unspecified.

The distinction between unipolar and bipolar depression is important as periodic phenomena are more likely in bipolar than unipolar illnesses. A bipolar disorder is characterized by episodes of mania or hypomania as well as episodes of depression. A unipolar disorder is characterized by recurrent episodes which are always depressive.

The older terms manic depressive psychosis and depressive neurosis are excluded from DSM III and from the RDC but they are referred to in several of the papers

Table 9.2 DSM III criteria for major depression with and without melancholia

Diagnostic criteria for major depressive episode (From Diagnostic and Statistical Manual, Third Edition, 1980)
A. Dysphoric mood or loss of interest or pleasure in all or almost all usual activities and pastimes. The dysphoric mood is characterized by symptoms such as the following: depressed, sad, blue, hopeless, low, down in the dumps, irritable. The mood disturbance must be prominent and relatively persistent, but not necessarily the most dominant symptom, and does not include momentary shifts from one dysphoric mood to another dysphoric mood, e.g. anxiety to depression to anger, such as are seen in states of acute psychotic turmoil. (For children under 6, dysphoric mood may have to be inferred from a persistently sad facial expression.)
B. At least four of the following symptoms have each been present nearly every day for a period of at least 2 weeks (in children under 6, at least three of the first four):
　(1) poor appetite or significant weight loss (when not dieting) or increased appetite or significant weight gain (in children under 6, consider failure to make expected weight gains)
　(2) insomnia or hypersomnia
　(3) psychomotor agitation or retardation (but not merely subjective feelings of restlessness or being slowed down) (in children under 6, hypoactivity)
　(4) loss of interest or pleasure in usual activities, or decrease in sexual drive not limited to a period when delusional or hallucinating (in children under 6, signs of apathy)
　(5) loss of energy; fatigue
　(6) feelings of worthlessness, self-reproach, or excessive or inappropriate guilt (either may be delusional)
　(7) complaints or evidence of diminished ability to think or concentrate, such as slowed thinking, or indecisiveness not associated with marked loosening of associations or incoherence
　(8) recurrent thoughts of death, suicidal ideation, wishes to be dead, or suicide attempt.
C. Neither of the following dominate the clinical picture when an affective syndrome is absent (i.e. symptoms in criteria A and B above):
　(1) preoccupation with a mood-incongruent delusion or hallucination (see definition below)
　(2) bizarre behaviour.
Fifth-digit code numbers and criteria for subclassification of major depressive episode
(When psychotic features and melancholia are present the coding system requires that the clinician record the single most clinically significant characteristic.)
6- In Remission. This fifth-digit category should be used when in the past the individual met the full criteria for a major depressive episode but now is essentially free of depressive symptoms or has some signs of the disorder but does not meet the full criteria.
4- With Psychotic Features. This fifth-digit category should be used when there apparently is gross impairment in reality testing, as when there are delusions or hallucinations, or depressive stupor (the individual is mute and unresponsive). When possible, specify whether the psychotic features are mood-congruent or mood-incongruent. (The non-ICD-9-CM fifth-digit 7 may be used instead to indicate that the psychotic features are mood-incongruent; otherwise, mood-congruence may be assumed.)
　Mood-congruent Psychotic Features. Delusions or hallucinations whose content is entirely consistent with the themes of either personal inadequacy, guilt, disease, death, nihilism, or deserved punishment; depressive stupor (the individual is mute and unresponsive).
　Mood-incongruent Psychotic Features. Delusions of hallucinations whose content does not involve themes of either personal inadequacy, guilt, disease, death, nihilism, or deserved punishment. Included here are such symptoms as persecutory delusions, thought insertion, thought broadcasting, and delusions of control, whose content has no apparent relationship to any of the themes noted above.
3- With Melancholia. Loss of pleasure in all or almost all activities, lack of reactivity to usually pleasurable stimuli (does not feel much better, even temporarily, when something good happens), and at least three of the following:
　(a) distinct quality of depressed mood, i.e. the depressed mood is perceived as distinctly different from the kind of feeling experienced following the death of a loved one
　(b) the depression is regularly worse in the morning
　(c) early morning awakening (at least 2 hours before usual time of awakening)
　(d) marked psychomotor retardation or agitation
　(e) significant anorexia or weight loss
　(f) excessive or inappropriate guilt
2- Without Melancholia
0- Unspecified

that will be reviewed. Manic depressive psychosis as used in the older variations of the International Classification of Diseases (e.g. ICD - 9) includes illnesses that would meet DSM III criteria for bipolar disorder, mania, hypomania, and major depression, particularly when seen with melancholia. Depressive neurosis includes cases of major and minor depression in the absence of melancholia.

Clinical characteristics of affective disorders that suggest a disturbance of biological rhythms

The following features which imply a relationship to biological rhythms are characteristic of the affective disorders. They are unusual in other psychiatric disorders unless these are related to the affective disorders. Thus schizoaffective illness [4,5] and the Klein–Levin Syndrome [6] meet the first of the following characteristics, but depression is seen in both conditions.

1. The episodic nature of the illness first led to the separation of the manic depressive psychoses from other psychoses [1]. Even though some other psychoses follow an episodic course, and even though a few affective illnesses follow a continuous rather than episodic course, most affective illnesses are episodic. Anybody who suffers one episode of depression or mania is likely to experience another [7].
2. Among patients with frequent episodic illnesses are to be found some in whom the illness follows a regular periodic course. Periodicity is particularly characteristic of bipolar illnesses but even here it is the exception rather than the rule [8].
3. Extreme examples of periodicity are those illnesses with a period of 48 h. According to von Zerssen *et al.* [9] 80 such cases have been reported in the world literature. In these illnesses days are alternately spent in depression and either normality or hypomania. In one well-described case this 48-h period persisted in temporal isolation even though the period of the sleep/wake cycle shortened to 19.5 h; as the period of temperature and cortisol rhythms remained at 24 h it appeared that the manic depressive illness was entrained to the same oscillator that drove the rhythms of plasma cortisol and body temperature [10]. In a second case, 48-h periodicity of mood persisted during a much shorter period of temporal isolation when the sleep/wake cycle appeared to shorten [11]. In another case, a 48-h cycling illness assumed a 44-h periodicity when subjected to an artificial day of 22 h [12].
4. The term 'rapid cycler' refers to any patient with a bipolar disorder who has experienced at least four episodes of affective disorder each year. Among the characteristics of rapid cycling illnesses is the phenomenon of *mood switch*. The term is appropriate as within hours or even minutes mood changes completely from severe depression to mania or back again. When a rapid cycling illness follows a regular periodic course mood switches into mania occur at night [13] whereas if the illness follows a sporadic course mood switches can occur at all times of the day or night. (The author has observed a mood switch from hypomania to stuporose depression take place while a patient with a sporadic illness was playing tennis.) A switch into mania is often preceded by a night of partial or total insomnia [14].
5. Tricyclic antidepressants have been reported to initiate, and thyroxine has been

reported to terminate episodes of rapid cycling. However, such observations are infrequently made and so far none has been made under placebo-controlled conditions [15].

6. Some patients regularly become depressed at the same time of year. Such annual depressions can recur in spring, summer, autumn or winter. Seasonal rhythms in affective disorder may be under the influence of the length of daylight as are some seasonal rhythms of behaviour in the animal kingdom. Winter depression will be discussed in more detail later on, as will seasonal rhythms in the incidence of depression.

7. Seasonal rhythms have been reported for the presentation of depression to general practitioners, to community psychiatric services and to psychiatric hospitals. In all reports a spring peak is evident and in some an autumn peak is also significant. Similarly, most studies of suicide throughout the year report a spring peak and some find one in autumn also. Although climate influences many medical conditions and so results in seasonal rhythms for their presentation to general practitioners, among psychiatric disorders seasonal rhythms have only been reported for the affective disorders.

8. Circadian variation in the severity of depression. Similarly among functional psychiatric disorders it is only within the affective disorders that can be seen a circadian variation in the severity of a psychiatric disorder. Typically endogenous depression is worse in the morning and hypomania is often worst in the evening. In extreme cases a depressed patient can be mute and retarded in the morning but free of depression in the evening. In one chronobiological study that was conducted under entrained conditions, there was a highly significant correlation in patients between the timing of the rhythm of urinary free cortisol and the timing of the circadian variation of mood [16].

9. Early morning wakening is a common subjective complaint in patients with endogenous depression but is only one of many abnormalities in sleep architecture which will be discussed later.

A brief account will now be given of some of the hypotheses which have sought to explain the above observations in terms of what is known about the circadian system.

Circadian, circannual and photoperiodic hypotheses concerning the affective disorders

1. The internal desynchronization hypothesis [17] proposed that the periodicity of rapid cycling illness is generated by an interaction between two circadian pacemakers at least one of which is free-running. According to this hypothesis the temporary coincidence between the maxima of two independent rhythms generates a 'beat' phenomenon which triggers the episodes of illness. This hypothesis predicts that the difference between the periods of the two rhythms can be calculated from the period of the illness. If the patient becomes depressed every 6 days the faster rhythm must be gaining on the slower rhythm by 4 h every day. The hypothesis also predicts that internal desynchronization should be evident whenever a rapid cycler is put in temporal isolation and that a mood switch should occur whenever coincidence is seen between the sleep/wake cycle and the rhythms of cortisol concentration and temperature.

2. The phase advance hypothesis [18] implies a partial desynchronization between two oscillators but a resynchronization each night. As each day proceeds the temperature and cortisol rhythms are thought to gain on the sleep/wake cycle so that by the evening the advance of their phase is maximal. A resynchronization of the circadian system thought to occur at night prevents a complete internal desynchronization.

   This hypothesis assumes that the cortisol and temperature rhythms will show a phase advance in the evening. Depending on the time and mechanism of resynchronization the phase position in the morning should either be normal or advanced: a delay in the phase position of the temperature and cortisol rhythms in the morning is incompatible with the phase advance hypothesis. The phase advance hypothesis implies a shortened intrinsic period of the temperature and cortisol rhythms which should become evident under conditions of temporal isolation.

3. The phase delay hypothesis for the mechanism of action of antidepressant drugs [19] is an extension of the phase advance hypothesis. It has been found that many antidepressant treatments alter the circadian rhythms either of motor activity or of neuroreceptor number. In animals a phase delay of these rhythms has been reported following chronic treatment with antidepressant drugs. Consequently it has been proposed that antidepressant drugs may act primarily to reverse the phase advance of circadian rhythms that may be characteristic of depression.

Clinical features of the affective disorders that appear unrelated to biological rhythms

The following section is needed in order to obtain a balanced view of the importance of biological rhythms in the pathogenesis of depression.

1. The most common form of depression is the mild self-limiting state that is usually seen and treated in general practice and which affects at least 10% of the female population [20]. Social factors are the principal aetiological factors and it has been estimated that life events (e.g. bereavement or loss of a job) can result in depression occurring 10 years earlier than it would have done if it were simply an expression of the patient's constitutional predisposition [21]. In the case of bipolar illnesses genetic factors are the principal predisposing factor. On the basis of earlier twin studies it has been estimated that heredity may account for 70% of the likelihood of a proband becoming depressed if his or her (monozygous) co-twin has a bipolar illness [22]. More recent twin studies report a 100% concordance between the presence of bipolar illness in identical twins (A. Reveley personal communication, 1988). It is interesting to note that the patients in whom circadian and circannual rhythms may be most influenced are the same patients in whom genetic factors are the most important.

2. Many of the symptoms of depression (Table 9.2) would seem to defy chronobiological explanation, except insofar as a circadian variation of the severity of *all* symptoms is seen in some patients.

3. Negative and self-deprecatory thoughts are a characteristic feature of depression and account for suicidal behaviour being much commoner in depression than in other psychiatric conditions. No circadian mechanism has been proposed for

these cognitive abnormalities even though the timing of suicide is linked to the circadian variation in depressed mood.

Experimental tests of chronobiological hypotheses of the affective disorders

The first studies to be reviewed will be those in which circadian rhythms of plasma cortisol and body temperature are measured. Both the phase advance hypothesis [18] and the internal desynchronization hypothesis [17] predict a shortening of the period of these rhythms, under both entrained and free-running conditions.

Overt rhythms of plasma cortisol in depressed patients under entrained conditions

The control of cortisol secretion is relatively well understood and the following methodological issues must be addressed in any clinical study of cortisol rhythms.

1. Cortisol secretion is increased by 'stress', venepuncture and the ingestion of food. Consequently patients should be investigated after acclimatization to a research ward. Blood samples must be taken through indwelling cannulae and meals must be given at controlled times.
2. As age has been reported to advance the timing of the cortisol rhythm [23] patients and controls must be matched for age.
3. Since in animals tricyclic antidepressants and lithium have been reported to alter the period of circadian rhythms [19] patients should be studied in a drug-free state.
4. Since cortisol secretion is altered particularly in patients with endogenous depression [3], it is wise to restrict studies to patients with this form of depression.
5. In view of the episodic secretion of cortisol it is necessary to measure plasma cortisol at least every 30 min. Computer programs are available for the objective identification of episodes of cortisol secretion (see also Chapters 3 and 14).
6. The episodic nature of cortisol secretion makes the measurement of cortisol rhythms difficult. The fitting of plasma cortisol values to sine curves results in the loss of 50% of the variance of change in plasma cortisol over time [24] as episodic secretion is ignored and as the acrophase (or peak) is forced to be 12 h after the nadir (a trough): in fact the acrophase of the cortisol rhythm is 8 h after the nadir. To avoid this problem the nadir can be defined as the mean of the lowest three consecutive values [25] and the onset of cortisol secretion can be defined as the time when plasma cortisol first exceeds the nadir by two standard deviations of the value of the nadir.

To date only four studies have been reported which adequately control for issues (1)–(5) above. Their results can be summarized as follows:

1. The usual episodic release of ACTH and cortisol is found in endogenous depression. The number of secretory episodes is probably normal [26,27] although one group reported a reduced number [24]. All groups reported an increased duration and amplitude of the secretory episodes.
2. In a few individual patients no circadian rhythm of plasma cortisol was statistically significant [24,28]. However, in all four reported studies a significant

circadian rhythm was detected for the group of depressed patients studied [24,25,27,29], and in all four studies the absolute amplitude of the cortisol rhythm (the difference between acrophase and nadir) was the same as that of the controls.

3. All groups reported an increase in mean plasma cortisol and, although the differences between patients and controls were often small, they were present at all times of the day in all four studies.

4. Inspection of the curves of mean plasma cortisol against time revealed that in all studies there was at least a tendency for the nocturnal surge of cortisol secretion to start earlier and to stop later in the depressed patients. In view of the points made in (6) above, it is not surprising that the four studies diverge principally in the interpretation of whether the cortisol rhythm is phase advanced or not. As measured from absolute values the timing of the nadir was significantly advanced in three studies [24,27,29] but not in the fourth [25]. As tested by curve fitting a significant phase advance was noted by Pfohl [29] but not by Halbreich [24]. Linkowski [27] noted a significant advance of the timing of the acrophase but curiously this was only significant in his unipolar but not his bipolar patients. Rubin [25] decided that curve fitting would introduce an unacceptable distortion to his data.

Of the four groups only Linkowski's [27] reported data on the time of onset of sleep in relation to the onset of cortisol secretion. As his unipolar patients went to sleep an hour later than his controls the phase advance of the cortisol rhythm in those patients was enhanced when measured with respect to the sleep/wake cycle. Similar findings had earlier been reported by Jarrett et al. [30].

It can be seen that attention has been focused upon the onset of cortisol secretion which is earlier in some depressed patients. No attention has been given to the timing of the decline in cortisol secretion which is apparently later in depressed than in normal volunteers. There is no doubt that total secretion is increased in depression but whether there is a phase advance of the cortisol rhythm is hard to determine from studies conducted under entrained conditions. In all of the studies there is an apparent change in the shape of the cortisol rhythm which is 'splayed out' in depressed patients: it would be possible to use an analysis of variance with repeated measures to test whether or not such a change in shape were statistically significant.

Cortisol rhythms under free-running conditions

The technical problem of measuring the onset of cortisol secretion should be eased by studying cortisol rhythms under free-running conditions. Under these conditions both the phase advance and the internal desynchronization hypotheses predict that the period of the cortisol rhythm should be less than around 24 h. The principal limitations of these studies are the small number of patients who have so far been studied in temporal isolation and uncertainty as to whether all zeitgebers were successfully excluded.

The most informative single case study is of a 66-year-old man who, for 13 years, had suffered from a recurrent unipolar depressive illness with a regular period of 48 h [10]. He was studied in a drug-free state for 62 days on a research ward under entrained conditions and then for 15 days in a temporal isolation unit [31]. Patients with severe mental illness cannot be left alone for long periods of time but his nursing care was arranged so that six care assistants visited him for periods between 2 and 6 h at random times of the day and night. Urinary free cortisol was measured from urine voided at 3-hourly intervals under entrained conditions and at random periods under free-running conditions.

Under free-running conditions the rest/activity cycle, as measured by timing of lights on to lights off, was reduced to about 19.5 h. However, the rhythms for body temperature and urinary free cortisol persisted at about 24 h. Perhaps the most interesting finding was that the period of the affective illness remained at 48 h. This is probably the strongest evidence available to show that manic depressive illness can be entrained to truly endogenous circadian rhythms.

However, as mood affects cortisol secretion it is impossible to exclude a masking effect of mood on cortisol, and indeed power spectral analysis revealed a 48-h, as well as a 24-h, rhythm for cortisol. This interesting and carefully controlled study permits three conclusions.

1. The periodicity of this 48-h affective disorder persisted under apparently free-running conditions in temporal isolation.
2. The periodicity of this illness could not be explained by the internal desynchronization hypothesis [17] as this would have required coincidence of cortisol and sleep/wake cycles every 48 h.
3. The phase advance hypothesis [18] predicted that the period of the cortisol rhythms should be less than 24 h. Again this prediction was not confirmed although in the case of the cortisol rhythm a masking effect of the mood cycle could not be excluded.

In view of the interest of this case study, it is of the greatest importance that cortisol rhythms from other patients be studied under free-running conditions. At the time of writing, it cannot be accepted that there is any abnormality of the cortisol rhythm in depression beyond the well-established hypersecretion of cortisol throughout the 24 h.

Temperature rhythms in depressed patients studied under entrained conditions

As oral temperature is subject to many artefacts, this review will be restricted to the six studies that have monitored core body temperature using rectal probes. Four studies have compared the temperature rhythms of endogenous depressives with those of controls matched for age and sex [16,32,33,34] and two studies compared the temperature rhythms of depressed patients subdivided by REM latency [35,36].

In the most detailed of the studies a computerized averaging procedure was used [37] to obtain temperature curves from the raw data. In this study 16 drug-free patients with endogenous depression had significantly higher temperature minima than did 10 normal controls [16]. There was also a significant reduction in the amplitude of the temperature rhythm in the patients and a non-significant trend towards a phase advance of the temperature rhythm.

A more striking apparent phase advance of the temperature rhythm of 11 endogenous depressives as compared to five controls was reported by Wehr et al. [14]. This analysis, which was restricted to patients with only one temperature minimum, reported an apparently bimodal distribution of the timing of the temperature minimum: the depressed patients had early and late minima whereas the controls had late (04:00–07:00 h) minima. Although Wehr and Goodwin [14] fitted their data to a sine curve, Avery *et al.* [33] and Dietzel *et al.* [34] simply examined raw data. Avery found no evidence for a phase advance of the temperature minima of his nine patients as compared to 17 controls whereas Dietzel's data suggested a phase advance of the temperature curves of 10 patients as compared to 20 controls.

Comparisons between the temperature rhythms of depressed and recovered patients were reported by Avery·*et al.* [33] and by Lund *et al.* [38]. Four out of seven of Avery's patients had an earlier timing of the apparent temperature minimum in the depressed as compared to the recovered state while Lund could find no difference between the educed temperature curves of seven endogenous depressives who were later retested on clinical recovery.

Temperature rhythms have been compared between depressed patients with REM sleep within 20 min of sleep onset and depressed with a later onset of the first REM cycle. As the rhythms for REM and body temperature are coupled [39], it was argued that a phase advance of the temperature rhythm should be particularly evident in patients with sleep onset REMs. Contrary to this prediction no such difference could be found by two independent groups [35,36]. Both authors, like von Zerssen *et al.* [16] reported a reduced amplitude of the temperature rhythm in depression. However, this effect could be due to a masking effect of sleep on the temperature rhythm [31] since it was not evident during a night of sleep deprivation [35].

It is apparent that temperature rhythms are just as difficult to measure in depressed patients under entrained conditions as are cortisol rhythms. Mean plasma cortisol and mean body temperature are elevated in depression. Some depressed patients have no significant rhythm for plasma cortisol [24,28] and others have no significant rhythm for body temperature. Both cortisol [40] and temperature [31] rhythms are directly affected by sleep which itself is disturbed in depression. In an attempt to avoid these difficulties temperature rhythms have been monitored under free-running conditions in isolation from time cues.

Temperature rhythms in depressed patients studied in temporal isolation

The 48-h cycling patient studied by Dirlich *et al.* [10] has already been discussed. It will be recalled that a 24-h periodicity of the depressive illness persisted in temporal isolation even though the period of the sleep/wake cycle apparently shortened to 19.5 h. Body temperature, like urinary free cortisol, continued to have periodicities of 24 and 48 h in temporal isolation. As depression directly affects body temperature it is possible that the temperature rhythms had become entrained to the mood cycle. In any case the findings are opposed to the phase advance [18] and the internal desynchronization [17] hypotheses, both of which predict a shortened period of the temperature rhythm under free-running conditions.

Wehr *et al.* [41] have also reported circadian rhythms in four patients with affective illness studied in a temporal isolation unit. Although they were not able to exclude the possible influence of all external zeitgebers, in two patients free-running temperature and cortisol rhythms were obtained. The first of these patients remained depressed throughout the isolation experiment: the temperature rhythm had a period of 24.28–24.57 h and remained synchronized with the sleep/wake cycle. The second patient cycled from depression to hypomania throughout the isolation experiment with a period of roughly 6 days: the temperature rhythm of this patient was 24.84–25.07 h and this also remained synchronized with the sleep/wake cycle.

The synchronization between the temperature rhythm and sleep/wake cycle in this second patient is directly opposed to the hypothesis [17] that rapid cycling is due to internal desynchronization.

Internal desynchronization between the temperature rhythm and the sleep/wake cycle was noted in the fourth patient studied by Wehr *et al.* [41] but contrary to theory this patient's mood remained unaltered (and hypomanic) throughout the period of internal desynchronization in temporal isolation. Thus no evidence for the internal desynchronization hypothesis has been found from the study of three rapidly cycling patients studied in temporal isolation.

The phase advance hypothesis [18] has not fared any better. It predicted a shortened period of the temperature and cortisol rhythms, but these remained at 24 h in Dirlich's patient and at more than 24 h in the depressed patients studied by Wehr. A shortened period of the sleep/wake cycle was noted in Wehr's third patient but only when she was manic.

Sleep abnormalities

Before discussing the possibility that a disturbance in circadian mechanisms might explain sleep abnormalities in depression it is firstly necessary to summarize those abnormalities. It is convenient to discuss separately abnormalities in non-REM and REM sleep.

1. Although some depressed patients experience hypersomnia [42], most have a reduced total sleep time [43]. Typically sleep onset is delayed, it is interrupted unusually frequently and it ends earlier than usual [43].
2. The sleep of a depressed patient is lighter than normal with more time in stage 1 sleep and less time in stages 3 and 4 [44,45]. The threshold for waking in response to sensory stimulation is raised [46].
3. Among the many changes in REM sleep a reduced latency from sleep onset to the first episode of REM is the most consistent finding [47] and is seen in patients with increased as well as reduced total sleep time [44]. The distribution of REM cycles throughout the night is changed, with an increased proportion of the first third of the night being spent in REM sleep and a corresponding decrease in REM during the third third of the night. The first REM period is usually longer than normal and it has more eye movement each minute than is normal [45,48].

The hypothesis that the REM cycle is phase advanced in depression

There is good evidence for believing that there is a circadian rhythm for REM latency and other measures of propensity to REM sleep [39,49] and there is some evidence that this rhythm is coupled to the rhythm of body temperature [39,50]. All of the changes in REM sleep that have been reviewed (above) might therefore be due to a phase advance of such a rhythm for REM propensity [51].

The most strict test of this hypothesis would be to measure REM latency during brief naps taken at regular intervals throughout the 24 h. Such a study has not been described but REM latency has been measured in depressed patients woken at

02:30 h [52]. As REM latency may normally be shortest at between 04:00 and 08:00 h [53], had there been a phase advance of this rhythm, then REM latency at 02:30 h should be longer than at sleep onset. Unfortunately Schultz and Tetzlaff [52] did not present REM latency data under both conditions but they did show that some depressed patients still had very short REM latencies (of less than 20 min) even when woken at 02:30 h. Furthermore, patients with sleep-onset REMs at the beginning of the night were more likely to have sleep-onset REMs after returning to sleep after 02:30 h than were the patients without sleep-onset REMs.

The hypothesis of a phase advance of the rhythms for REM latency and body temperature would predict that those depressed patients with very short REM latencies should be the patients with particularly advanced temperature rhythms. Contrary to this prediction, neither van den Hoofdakker and Beersma [35] nor Schulz and Lund [36] could find differences between the temperature rhythms of depressed patients with and without very short REM latencies. These studies do not support the hypothesis that there is a phase advance of the rhythm of REM latency in depression. To date no study has been reported in which the circadian rhythm of REM latency has been studied under free-running conditions.

The hypothesis of a deficient accumulation of Borbely's hypothetical sleep factor S (process S)

Using power spectral analysis of the sleep EEG, Borbely [54] has shown an exponential decline of slow wave activity through successive sleep cycles. Following sleep deprivation there is an accumulation of slow wave activity which again declines exponentially with the onset of sleep; whereas slow wave sleep is principally determined by the length of wakefulness, REM sleep is much less affected by sleep deprivation but instead is strongly influenced by a circadian rhythm which is linked to that for body temperature and plasma cortisol. Borbely [54] has proposed that the regulation of sleep depends upon an interaction between process S (which generates slow wave sleep) and process C (the circadian variation of physiological variables such as REM).

Furthermore, Borbely and Wirz-Justice [55] have proposed that the sleep disturbance in depression is due to a deficient accumulation of process S. A deficiency of process S at sleep onset would explain prolonged sleep latency, increased waking throughout the night and an overall reduction in the time spent in slow wave sleep. Since there is thought to be a reciprocal interaction between slow wave sleep and REM sleep [54] a reduction in slow wave sleep at sleep onset could also explain the increased propensity of REM sleep during the first half of the night. Finally as sleep deprivation leads to the accumulation of slow wave sleep (process S) and as sleep deprivation has an antidepressant effect which is abolished by sleep [56], Borbely and Wirz-Justice have proposed that a deficiency of process S may be 'causally related to the disease process'. The phenomenon of diurnal variation of mood might also be explained by a maximum deficiency of process S on waking.

Borbely's model for understanding sleep itself requires further investigation, and its application to depression might seem premature but some encouraging findings have been reported. Borbely and Wirz-Justice's model predicts that as measured by spectral analysis the sleep EEG of depressed patients should have less slow wave activity than that of normal subjects at all times of the night. An exponential decline in slow wave activity should be evident both in patients and in controls but the depressed patients should always have less slow wave activity than the controls. Such data have been presented by Borbely et al. [57] and also by Kupfer et al. [58], although Mendelson et al. [59] could find no difference between eight depressed patients and eight controls for the amount of slow wave activity at any time of the night. The discrepancies between these studies may be due to the small samples studied by Borbely and Mendelson: clearly further studies are needed. The effect of sleep deprivation and day time naps should also be studied to test whether there is a constant relationship between reduced slow wave activity and depressed mood. A patient with diurnal variation of mood should feel worse after an early morning nap.

Effects of sleep deprivation

There is general agreement that many depressed patients experience a transient alleviation of depressive symptoms following a night of total sleep deprivation [60]. The effect is short lived and usually is abolished by a night's sleep [61–63] or even after a brief nap [56].

Although it might be thought that sleep deprivation might alter the phase position of circadian rhythms, no such effect has been found in experimental animals [64]. Nor was it possible to detect any effect of sleep deprivation upon the temperature rhythms of depressed patients other than the effect of removing the masking effect of sleep on temperature [35]. One plausible explanation for the mechanism of action of sleep deprivation would be an accumulation during wakefulness of process S [64] which regulates slow wave activity in the sleep EEG. It should be possible to test the prediction that the antidepressant effect of sleep deprivation is proportional to the accumulation of slow wave activity, but this has yet to be reported.

Effects of psychotropic drugs upon circadian rhythms

Effects of lithium

Lithium is used principally for the prevention of recurrent affective disorders [65,66]. It is also of some value in the acute treatment of hypomania [67], and in combination with tricyclic antidepressants it is effective in the treatment of severe depressive illnesses that have not responded to other treatments [68].

It is therefore of interest to note that lithium has been shown to lengthen the intrinsic period of free-running circadian rhythms in plants, insects, rodents and even in man [69]. Normal volunteers have been investigated in relatively time-free conditions in the Arctic winter: in four such subjects lithium treatment lengthened the intrinsic period of the circadian system and altered the coupling between the temperature rhythm and the sleep/wake cycle; in four other subjects no such change was seen. Lithium may advance the phase of the temperature rhythm in some manic depressives [70,71] but so far only oral temperature has been measured in these studies.

Lithium is only of therapeutic value in some patients and it would be of interest to know if there was a relationship between the effect of lithium on mood and the effect of lithium on circadian rhythms. A central problem in understanding the mechanism of action of lithium is its multiplicity of clinical effects (as outlined above) and an equal multiplicity of biological effects which might underlie any or none of the clinical effects. Whether any effect on lithium of circadian mechanisms is related to one of its therapeutic effects is at present unknown.

Effects of tricyclic antidepressants

Tricyclic antidepressants are the drugs of first choice in the treatment of depression [72]. The tricyclic antidepressant imipramine lengthens the period of the activity rhythm of free-running hamsters and promotes dissociation of activity components of the rest/activity cycle [73]. Imipramine also delays the phase of the 24-h rhythms of a range of neuroceptors [19]. However, the tricyclic antidepressant desipramine does not cause a similar delay in the phase of plasma cortisol and plasma melatonin rhythms in depressed patients and in normal subjects [74].

An earlier onset of melatonin secretion was seen in depressed and normal subjects treated with desipramine and also in normal subjects treated with the stereoselective inhibitor of noradreanline uptake, (+)-oxaprotiline [75]. However, this effect could be attributed to a direct effect of the drugs on the noradrenergic innervation of the pineal. No evidence was found for a delay in the phase of melatonin rhythms in a number of studies of established or putative antidepressants [74–76].

Effects of monoamine oxidase inhibitors

Although not as effective as tricyclic antidepressants [77], monoamine oxidase inhibitors (MAOIs) are used in the treatment of depression. The effect of the MAOI clorgyline on the rest/activity cycle of free-running hamsters was more marked than that of imipramine [69], but no clinical testing has yet been reported of the effects of MAOIs upon circadian rhythms in depression.

Effects of a benzodiazepine

Even more marked phase shifts of the activity rhythms of free-running hamsters have been reported following treatment with the benzodiazepine, triazolam [78]. At present the sedative rather than the antidepressant properties of a drug may be more relevant to its ability to cause phase shifts in the activity rhythms of experimental animals. As far as humans are concerned, only lithium has so far been shown to modify the period of a circadian rhythm and whether this effect is of therapeutic relevance is at present unknown.

Annual rhythms in the incidence of affective disorders

Seasonal rhythms in the incidence of manic depressive illness were noted by Aretaeus, Hippocrates and Socrates as reviewed by Rosenthal *et al.* [79]. Modern studies have almost always shown a peak of presentations of depressive illness in spring: many studies have also shown a smaller autumnal peak [79]. Seasonal rhythms have been reported for the following indirect and direct measures of the incidence of affective disorder.

1. Depression is the major cause of suicide [80] and both spring and autumn peaks for suicide rates have been reported in many studies [81].
2. ECT, which is the most effective treatment for severe depression [77], is used more frequently in spring and autumn [82].
3. Hospital admissions with a diagnosis of depression are more frequent in spring and autumn than at other times of the year (see 14 studies reviewed by Rosenthal et al. [79]).
4. The incidence of depression can be measured more directly by using a register of all cases seen within the community services of a defined geographical area. Only one such case register study has been published [83]. In this study, spring and autumn peaks were evident for both males and females although only in the males did this rhythm reach statistical significance.

Possible causes of seasonal rhythms in the incidence of affective disorders

It will never be ethically or practically possible to study seasonal rhythms of mood in temporal isolation. Consequently we may never know whether the seasonal incidence of affective disorder depends upon a truly endogenous annual rhythm of mood.

We can, however, ask whether or not the seasonal incidence of depression is due to a seasonal rhythm of life events or other forms of social difficulty. Seasonal rhythms for example have been reported for rape and other violent crimes [84,85] and although the causes of such rhythms are not known, it would seem likely that they might reflect or even cause seasonal variations in social behaviour. If depression were affected by seasonal variations in social stress, then this effect should be seen for depressive neurosis more than for manic depressive psychosis, since life events are probably more important in precipitating depressive neurosis than manic depressive psychosis [86].

Contrary to this prediction, seasonal rhythms are evident for manic depressive psychosis much more than for depressive neurosis. In the case register study from South Verona, significant seasonal rhythms were found for manic depressive psychosis but not for depressive neurosis [83]. Similarly in studies of admissions to psychiatric hospitals seasonal rhythms have been detected for manic depressive psychosis but not for depressive neurosis [87]. For these reasons it is unlikely that the seasonal incidence of affective disorders is a consequence of seasonal variations in life events or other social difficulties.

Seasonal affective disorder (SAD)

The term seasonal affective disorder or winter depression refers to major depression (DSM III) that is exclusively restricted to the winter months. For inclusion within this category patients should be depressed for at least two successive winters without social precipitants for those depressions: similarly the patients should not be depressed in summer except in the presence of an exceptional social stress [88].

There is surprising agreement about the clinical features of patients who meet these criteria and who find their way to research centres usually as a result of media interest in this condition [88–91].

1. The patients have long histories of recurrent depression which starts usually between the ages of 20 and 30 and then continues throughout most successive winters.
2. At least half of the patients report that the winter depression is terminated by a self-limiting period of mild hypomania in the spring or early summer. This observation is of theoretical importance since it places the SAD entity within the bipolar rather than the unipolar subdivision of the affective disorders. It will be recalled that life events have less effect upon bipolar illnesses than upon depressive neurosis, whereas genetic factors are of paramount importance in bipolar affective disorders. Although no study has yet interviewed every first-degree relative of a group of patients with SAD, the patients themselves report relatively high rates of affective illness in their first-degree relatives and this finding also places SAD within the more biological subtypes of affective disorder.
3. Patients with winter depression describe most of the common depressive symptoms such as sadness, anxiety, lethargy and poor concentration. They also report the more atypical depressive symptoms of carbohydrate craving, increased eating and increased sleeping. Interestingly such symptoms are found in other bipolar patients.
4. The peak incidence of winter depression is in December whereas the month for peak incidence of all depression is March. Consequently winter depression is seasonally distinct from other forms of depression. Slater [92] noted that Kraeplin's original group of patients tended to relapse at the same time of year. Presumably spring depressions are more common than autumn depressions and presumably both are more common than winter and summer depressions. Ironically it is winter [88] and summer [33] depressions that have attracted attention. The more frequent spring and autumn cases have yet to be studied.
5. Some patients with winter depression report that their illness started on moving from a tropical to a temperate climate. Others report that a winter depression has been suppressed throughout the duration of a visit to a tropical country. These observations [88-91] suggest that winter depression may be a photoperiodic phenomenon.

The photoperiod is the interval between the first and last exposure to light each day. Since the duration of the photoperiod is the trigger to much seasonal behaviour in the animal kingdom [93], it was reasonable to propose that winter depression is a photoperiodic phenomenon, whose onset is triggered by the shortening of photoperiod in autumn, and whose spontaneous recovery waits for the lengthening of photoperiod in spring. In support of this hypothesis are the observations that winter depression is common in December and that a trip to brighter climes results in a temporary loss of symptoms [88]. The treatment of winter depression with artificial daylight was designed on this basis. Patients were exposed to artificial daylight, 2500 lux in intensity, from 07:00 to 10:00 h and from 20:00 to 23:00 h for 5 successive days to create a summer photoperiod in winter. The apparent success of this treatment lent support to the hypothesis that photoperiodic mechanisms underlay the mode of action of the treatment.

It is difficult to test the hypothesis that the onset of winter depression is triggered by the shortening of photoperiod but it is relatively easy to test the slightly different hypothesis that phototherapy for winter depression acts by creating a summer photoperiod in winter.

According to the latter hypothesis phototherapy given within the winter photoperiod should not be effective treatment. Contrary to this prediction seven patients reported a similar antidepressant response to light given within a winter photoperiod (from 09:00 to 12:00 h and from 14:00 to 17:00 h) to light given within a summer photoperiod (from 07:30 to 10:30 h and from 20:00 to 23:00 h) [76].

Another prediction can be made from the hypothesis that phototherapy acts by lengthening photoperiod: all treatments that present the same photoperiod should have the same antidepressant response regardless of the total amount of light given. To test this prediction we gave the following treatments for 5 days each with a 9-day washout in between:

1. Artificial daylight (2500 lux) from 07:00 to 10:00 h and from 20:00 to 23:00 h;
2. Red light (400 lux) for the same time as a placebo treatment;
3. Artificial daylight (2500 lux) from 07:00 to 08:00 h and from 22:00 to 23:00 h.

Although treatments (1) and (3) presented an identical photoperiod only treatment (1) was superior to the placebo. Mean percentage reduction in Hamilton Rating Scores for depression following the three treatments were 52.9%, 25.2% and 25.4% respectively [76].

Similarly phototherapy has been given in the middle of the day and found to be effective in the treatment of SAD even though overt melatonin rhythms were unchanged [33].

For these reasons it is unlikely that phototherapy acts through photoperiodic mechanisms. It is still possible that shortening of photoperiod might precipitate depression and this could be tested by the prophylactic administration of skeleton photoperiods as in treatment (3) above.

If phototherapy were to act through photoperiodic mechanisms then it might be expected to do so by influencing the secretion of melatonin. In the animal kingdom melatonin secretion mediates the effect of photoperiod on seasonally determined behaviour [93]. In the above-mentioned experiment hourly plasma samples for melatonin were taken before treatment and on the last day of each treatment. As expected, light treatment suppressed melatonin secretion and as expected the two

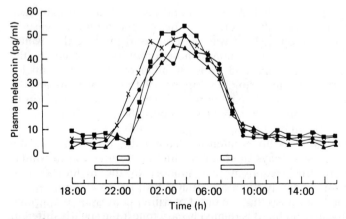

Figure 9.1 Mean plasma melatonin concentrations in seven patients with winter depression before treatment (×) and after treatments (1) (▲), (2) (■) and (3) (●) as described in the text. Unpublished data of Winton, Corn, Franey, Arendt and Checkley

treatments (1) and (3) that presented the same photoperiod had similar effects upon melatonin. The fact that only treatment (1) was superior to the placebo is also evidence that melatonin does not mediate the effect of phototherapy on winter depression (Figure 9.1).

The phase delay hypothesis of seasonal affective disorder

Lewy has proposed that 'the circadian rhythms of most patients with winter depression are abnormally phase delayed and that most of these patients should preferentially respond to morning light which would provide a corrective phase advance' [94]. In support of this hypothesis Lewy measured the onset of melatonin secretion in eight patients with SAD studied under dim light. The onset of melatonin secretion was about 90 min later in the patients than in the controls. After 1 week of phototherapy given in the morning, melatonin secretion started earlier. However, if the patients and normal controls were given phototherapy in the evening then the onset of melatonin secretion of the controls coincided with that of patients. Phototherapy given in the morning had a significant antidepressant effect whereas phototherapy in the evening did not. Phototherapy in the morning and evening had an intermediate effect both upon melatonin onset and upon mood.

Our own data (Figure 9.2) are somewhat different. We measured plasma concentrations every hour in 10 patients with winter depression and in 10 controls

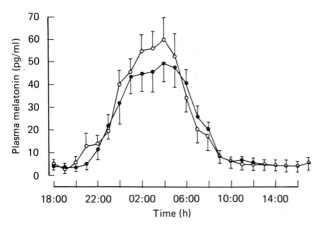

Figure 9.2 Mean melatonin concentrations (± S.E.M.) in 10 patients with winter depression (●) and in 10 volunteers (○) matched for age, sex and months of investigation (Checkley, Winton, Murphy, Abas, Franey and Arendt, unpublished data)

matched for age, sex and month of study. The curves of plasma melatonin against time were fitted to sine curves and the acrophase in the patients was only 10 min later than in the controls. This difference was not statistically significant and reflected a difference between the curves of only one pair of patients and controls.

Similarly plasma melatonin curves were plotted in 10 patients and 10 controls after 5 days of treatment with artificial daylight from 07:00 to 10:00 h and from 20:00 to 23:00 h. In neither case was a significant advance of the melatonin curves detected even though a 50% reduction in Hamilton Depression Rating Scores was obtained within the patient group. Thus not only have we found winter depressives without a significant delay in melatonin rhythms but we have successfully treated them without causing a significant phase advance. Our findings do not exclude the possibility that a small subgroup of patients may have a phase delay of melatonin rhythms.

The seasonality of affective disorders: conclusions

Recent epidemiological studies have strengthened the classical view that the affective disorders are sensitive to the season of year. They have shown that seasonality is a feature of manic depressive illness rather than of depressive neurosis. Seasonal affective disorder is more related to manic depressive illness than to depressive neurosis. Thus, in general, the seasonality of affective disorder would seem to be related to the genetically influenced manic depressive disorder rather than to the more environmentally determined depressive neurosis.

Beyond this statement the cause of the seasonality of affective disorder is unknown. Anecdotal accounts suggest that seasonal affective disorder may be a photoperiodic phenomenon although its treatment with phototherapy does not involve photoperiodic mechanisms.

Available experimental approaches for understanding the seasonality of depression are limited and only in animals can annual rhythms be studied under time-free conditions. The effects of seasonality upon animal models of depression have not been studied and little is known of the effects of phototherapy on brain function in animals. The photoperiodic and phase delay hypotheses for seasonal affective disorders have been questioned and new hypotheses are required for testing in patients with seasonal affective disorder.

At present it is not possible to say whether the seasonality of depression is due to passive response to season of year or whether it reflects the activity of an endogenous circannual oscillator whose rhythm is expressed in temperate but not in tropical climes. In either case manic depressive illness is more sensitive than other forms of mental illness to season of year.

Circadian rhythms in depression: concluding remarks

The previous sections can be summarized in the following ways:

1. Although sleep architecture is profoundly disrupted in depression, experimental data do not support the view that sleep disruption is due to a phase advance of the rhythm of REM latency. Some published data do support Borbely and Wirz-Justice's views that there may be a deficient accumulation of process S which regulates slow wave activity.

2. Mean plasma cortisol and mean body temperature are elevated in some patients with endogenous depression partly as a result of physiological arousal. For technical reasons it is difficult to measure the phase position of these rhythms under entrained conditions. In old age a clear phase advance of both rhythms is seen. Although depressed patients do not have a similar phase advance it cannot be excluded that a smaller phase advance exists. The matter can best be resolved by studying temperature and cortisol rhythms under free-running conditions. Although very few patients have been investigated in this way so

far, the rhythms that have been published support neither the phase advance hypothesis [18] nor the internal desynchronization hypothesis [17].
3. The amplitude of the cortisol rhythm is probably normal in depression and although the amplitude of the temperature rhythm is often reduced this may be due to a masking effect of interrupted sleep.
4. In animals, tricyclic antidepressants delay the timing of many circadian rhythms, but in man, cortisol and melatonin rhythms are not apparently phase delayed by tricyclic antidepressants.

Within the limitation of the clinical studies that have been reviewed, circadian mechanisms would appear to function well in depression. It seems unlikely that depression is primarily a disorder of the circadian system. On the contrary, clinical evidence suggests that normally functioning oscillators have a greater influence on affective disorder than on other psychiatric states.

1. The clearest evidence is provided by cases of 48-h rapidly cycling affective illness which retain a periodicity of 48 h under free-running conditions [10,11].
2. The phenomenon of circadian variation of depressed and manic mood could similarly be due to an entrainment of affective disorder to a circadian rhythm. This view, which requires testing in temporal isolation, finds support from the evidence of von Zerssen et al. [16]. In their depressed patients studied under entrained conditions, there was a significant between-patient correlation for the timing of the acrophases of the rhythms of mood and of urinary free cortisol excretion.
3. A similar explanation could apply to the regularity in the timing of the switch process in rapid cycling illnesses which follow a regularly periodic course. Switches from depression to hypomania take place at night regardless of whether the patient is awake or asleep [10,13,95,96]. The switch process would appear to be sensitive to an oscillator.
4. Manic depressive illness is apparently more sensitive to season of year than are other psychiatric disorders including depressive neurosis.

References

1. Kraeplin, E. Manic Depressive Insanity and Paranoia. E and S Livingstone, Edinburgh (1921)
2. Spitzer, R.L., Endicott, J. and Robins, E. Research Diagnostic Criteria (RDC) for a Selected Group of Functional Disorders. New York State Psychiatric Institute, New York (1977)
3. Checkley, S.A. Biological markers in depression. In: Recent Advances in Clinical Psychiatry Volume 5, (ed. K. Granville-Grossman), Churchill Livingstone, Edinburgh, pp. 201–224 (1985)
4. Kasanin, J. The acute schizoaffective psychosis. Am. J. Psychiatry, 90, 97–126 (1933)
5. Brockington, I.F. and Leff, J.P. Schizoaffective psychosis: definitions and incidence. Psychol. Med., 9, 91–99 (1979)
6. Critchley, M. Periodic hypersomnia and megaphagia in adolescent males. Brain, 85, 627–656 (1962)
7. Bebbington, P. The course and prognosis of affective psychoses. In: The Handbook of Psychiatry, 3, (eds J.K. Wing and L. Wing), Cambridge University Press, Cambridge, pp. 120–128 (1982)
8. Goodwin, F.K. and Jamison, K.R. The natural course of manic depressive illness. In: Neurobiology of Mood Disorders, (eds R.M. Post, J.C. Ballenger), Wilkins & Wilkins, Baltimore pp. 20–37 (1984)
9. Zerssen, D. von, Lund, R., Doerr, P., Fischler, M., Emrich, H.M. and Ploog, D. 48-hour cycles of depression and their biological concomitants with and without zeitgebers. In: Recent Advances in Neuropsychopharmacology (eds B. Saletu, P. Berner and L. Hollister), Pergamon Press, New York, pp. 233–245 (1979)

180   The relationship between biological rhythms and the affective disorders

10. Dirlich, G., Kammerloher, A., Schulz, H., Lund, R., Doerr, P. and von Zerssen, D. Temporal co-ordination of rest-activity cycle, body temperature, urinary free cortisol, and mood in a patient with 48-hour unipolar depressive cycles in clinical and time-cue-free environments. *Biol. Psychiatry*, **16**, 163–179 (1981)
11. Welsh, D.K., Nini-Murcia, G., Gander, P.H., Keenan, S. and Demont, W.C. Regular 48-hour cycling of sleep duration and mood in a 35-year-old woman's use of lithium in time isolation. *Biol. Psychiatry*, **21**, 527–537 (1986)
12. Jenner, F.A., Goodwin, J.C., Sheridan, M., Tauber, I.J. and Labban, M.C. The effect of an altered time regime on biological rhythms in a 48-hour periodic psychosis. *Br. J. Psychiatry*, **114**, 215–224 (1968)
13. Sitaram, N., Gillin, J.C. and Bunney, W.E. Circadian variation in the time of switch of a patient with 4-hour manic depressive cycles. *Biol. Psychiatry*, **13**, 567–574 (1978)
14. Wehr, T.A. and Goodwin, F.K. Biological rhythms in manic depressive illness. In: *Circadian Rhythms in Psychiatry* (eds T.A. Wehr and F.K. Goodwin), Boxwood Press, California, pp. 129–184 (1988)
15. Wehr, T.A. and Goodwin, F.K. Can antidepressants cause mania and worsen the course of affective illness? *Am. J. Psychiatry*, **144**, 1403–1411 (1987)
16. Zerssen, D. von, Barthelmes, H., Dirlich, G., Doerr, P., Emrich, H.M., von Lindern, L., Lund, R. and Pirke, K.M. Circadian rhythms in endogenous depression. *Psychiatry Res.*, **16**, 51–63 (1985)
17. Halberg, F. Physiological considerations underlying rhythmometry with special reference to emotional illness. In: *Cycles Biologiques et Psychiatrie*, (ed. J. Ajuriaguerra), Georg, Geneve & Masson, Paris (1968)
18. Papousek, M. Chronobiologische Aspekte der Zyclothymic. *Fortsch. Neurol. Psychiatr.*, **43**, 381–390 (1975)
19. Wirz-Justice, A. Circadian rhythms in mammalian neurotransmitter receptors. *Prog. Neurobiol.*, **29**, 219–259 (1987)
20. Bebbington, P., Hurry, J., Tennant, C., Sturt, E. and Wing, J.K. Epidemiology of mental disorders in Camberwell. *Psychol. Med.*, **11**, 561–570 (1981)
21. Brown, G., Harris, T.O. and Peto, J. Life events and depression. Part II: The nature of the causal link. *Psychol. Med.*, **3**, 159–176 (1973)
22. McGuffin, P. and Katz, R. Nature, nurture and affective disorder. In: *The Biology of Depression* (ed. J.F.W. Deakin), Gaskell, London, pp. 26–52 (1986)
23. Sherman, B., Wysham, C. and Pfohl, B. Age-related changes in the circadian rhythm of plasma cortisol in man. *J. Clin. Endocrinol. Metab.*, **61**, 439–443 (1985)
24. Halbreich, U., Asnis, G.M., Schindledecker, R., Zumoff, B. and Nathan, S. Cortisol secretion in endogenous depression II. Time related functions. *Arch. Gen. Psychiatry*, **42**, 909–914 (1985)
25. Rubin, R.T., Poland, R.E., Lesser, I.M., Winston, R.A. and Blodgett, A.L.N. Neuroendocrine aspects of primary endogenous depression. I Cortisol secretory dynamics in patients and matched controls. *Arch. Gen. Psychiatry*, **44**, 328–336 (1987)
26. Sherman, B.M. and Pfohl, B. Rhythm related changes in pituitary adrenal function in depression. *J. Affective Disord.*, **9**, 55–61 (1985)
27. Linkowski, P., Mendlewicz, J., Leclercq, R., Brasseur, M., Hubain, P., Golstein, J., Copinschi, G. and van Cauter, E. The 24-hour profile of adrenocorticotrophin and cortisol in major depressive illness. *J. Clin. Endocrinol. Metab.*, **61**, 429–437 (1985)
28. Sherman, B., Pfohl, B. and Winokur, A. Circadian analysis of plasma cortisol levels before and after dexamethasone administration in depressed patients. *Arch. Gen. Psychiatry*, **41**, 271–275 (1985)
29. Pfohl, B., Sherman, B., Schlechte, J. and Stone, R. Pituitary adrenal axis rhythm disturbances in psychiatric depression. *Arch. Gen. Psychiatry*, **42**, 897–903 (1985)
30. Jarrett, D.B., Coble, P.A. and Kupfer, D.J. Reduced cortisol latency in depressive illness. *Arch. Gen. Psychiatry*, **40**, 506–511 (1983)
31. Wever, R. The circadian systems of man: results of experiments under temporal isolation. Springer-Verlag, New York (1979)
32. Wehr, T.A., Sack, D.A. and Rosenthal, N.E. Seasonal affective disorder with summer depression and winter hypomania. *Am. J. Psychiatry*, **144**, 1602–1603 (1987)

33. Avery, D.H., Wildschiodtz, G. and Rafaelson, D.J. Nocturnal temperature in affective disorder. *J. Affective Disord.*, **4**, 61–71 (1982)

34. Dietzel, M., Saletu, B., Lesch, O.M., Sieghart, W. and Schjerve, M. Light treatment in depressive illness. Polysomnographic psychometric and neuroendocrinological findings. *Eur. Neurol. Suppl.*, **2**, 93–103 (1986)

35. Van den Hoofdakker, R.H. and Beersma, D.G.M. On the explanation of short REM latencies in depression. *Psychiatry Res.*, **16**, 155–163 (1985)

36. Schulz, H. and Lund, R. On the origin of early REM episodes in the sleep of depressed patients: a comparison of three hypotheses. *Psychiatry Res.*, **16**, 65–77 (1985)

37. Czeisler, C.A. Human circadian physiology: Internal organisation of temperature, sleep-wake and neuroendocrine rhythms monitored in an environment free of time cues. Doctoral dissertation, Stanford University (1978)

38. Lund, R., Kammerloher, A. and Dirlich, G. Body temperature in endogenously depressed patients during depression and remission. In: *Circadian Rhythms in Psychiatry* (eds T.A. Wehr and F.K. Goodwin), The Boxwood Press, California, pp. 77–88 (1983)

39. Czeisler, C.A., Weitzman, E.D., Moore-Ede, M.C., Zimmerman, J.C. and Knauer, R.S. Human sleep: Its duration and organisation depend on its circadian phase. *Science*, **210**, 1264–1267 (1980)

40. Weitzman, E.D., Czeisler, C.A. and Moore-Ede, M.C. Sleep-wake endocrine and temperature rhythms in man during temporal isolation. In: *Advances in Sleep Research*, Volume 7, SP Medical and Scientific Books, New York, pp. 75–93 (1979)

41. Wehr, T.A., Sack, D.A., Duncan, W.C., Mendelson, W.B. and Goodwin, F.K. Sleep and circadian rhythms in affective patients isolated from external time cues. *Psychiatry Res.*, **15**, 327–339 (1985)

42. Kupfer, D.J., Detre, T.P., Foster, F.G., Tucker, G.J. and Delgado, J. The application of Delgado's telemetric mobility recorder for human studies. *Behavioural Biology*, **7**, 585–590 (1972)

43. Gillin, J.C., Duncan, W., Pettigrew, K.D., Frankel, B.L. and Snyder, F. Successful separation of depressed, normal and insomniac subjects by EEG sleep data. *Arch. Gen. Psychiatry*, **36**, 85–90 (1979)

44. Kupfer, D.J., Himmelhock, J., Schwartzburg, M., Anderson, C., Byck, R. and Detre, J.P. Hypersomnia in manic-depressive disease. *Dis. Nerv. System*, **33**, 720–724 (1972)

45. Gillin, J.C., Duncan, W., Murphy, D.L., Post, R.M., Goodwin, F.K., Wyatt, R.J. and Bunney, W.E. Age related changes in sleep in depressed and normal subjects. *Psychiatry Res.*, **4**, 73–78 (1981)

46. Zung, W.W.K. Effect of antidepressant drugs on sleeping and dreaming III. On the depressed patient. *Biol. Psychiatry*, **1**, 283–287 (1969)

47. Kupfer, D.J. REM latency: a psychobiological marker for primary depressive illness. *Biol. Psychiatry*, **11**, 159–162 (1976)

48. Kupfer, D.J., Brondy, D., Coble, P.A. and Spiker, D.G. EEG sleep and affective psychosis. *J. Affective Disord.*, **2**, 17–25 (1980)

49. Hume, K.I. and Mills, J.N. Rhythms of REM and slow wave sleep in subjects living on abnormal time schedules. *Waking Sleeping*, **1**, 291–295 (1977)

50. Zulley, J., Wever, R. and Aschoff, J. The dependence of onset and duration of sleep on the circadian rhythms of rectal temperature. *Pflugers Arch.*, **391**, 314–318 (1981)

51. Wehr, T.A., Wirz-Justice, A., Goodwin, F.K., Duncan, W. and Gillin, J.C. Phase advance of the circadian sleep wake cycle as an antidepressant. *Science*, **206**, 710–713 (1979)

52. Schulz, H. and Tetzlaff, W. Distribution of REM latencies after sleep interruption in depressive patients and control subjects. *Biol. Psychiatry*, **17**, 1367–1376 (1982)

53. Hume, K.I. and Mills, J.N. Rhythms of REM and slow wave sleep in subjects living on abnormal time schedules. *Waking Sleeping*, **1**, 291–295 (1977)

54. Borbely, A.A. A two process model of sleep regulation. *Hum. Neurobiol.*, **1**, 195–204 (1982)

55. Borbely, A.A. and Wirz-Justice, A. Sleep, sleep deprivation and depression. *Hum. Neurobiol.*, **1**, 205–210 (1982)

56. Knowles, J.B., Southmayd, S.E., Delva, N., Maclean, A.W., Cairns, J. and Letemendia, F.J. Five variations of sleep deprivation in a depressed patient. *Br. J. Psychiatry*, **135**, 403–410 (1979)

57. Borbely, A.A., Tobler, IK., Loepte, M., Kupfer, D.J., Ulrich, R.F., Grochocinski, V., Doman,

J. and Matthews, G. All-night spectral analysis of the sleep EEG in untreated depressives and normal controls. *Psychiatry Res.*, **12**, 27–33 (1984)

58. Kupfer, D.J., Ulrich, R.F., Coble, P.A., Jarrett, D.B., Grochocinski, V.J., Doman, J., Matthews, G. and Borbely, A.A. Application of automated REM and slow-wave sleep analysis II. Testing the assumptions of the two-process model of sleep regulation in normal and depressed subjects. *Psychiatry Res.*, **13**, 335–340 (1984)

59. Mendelson, W.B., Sack, D.A., James, S.P., Martin, J.V., Wagner, R., Garnett, D., Mitton, J. and Wehr, T.A. Frequency analysis of the sleep EEG in depression. *Psychiatry Research*, **21**, 89–94 (1987)

60. Pflug, B. and Tolle, R. Disturbance of the 24-hour rhythm in endogenous depression and the treatment of endogenous depression by sleep deprivation. *Int. Pharmacopsychiatry*, **6**, 187–196 (1971)

61. Matussek, N., Ackenheil, M., Athen, D., Beckman, H., Benkert, D., Dittmer, T., Hippius, H., Loosen, P., Ruther, E. and Scheller, M. Catecholamine metabolism under sleep deprivation therapy of improved and not improved depressed patients. *Pharmacopsychiatry*, **7**, 108–114 (1974)

62. Van Den Burg, and Van Den Hoofdakker, R.H. Total sleep deprivation on endogenous depression. *Arch. Gen. Psychiatry*, **32**, 1121–1125 (1975)

63. Larsen, I.K., Lindberg, M.L. and Skougaard, B. Sleep deprivation as treatment for endogenous depression. *Acta. Psychiat. Scand.*, **54**, 167–173 (1976)

64. Borbely, A.A. Sleep regulation: circadian rhythm and homeostasis. In: *Sleep. Clinical and experimental aspects* (eds D. Ganten and D. Pfaff), Springer, Berlin, Heidelberg, New York, pp. 83–163 (1987)

65. Coppen, A., Noguera, R., Bailey, J., Burns, B.H., Swan, M.S., Hare, E.H., Gardner, R. and Maggs, R. Prophylactic lithium in affective disorders: controlled trial. *Lancet*, **ii**, 275–279 (1971)

66. Abou-Saleh, M.T. and Coppen, A. Who responds to prophylactic Lithium? *J. Affective Disord.*, **10**, 115–125 (1986)

67. Goodwin, F.K. and Zis, A.P.C. Lithium in the treatment of mania. *Arch. Gen. Psychiatry*, **36**, 840–844 (1979)

68. Heninger, G.R., Charney, D.S. and Sternberg, D.E. Lithium carbonate augmentation of antidepressant treatment – an effective prescription for treatment of refractory depression. *Arch. Gen. Psychiatry*, **40**, 1335–1342 (1983)

69. Wirz-Justice, A. Antidepressant drugs: effects on the circadian system. In: *Circadian Rhythms in Psychiatry* (eds T.A. Wehr and F.K. Goodwin), The Boxwood Press, California, pp. 235–264 (1983)

70. Tupin, R.J.P. Certain circadian rhythms in manic-depressives and their response to lithium. *Int. J. Pharmacopsychiatry*, **5**, 227–232 (1970)

71. Mellerup, E.T., Widding, A., Wildschiodtz, G. and Rafaelson, O.J. Lithium effect on temperature rhythm in psychiatric patients. *Acta Pharmacol. Toxicol.*, **42**, 125–129 (1978)

72. Paykel, E.S. and Hale, A.S. Recent advances in the treatment of depression. In: *The Biology of Depression* (ed. J.F.W. Deakin), Gaskell, London, pp. 153–173 (1986)

73. Wirz-Justice, A., Kafka, M.S., Naber, D., Campbell, I., Marangos, P.J., Tamarkin, L. and Wehr, T.A. Clorgyline delays the phase-position of circadian neurotransmitter receptor rhythms. *Brain Res.*, **241**, 115–112 (1982)

74. Thompson, C., Mezey, G., Corn, T., Franey, C., English, J., Arendt, J. and Checkley, S.A. The effect of desimipramine upon melatonin and cortisol secretion in depressed patients and normal subjects. *Br. J. Psych.*, **147**, 389–393 (1985)

75. Palazidou, E., Papadopolous, A., Sisten, A., Stahl, S. and Checkley, S.A. An alpha$_2$ antagonist, ORG 3770, enhances nocturnal melatonin secretion in man. *Psychopharmacology*, **97**, 115–117 (1989)

76. Checkley, S.A., Winton, F., Corn, T.H., Franey, C. and Arendt, J. Neuroendocrine studies of the mechanism of action of phototherapy. In: *Seasonal Affective Disorders* (eds C. Thompson and T. Silverstone), CNS Neuroscience, London (1988)

77. Medical Research Council Clinical trial of the treatment of depressive illness. *Br. Med. J.*, 881–886 (1965)

78. Turek, F.W. and Loosee-Olson, S. A benzodiazepine used in the treatment of insomnia phase-shifts the mammalian circadian clock. *Nature*, **321**, 167–168 (1986)

79. Rosenthal, N.E., Sack, D.A. and Wehr, T.A. Seasonal variation in affective disorders. In: *Circadian Rhythms in Psychiatry* (eds T.A. Wehr and F.K. Goodwin), The Boxwood Press, California, pp. 185–202 (1983)

80. Barraclough, B.M., Bunch, J., Nelson, B. and Sainsbury, P. A hundred cases of suicide: clinical aspects. *Br. J. Psychiatry*, **125**, 355 (1974)

81. Souetre, E., Salvati, E., Belugou, J.C., Douillet, P., Braccini, T. and Darcourt, G. Seasonality of suicides: environmental, sociological and biological covariations. *J. Affective Disord.*, **13**, 215–225 (1987)

82. Eastwood, M.R. and Peacocke, J. Seasonal patterns of suicide, depression and electroconvulsive therapy. *Br. J. Psychiatry*, **129**, 472–475 (1976)

83. Williams, P., Balestrieri, M. and Tansella, M. Seasonal variation in affective disorders: a case register study. *J. Affective Disord.*, **12**, 145–152 (1987)

84. Michael, R.P. and Zumpe, D. Sexual violence in the United States: the role of season. *Am. J. Psychiatry*, **140**, 883–886 (1983)

85. Michael, R.P. and Zumpe, D. An annual rhythm in the battering of women. *Am. J. Psychiatry*, **143**, 637–640 (1986)

86. Dunner, D.L., Patrick, V. and Fieve, R.R. Life events at the onset of bipolar affective illness. *Am. J. Psychiatry*, **136**, 508–522 (1979)

87. Hare, E.H. and Walter, S.D. Seasonal variation in admissions of psychiatric patients and its relation to seasonal variation in their birth. *J. Epidemiol. Community Health*, **32**, 47–52 (1978)

88. Rosenthal, N.E., Sack, D.A., Gillin, J.C., Lewy, A.J., Goodwin, F.K., Davenport, Y., Mueller, P.S., Newsome, D.A. and Wehr, T.A. Seasonal affective disorder: a description of the syndrome and preliminary findings with light therapy. *Arch. Gen. Psychiatry*, **41**, 72–78 (1984)

89. Wirz-Justice, A., Bucheli, C., Grav, P., Fisch, H.U. and Woggan, B. Light treatment of seasonal affective disorder in Switzerland. *Acta. Psychiat. Scand.*, **74**, 193–204 (1986)

90. Thompson, C. and Isaacs, G. Seasonal Affective Disorder 3. A British Sample: influence of referral source and diagnostic group in symptomatology. *J. Affective Disord.*, **14**, 1–12 (1988)

91. Winton, F. and Checkley, S.A. Clinical characteristics of patients with seasonal affective disorder. In: *Seasonal Affective Disorders* (eds C. Thompson and T. Silverstone) CNS Neuroscience, London (1988, in press)

92. Slater, E. Zur periodik des manisch-depressiven irreseins. *Z. Neurol. Psychiat.*, **162**, 794–801 (1938)

93. Arendt, J. Role of the pineal gland and melatonin in seasonal reproductive function in mammals. *Oxford Reviews of Reproductive Biology*, **8**, 266–320 (1986)

94. Lewy, A.J., Sack, R.L., Miller, E.S. and Hoban, T.M. Antidepressant and circadian phase-shifting effects of light. *Science*, **235**, 352–354 (1987)

95. Hanna, S.M., Jenner, F.A. and Souster, P.L. Electro-oculogram changes at the switch in a manic depressive patient. *Br. J. Psychiatry*, **149**, 229–232 (1986)

96. Trapp, G., Eckert, E.D., Vestergaard, P., Southern, R.B. and Halberg, F. Psychobiological rhythmometry on manic-depressive twins. *Chronobiologia*, **6**, 387–396 (1979)

97. *Diagnostic and Statistical Manual of Mental Disorders*, Third Edition (DSM III) (1980). The American Psychiatric Association

Chapter 10

Melatonin and the pineal gland

J. Arendt

Introduction

In 1958, the American dermatologist Aaron Lerner [1] isolated from many thousands of beef pineal glands the most potent known amphibian skin-lightening factor. This compound was characterized as N-acetyl-5-methoxytryptamine. Lerner named it melatonin from its ability to cause pigment contraction of amphibian melanophores. It has often been said that this project would be very unlikely to attract funding in today's climate yet it has led to an explosion of research defining the function of the pineal gland, to a re-evaluation of human circadian biology, to new treatments for depression and rhythm disturbance, possibly for some hormone-dependent cancers and to improvements in the breeding of domestic animals. After years of disregard, the pineal has taken its place in mainstream biology and medicine. It is an organ of particular fascination in that it serves as an interface between the environment and the body. Its primary functions subserve the effects of light/dark cycles on physiology via the secretion of melatonin.

Any discussion of the possible physiological role of melatonin in man requires an introduction to the basic physiology and biochemistry of the pineal and its functions in animals.

Structure of the pineal

In lower vertebrates, the pineal has been referred to as the 'third eye'. It is an organ of direct photoreception [2]. In birds and reptiles it appears to have a mixed photoreceptor and secretory function. In mammals the gland is entirely secretory in nature. Typically it consists of pinealocytes which are effectively modified photoreceptor cells, and glial cells.

The pineals of different mammals all originate from the posterodorsal region of the diencephalic roof, but are heterogeneous in shape, size and position. In man it occupies the depression between the superior colliculi of the mesencephalon. Relative to total body weight the pineal is small (50–150 mg in man; 1 mg in the rat), but its blood flow is second only to the kidney. There is some evidence in animals for increasing pineal size relative to body weight with distance from the equator, an interesting observation as the gland's primary function is concerned with changing day length. In humans, the pineal exhibits calcification relatively early in life, but this does not appear to have functional significance as far as melatonin production is concerned (see for example, ref. [4] for a review of this phenomenon). Vollrath [3] has published an extensive review of pineal gross and microscopic anatomy.

In mammals the pineal is innervated by sympathetic input from the superior cervical ganglion [5]. Parasympathetic input has been identified in some species and, in addition, there are fibres from the posterior and habenular commissures [3]. A pineal nerve with both efferent and afferent fibres has been found in fetal mammals but not adults [3]. The sympathetic innervation of the pineal is essential for its function in relation to light/dark cycles in mammals. The significance of other neural inputs has yet to be determined.

Although melatonin is referred to as the hormone of the pineal, there is no doubt that the gland produces many other active principles, both indolic and peptidergic. So far, however, evidence for the physiological importance of non-melatonin pineal products has been slow to accumulate.

Synthesis and metabolism of melatonin

Melatonin is synthesized from tryptophan within the pineal (Figure 10.1) via hydroxylation and decarboxylation to serotonin (5-hydroxytryptamine) [6]. Subsequent N-acetylation of serotonin by serotonin N-acetyltransferase (SNAT) appears in most cases to be the rate-limiting step in melatonin synthesis [7]. The activity of this enzyme is increased 30–70-fold during the dark phase of the day leading to melatonin production almost exclusively at night in normal conditions. The final enzyme in this pathway, hydroxyindole O-methyltransferase (HIOMT), is usually higher at night but to a lesser extent [7]. This light/dark variation in melatonin synthesis is the essential feature of the role of the pineal in physiology.

The pineal is not the only site of melatonin synthesis. Rhythmic production also occurs in the retina [8,9] although a function for retinal melatonin has yet to be defined. Pinealectomy in mammals leads to undetectable plasma levels of melatonin (see Arendt [10] for a review) although this is not true of some birds and lower vertebrates. Hence the function of retinal melatonin in mammals is probably local. Other reported sites of synthesis include the Harderian gland [8] and the gut [11] although, once again, their contribution to plasma levels must be small in mammals. Melatonin appears to be secreted from the pineal primarily into the circulation rather than the cerebrospinal fluid [12]. It is quite clear that events affecting melatonin synthesis are rapidly reflected (minutes) in the plasma [13]. At present little is known of the mode of melatonin secretion. Certainly there does not appear to be a large storage pool in the pineal available for release.

The primary metabolic routes followed by melatonin vary from species to species. In humans and rodents 6-hydroxylation in the liver is followed by sulphate and glucuronide conjugation, with 6-sulphatoxymelatonin (aMT6s) being the major urinary metabolite [14,15], providing a faithful reflection of melatonin production [16]. A very close correlation is found between plasma melatonin levels and both plasma and urinary aMT6s in humans (Figure 10.2). Measurement of urinary aMT6s provides a simple non-invasive method for assessing melatonin rhythms in man.

186

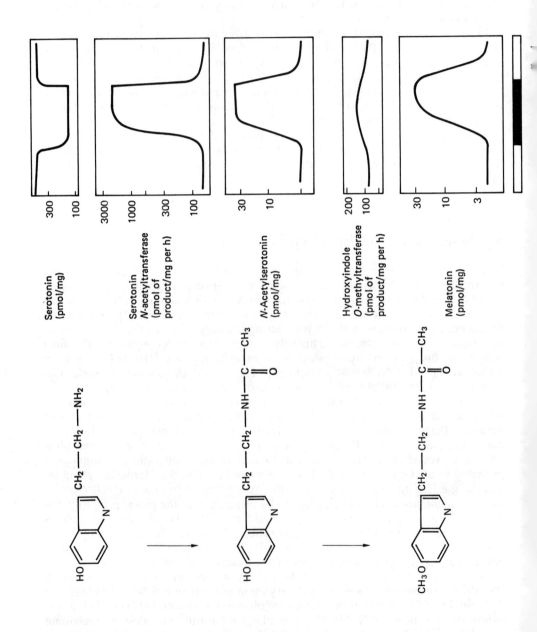

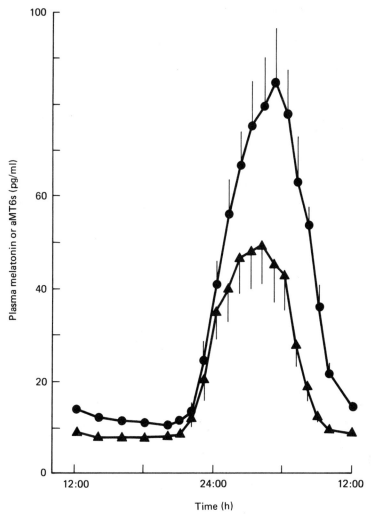

Figure 10.2 Profiles (24 h) of plasma aMT6s (●) and melatonin (▲) measured by direct radioimmunoassay in 22 normal subjects (16 men, 6 women). Results are given ± s.e.m. aMT6s is the major metabolite of melatonin in humans. Both plasma and urine levels closely reflect the plasma levels of melatonin itself. (Reproduced from ref. [85] with permission)

Control of melatonin synthesis

Melatonin synthesis is initiated by noradrenergic stimulation from postganglionic sympathetic fibres terminating on B_1 receptors (at least in rodents [17]). This is followed in a classic sequence by a rise in cAMP [6]. α_1 stimulation potentiates β_1 stimulation in the rat [17] and there is good evidence in humans for involvement of sympathetic innervation [18], β_1 receptors [19], α_1 receptors and cAMP [20] in stimulation of synthesis. Further reference to the adrenergic control of the human pineal is found in the section on psychiatric studies.

Noradrenaline and β-receptors are coupled rhythmically in melatonin production. β-Receptor numbers rise during the second half of the light phase: noradrenergic stimulation is initiated in the dark phase and is followed by a decrease (down-regulation) of β-receptors in the course of the night [21]. It is possible that α_2 presynaptic receptors are involved in human melatonin synthesis [22] but the results are not consistent [23].

The rhythm of melatonin production is strongly endogenous, i.e. it persists in the absence of a light/dark cycle and runs slightly out of phase with 24 h [24]. The rhythm, like many other circadian rhythms, is generated in the suprachiasmatic nucleus (SCN) of the hypothalamus (at least in rats and primates [17]). It is entrained (synchronized) to 24 h by the light/dark cycle acting, in mammals, via the retina and the retinohypothalamic projection to the SCN and subsequently the paraventricular nucleus (PVN) [17]. Light of suitable intensity and spectral composition is able to suppress melatonin production at night [25,26]. Hence light both entrains and suppresses melatonin.

As a result of these various phenomena controlling melatonin production it can readily be appreciated that the hormone serves as a circadian rhythm marker, an

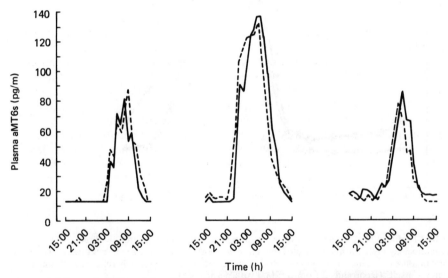

Time (h)

Figure 10.3 Reproducibility of the aMT6s rhythm in human plasma. Three male subjects were sampled at hourly intervals for 24 h, on two occasions, autumn and winter, in Antarctica. Night-time samples (23:00–08:00 h) were taken in dim red light. The solid line represents the first sampling and the dashed line the second sampling for each subject. These individual profiles are taken from the mean autumn and winter profiles referred to in ref. [37]

index of light sensitivity at night and reflects the functional status of the pineal noradrenergic synapse. The rhythm characteristics of melatonin and aMT6s are highly reproducible in the same individuals (Figure 10.3). Moreover, the duration of melatonin secretion reflects the length of the night in animals [10,27]; it can be considered to be a 'darkness' hormone. In order to appreciate the possible functions of the pineal in humans it is necessary to refer to basic studies in animals.

Role of the pineal in seasonal cycles: photoperiodism

Seasonal cycles in many species are controlled by the annually recurring changes in day length in non-equatorial regions. This phenomenon is known as photo-periodicity. The most obvious example is to be found in reproductive cycles whereby the birth of young is timed to occur at an appropriate time of year: many other functions such as changes in coat colour, coat growth and behaviour also show seasonal variations that are day length dependent.

Changes in day length act in such a way as to control the timing of these events. It is now quite clear that in a large number of species the pineal plays an essential role in the transmission of information about day length to body physiology [27,28]. Pinealectomy in, for example, sheep, hamsters and mink, *inter alia*, destroys the ability to perceive changes in day length (or photoperiod). In long-lived species there appear to be endogenous annual rhythms, which, in the absence of the pineal, persist but run out of phase with the precisely annual period (see, for example, ref. [29]). In consequence the effects of pinealectomy have required carefully designed long-term experiments to become manifest.

Humans are not considered to be a photoperiodic species. We exercise, particularly in urban situations, considerable control over our environment in terms of day length and temperature in particular. In Arctic regions, where day length effects should be greatest, seasonal variations in conception rate are found. One large study reported that conception took place throughout the year but with peaks in December during the Arctic night and April on the return of the sun [30]. In Northern Europe two peaks are also seen, a major peak in May–June and a minor peak in December [30]. Although it would seem reasonable to speculate that such variations are day length dependent, in fact in the United States the pattern is reversed [30]. It would appear that there are major cultural and economic influences on our cycles, unrelated (apparently) to the environment.

There are also seasonal influences on the onset of menarche [30] with a maximum number of first menstruations in summer. Any causal relationship to photoperiod is a matter for speculation. Many other seasonal variations both physiological and pathological exist in humans and it will be of interest to consider their possible relationship to day length and other seasonal synchronizers.

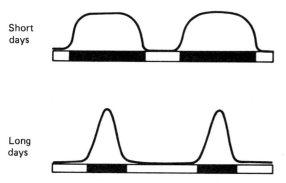

Figure 10.4 Diagrammatic representation of the secretion profiles of melatonin in different day lengths, in, for example, sheep. The duration of secretion appears to encode information about day length for the timing of day length-dependent functions (e.g. seasonal variations of reproductive function, coat changes, behaviour)

Day length change is perceived via the secretion of melatonin. In virtually all species studied, with the possible exceptions of humans and pigs, the length of dark-phase melatonin secretion is positively correlated to the length of the night (Figure 10.4) [27,28]. It is possible to administer melatonin in a variety of ways such as to mimic the long-duration secretion of a winter night or the short-duration secretion of summer. In these circumstances the physiological response is precisely that which would be given to an equivalent artificial night. For example, daily feeding of melatonin to intact ewes in the late afternoon from mid-June will, like artificial winter photoperiod, induce early onset of oestrus cycles. The oestrus advance induced is usually of the order of 6–8 weeks, leading to earlier lambing [27,31]. A constant-release implant, whether subcutaneous, intravaginal or intraruminal, has an identical short-day effect, i.e. oestrus advance [27,31]. This technique, which has considerable advantages over daily feeding, is about to be exploited commercially, to take advantage of the high price of early lamb, following successful field trials. An extra bonus is an increase in the number of lambs born per ewe, probably by advancing the seasonal peak in ovulation rate [31].

A long-day effect is difficult to achieve in intact animals as, at present, there is no well-characterized specific inhibitor of melatonin secretion. Such a technique would have considerable commercial interest in, for example, the breeding of racehorses.

Photoperiod-dependent variations in coat growth in a number of species may also be induced by manipulating melatonin levels [32]. Evidently commercial applications are under way, for example in the induction of early winter coat growth in the mink [32]. Melatonin is able to replicate the effects of photoperiod on prolactin secretion and it appears that prolactin mediates photoperiod-dependent coat changes [33].

Melatonin appears to be the photoperiodic signal whether the species be a long-day or a short-day breeder. In the long-day breeding hamster, short-duration melatonin induces reproductive activity [34] whereas in the short-day breeding sheep long-duration melatonin is inductive [35]. Both effects are fully reversible by appropriate administration of the non-inductive melatonin signal or through natural refractoriness to a sufficiently long-term constant signal. There is currently much debate as to whether the duration of melatonin secretion is the critical parameter for induction of a photoperiodic response or whether melatonin must be present at a specific time of day, i.e. whether there is a daily window (or windows) of melatonin sensitivity.

At present the most comprehensive interpretation of the action of melatonin in long-lived species is that it acts as a seasonal zeitgeber (synchronizer) of an underlying endogenous annual rhythm.

If the photoperiodic effects of melatonin have relevance to humans, then we might expect that modification of the duration of melatonin secretion would affect reproductive function. There is little evidence for such an effect, to date. There is no doubt, however, that photoperiod-related changes occur in the melatonin secretion pattern in humans in the course of the year (Figure 10.5). In both Northern temperate zones and in Antarctica there is a phase advance of the rhythm in summer compared to winter [36,37]. A steady change in the time of the rhythm in the course of the year, with a close correlation between peak time and day length, has been found [100]. A similar phase advance can be produced by treating subjects with an artificial bright light spring photoperiod during the Antarctic

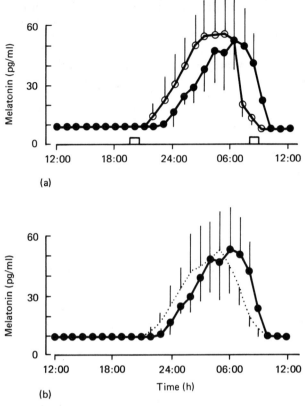

Figure 10.5 Human plasma melatonin response to bright (>2500 lux) light treatment for 2 h daily during the Antarctic winter. Two sessions of 1 h light were given daily for 6 weeks at the times shown by open blocks. The response to light treatment is comparable to the phase advance found in summer compared to winter. (a) 24 h mean plasma melatonin ($n = 5$), measured at the winter solstice (●) and after 6 weeks of light treatment following the winter solstice (○); (b) Measured at the winter solstice (●) as for (a) and at the summer solstice (····). Standard errors are shown. See text for details. A clear phase advance of ~2 h is seen ($P<0.0001$) following light treatment, similar to the phase-advance seen in summer. No significant effect of dim (<500 lux) light was found. (From ref. [37] with permission)

winter [37] (Figure 10.5). Presumably the seasonal phase advance is related to the higher intensity light perceived on waking in summer, compared to winter.

Puberty and development

There are undoubtedly photoperiodic influences on the timing of puberty in, for example, sheep [38], which can be attributed to the pineal in its role as photoneuroendocrine transducer. The pineal has also been attributed a role in pubertal development in humans and laboratory rats, neither of which are strongly photoperiodic. It is somewhat difficult to unravel the relevance of the pineal to puberty in these species. There is no doubt that administration of near-to-physiological doses of melatonin to both male and female juvenile rats in such a way as to create a long-duration (= long night) profile has delaying effects on the onset of puberty as judged by a number of different parameters [39]. Whether this represents a strict antigonadotropic action of melatonin or a photoperiodic signal remains unclear. No such experiments are possible in humans. Classically, pineal tumours are associated with both precocious and delayed puberty in man [40]. However, the effect of pineal tumours is complex and may not necessarily involve melatonin.

Much investigation has led to the conclusion that circulating melatonin levels decline in the course of human pubertal development, particularly at night [41]. Whilst this does suggest an inhibitory effect of melatonin it does not in any sense prove a cause–effect relationship and on the whole studies of delayed and precocious puberty have been disappointing. There are, moreover, insufficient data to draw conclusions from studies of melatonin in patients, either juvenile or adult, with pineal tumours. Although there are a number of reports in the literature showing little change in melatonin during human puberty, recent investigations using the major urinary metabolite aMT6s in children, and correcting for body weight, have served to confirm the consensus of a gradual decline in amplitude from infancy to adult [42]. A further decline is seen in old age [43].

It is worth noting at this point that blind girls may have slightly earlier menarche than sighted individuals [30]. Studies of the melatonin rhythm in blind adults suggest that the rhythm is not closely coupled to the 24-h day in some subjects [44]. The possible relationship of such uncoupling to gonadal development is worth exploring.

Menstrual and oestrus cycles

Many early reports have indicated that melatonin is inhibitory to ovulation (see [45] for a review). Findings of low melatonin prior to ovulation are somewhat controversial in humans [46] although this is clearly the case in rats [47]. Recent reports suggest possible phase shifts and/or a luteal phase increase in amplitude of the rhythm in normal women [48,49]. Following the clear definition of melatonin as a timing signal in seasonal cycles, it is time to rethink its possible role in ovulatory cycles. Evidence is accumulating that the pineal is involved in the timing of the lutropin surge [50,51]. Given that there appears to be a circadian basis for the lutropin surge in man [52,53], as well as in rodents, and the increasing interest in the possible circadian effects of melatonin, this approach would appear to be the most fruitful. Of particular interest in this respect are some anecdotal reports of the ability of light at night to modify the timing of menstrual cycles, and a seasonal difference in the timing of the lutropin surge in women [52]. Melatonin certainly has the potential to modify ovarian function and indeed testicular function, at many levels of the hypothalamic–pituitary–gonadal axis (see for example [27] for a review). Increased amplitude and duration of melatonin secretion are seen in hypothalamic amenorrhea, but any causal relationships remain to be established [53].

General endocrine relationships in humans

Although the pineal–reproductive axis is beginning to be understood, other observations related to the endocrine system remain difficult to interpret and are often inconsistent. A review by Vaughan [54] covers much of the literature. The most frequent observations concern cortisol secretion. For example, Wetterberg *et al.* [55] have proposed an inverse relationship between cortisol and melatonin levels in depressed patients and the administration of melatonin in both animals and humans may hasten the resynchronization of cortisol rhythms following an abrupt phase shift [56,57]. It is difficult to support a close physiological relationship between these two hormones, however, in the light of other observations. For example, the resynchronization of the melatonin rhythm following time-zone change is more rapid than that of cortisol [58].

Prolactin, a light- and melatonin-dependent hormone in animals, is undoubtedly influenced by exogenous melatonin in humans [59,60] but reports concerning melatonin levels in hyperprolactinaemia are inconsistent. Neither chronic nor acute milligram doses of melatonin were effective in influencing a large number of hormones (growth hormone, lutropin, follitropin, thyroxine, testosterone, cortisol) in two recent studies [59,60]. However, thyroid hormones are photoperiod-dependent in animals [61] and thus may be pineal-related in man. The acute modification of prolactin and growth hormone by sleep and the lack of such an effect on melatonin does not argue for a close relationship. If melatonin influences central rhythm-generating systems in man as it does in animals there is nevertheless considerable scope for modulatory effects on endocrine rhythms. Any hormone with a circadian rhythm may well show correlations with melatonin production, but this does not imply a causal relationship.

Problems in the interpretation of clinical observations concerning melatonin

It is the author's personal opinion that where the light/dark cycle has an important physiological role, as in seasonal and circadian rhythms (see the next section), the pineal gland is likely to be of physiological importance. The role of light in human endocrinology is poorly understood. Moreover the majority of clinical studies concerning melatonin have included little control over the light/dark environment. It is likely that many inconsistent reports in the literature are due firstly to methodological problems (see [62] and [63] for reviews and discussion) with melatonin assay and secondly to poor environmental control. In some animals the suppression of melatonin by different intensities of light is dependent on photoperiodic history [26]. In human populations many different lifestyles may be encountered, for example, outdoor versus office workers, habitual early risers and late risers, and these factors may contribute to the timing and amplitude of melatonin secretion. A great deal of clinical research merits a critical reassessment in view of these observations. It is, of course, very difficult to control the human environment, particularly when conducting long-term studies.

One curious observation is that a small percentage of apparently normal men have no detectable melatonin rhythm [10], implying that the pineal has no major functional importance in adult men. It is difficult, in the light of this phenomenon, to ascribe any major importance to findings of low melatonin in various clinical conditions.

Circadian rhythms and the pineal

General considerations

Light is the major synchronizer of circadian as well as seasonal (circannual) rhythms. Given the essential role of melatonin as the transducing signal for day length in photoperiodic species, one might assume that it has a similar role in the light/dark synchronization of circadian rhythms. Certainly in some birds and lower vertebrates the pineal has a major role in the organization of circadian rhythms, in some cases behaving like a master rhythm generator [64] and in others as a coupling agent [65]. One single cultured pinealocyte from the chicken pineal is capable of maintaining a rhythmic production of melatonin [66] *in vitro*, but such self-sustaining oscillations are not found in mammalian pineals.

There is sparse evidence at present to suggest a physiological role for the pineal in the mammalian circadian system. The central rhythm-generating system resides in the suprachiasmatic nucleus (SCN) and production of melatonin is a 'driven' rhythm from the SCN. Nevertheless, high-affinity melatonin receptors have been found in the SCN [67], pinealectomy in rats leads to a more rapid re-entrainment of some circadian rhythms following an abrupt phase shift [68], and daily timed administration of low pharmacological doses of melatonin to rats free-running (expressing their endogenous period of daily activity rhythms) in constant darkness will synchronize the free-running activity rhythm to a 24-h period (Figure 10.6) [69]. The period length of circadian rhythms free-running in the absence of time cues normally deviates slightly from 24 h. In man, most individuals assume a period length of about 25 h [70]; however, there are both species and individual variations. This ability to synchronize free-running rhythms is characteristic of the so-called zeitgebers, time cues that maintain circadian rhythms on a 24-h period.

The question as to whether melatonin has such zeitgeber properties in humans is important both from the point of view of academic interest and for therapeutic reasons. Disturbed circadian rhythms are reported in a large number of common conditions such as delayed (and advanced) sleep-phase insomnia, affective disease, old age, shift work, jet lag and in some blind subjects [44,71,72]. A simple means of resynchronizing rhythms with the external environment and with respect to each other would in principle have very considerable practical implications. Whilst there is some doubt as to the importance of abnormal rhythms in some clinical problems such as depression, there is no doubt that disturbed sleep can be a major problem in shift work [73] and jet lag [74]. Some preliminary reports suggest that melatonin is able to alleviate jet lag in humans, possibly via resynchronizing properties [75,76].

Pharmacological effects of melatonin in humans

It is important to recall that, whilst melatonin has potent, reversible, stimulatory and inhibitory effects on reproduction in photoperiodic seasonal breeders, humans are only marginally photoperiodic if at all. Chronic (1 month) timed (late afternoon) low doses (2 mg daily) of melatonin had no effect on growth hormone, lutropin, testosterone, thyroxine and cortisol concentrations [59]. The timing of prolactin secretion was slightly modified (idem). The major effect was to advance the time of self-rated 'fatigue' or actual sleep into the early evening (Figure 10.7) and to phase-advance its own endogenous rhythm (Figure 10.7) [63,77]. These results are consistent with the known mild hypnotic effects of melatonin [78,79] in man and animals but suggest that its effect is on the timing mechanisms of sleep, at least in low doses. Several reports suggest that in much higher doses melatonin may slightly decrease gonadotropin secretion and increase growth hormone and prolactin secretion in man [e.g. 60,80,81]. Overall, however, its endocrine effects in humans are slight, as is its ability to modify some performance tasks [82]. It has

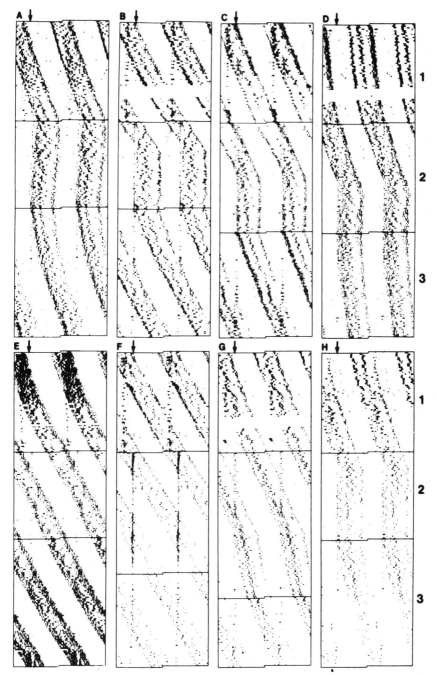

Figure 10.6 Double-plotted running-wheel activity records of rats housed under DD (continuous darkness) and free-running with periods greater than 24 h. Stage 1, pre-injection; stage 2, daily injections; stage 3, post-injection. (A–D) Melatonin injections (1 mg/kg) in stage 2. (E–H) Control injections (vehicle) in stage 2. Time of day of injection in stage 2 is indicated by the arrows at the top. Entrainment of the activity rhythm occurs when melatonin injections coincide with activity onset. (From ref. [68] with permission)

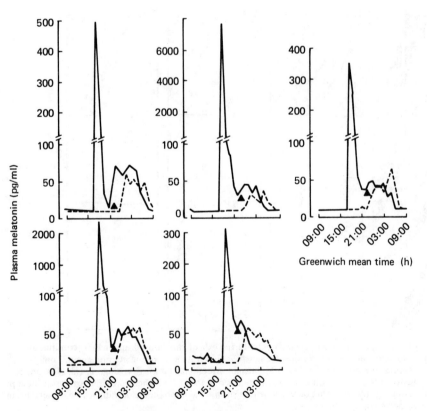

(a)

(b)

no known toxicity in humans, and in rodents toxicity was found to be extremely low even at very high doses [83] and so far there are no contraindications to its use, experimentally, in healthy humans. Enormous doses (up to 6 g/day) have been used (to little effect) in Parkinsonian patients [80]. In depression very large doses in the daytime caused exacerbation of symptoms [84].

Melatonin, jet lag and blindness
Armstrong *et al.* [75] have reported beneficial effects of melatonin on jet lag in uncontrolled studies. In a small placebo-controlled study over eight time-zones eastward, we have found an overall improvement in self-rated 'jet lag', sleep latency and quality, and mood in melatonin-treated subjects (Figure 10.8) [57,76]. Endogenous melatonin and cortisol rhythms resynchronized more rapidly in this group [57]. Treatment was timed in such a way as to induce a phase advance of the 'fatigue' rhythm prior to flight and to reinforce sleep on arrival at destination. A second similar study with a much larger number of subjects [52] travelling to Australia and back has reinforced these preliminary observations. Our subjects took melatonin in one direction and placebo in the other, the treatments being

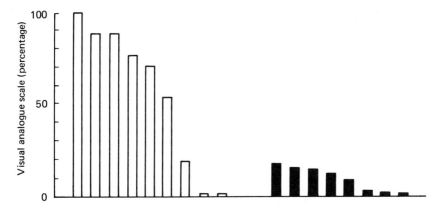

Figure 10.8 Visual analogue scores (0 = insignificant, 100 = very bad) showing severity of jet lag following a flight over eight time-zones eastwards among eight subjects given melatonin (■) and nine given placebo (□) (reproduced from ref. [76] with permission)

Figure 10.7 (a) Fatigue ratings at different times of day in volunteers taking 2 mg of melatonin (●) or placebo (■) daily at 17:00 h (arrows) for 1 month in spring (12 subjects, 10 men, 2 women) or 3 weeks in autumn (11 subjects, 9 men, 2 women). Fatigue was self-rated on a 10 cm visual analogue scale, 0 = rested, 100 = tired. Fatigue ratings are mean values for 1 month; bars show s.e. Analysis of variance indicated a highly significant increase in early-evening fatigue ($P<0.02$) in volunteers taking melatonin. (From ref. [63] with permission). (b) Profiles (24 h) of plasma melatonin concentrations in five subjects after either 3 weeks taking 2 mg of melatonin daily (——) or 3 weeks of placebo treatment (----) in autumn. Note that (i) there is a clear phase advance of the endogenous melatonin peak; (ii) individual peak levels of exogenous melatonin vary from 320 to 7500 pg/ml; (iii) there is a change of scale for the exogenous melatonin peak. The endogenous night-time rise following melatonin ingestion is indicated by arrowheads. (From ref. [63] with permission)

randomized and double-blind. A highly significant overall improvement in jet lag was noted, although four subjects felt distinctly worse on melatonin than on placebo. A small incidence of headache and nausea was reported (J. Arendt and M. Aldhous, unpublished results). Uncontrolled studies (using at least 60 subjects) also suggest that precisely timed melatonin treatment is helpful to most people. Most recently we [71] have been able to synchronize the free-running sleep/wake cycle of a blind man to the 24 h day with a daily melatonin capsule at normal bedtime. Although the sleep/wake cycle maintained a 24-h rhythm, core body temperature was not synchronized by melatonin. It is possible that melatonin acts on central rhythm-generating systems concerned with sleep but not those concerned with temperature. The improved well-being in this one subject was remarkable. It remains to be seen if equal benefit may be derived by other blind subjects with disturbed sleep.

Light as a rhythm synchronizer in humans

The role of light in the control of human circadian rhythms has aroused much recent interest, as a direct result of some observations on pineal function by Lewy *et al.* [25]. The intensity of light required to suppress melatonin production at night, in humans, is considerably higher than that in most animal species [26]. Specifically

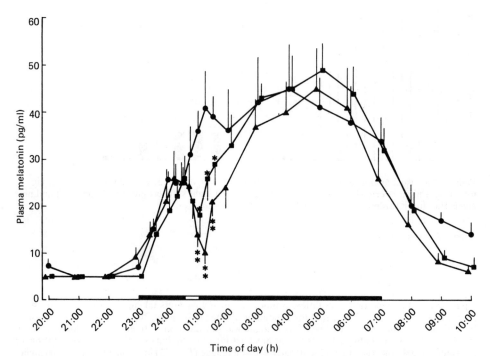

Figure 10.9 Lewy *et al.* [25] showed that >2500 lux of bright artificial incandescent light was necessary to suppress human melatonin production at night. Shown here is the suppression of melatonin in five normal individuals after exposure for 30 min to Vitalite (Duro-Test Corporation) at 2500 lux (▲), 300 lux (■) or <1 lux (●) from 24:30–01:00 h. The individual sensitivity to 300 lux was very variable with overall a significant partial suppression. This may depend on a number of factors including photoperiodic history and genetic make-up. From ref [85] with permission

2500 lux (approximately five times domestic intensity light) is required for complete suppression [25], although most individuals will respond partially to around 300 lux [85] (Figure 10.9). Previous experiments designed to assess the role of light in human circadian physiology had used a maximum of around 1000 lux and in general it was considered that light was not an important zeitgeber in man. Subsequent to Lewy's observation, Wever et al. [86] provided evidence that bright light (3500 lux) is a strong synchronizing agent in humans. Later we (see Figure 10.5) and others have demonstrated clearly the phase-shifting properties of light with respect to melatonin and other circadian rhythms in man [37,87,88]. Bright light is therefore a potential treatment for the rhythm disturbances previously described. Specifically, bright light in the late subjective night should phase-advance circadian rhythms and in the early subjective night should phase-delay according to a theoretical phase-response curve proposed by Lewy et al. [89], based on animal experiments [90]. It will be necessary to define the required light intensity, duration and timing clearly: there is evidence that rhythms are differentially responsive to different light intensities, and individual sensitivity variations may well be important.

It is of course possible that the entraining and synchronizing properties of bright light are closely related to its suppression of melatonin secretion but there is no evidence for this as yet.

Melatonin in psychiatric conditions

The rhythmic secretion of melatonin and its control by light and adrenergic neurones have proved of particular interest in psychiatric studies. Many reports suggest that night-time melatonin levels are low in depression, i.e. the amplitude of the rhythm is attenuated (see [91] for a recent review), and Wetterberg et al. [55] suggest an inverse relationship between melatonin and cortisol rhythms. A number of these studies have not been well controlled with respect to matching control subjects to patients by age, weight, height, reproductive status and season of sample collection. All of these factors have been reported to modify melatonin secretion, age being certainly the most important. In a recent well-matched study [92] we found no differences in either the timing or amplitude of secretion between patients and controls and the question remains open. In that various theories of depression have suggested reduced serotonergic and noradrenergic function, and both of these products are involved in the synthesis of melatonin as precursor and neurotransmitter, it would not in fact be at all surprising to find low melatonin in depression. One report suggests a high amplitude in mania [93] and another low amplitude in schizophrenia [94] but both remain to be confirmed.

The stimulation of melatonin secretion via adrenoceptors has provided a potent tool to investigate the mode of action of antidepressant drugs known to affect adrenergic and serotonergic function and cAMP. A relatively specific tricyclic noradrenaline-uptake inhibitor desmethylimipramine (DMI) advances the onset of production of melatonin if given in the late afternoon in normal subjects [95]. The stimulation is proportional to night-time endogenous secretion and thus provides a pineal function test (Figure 10.10). Checkley et al. [20] have concluded as a result of several such studies with noradrenaline-uptake inhibitors that their net effect is to increase noradrenergic transmission, at least at the level of the pineal gland. Reports of the effects of serotonin-uptake inhibitors [96] and precursors [97] are

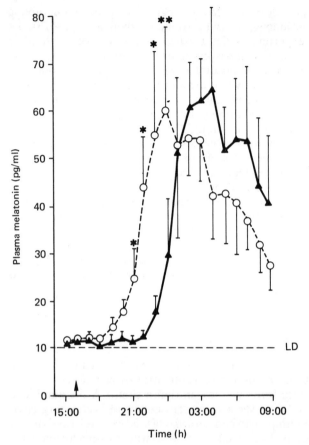

Figure 10.10 Mean hourly plasma melatonin concentrations (± s.e.m.) in eight normal male subjects (20–23 years old) after desmethylimipramine (100 mg) (○) or after placebo (▲), at 16:00 h. *$P<0.05$; **$P<0.01$. LD, limit of detection. (Reproduced from ref. [95] with permission)

scarce, but suggest increased melatonin production and possible changes in the timing of secretion. Rolipram, a phosphodiesterase inhibitor used as an antidepressant, also increases melatonin production, thus providing evidence for the involvement of cAMP in human melatonin production [20].

It is tempting to speculate that all antidepressants increase melatonin production whether this be meaningful or not. For an extended discussion of biological rhythms, including that of melatonin, in affective disorder, see Chapter 9.

At one time the most interesting potential involvement of the pineal with psychiatric disorders was in the syndrome of winter depression or seasonal affective disease (SAD). This is a recurring winter depression with atypical features such as weight gain, hypersomnia and carbohydrate craving [98]; such patients are sometimes described as hibernators. By analogy with photoperiodic seasonal effects, Lewy *et al.* [99] and Rosenthal and co-workers [98] reasoned that depression was induced by winter day length. They treated their patients with bright (>2500 lux) light in an artificial summer day length, 3 h in the evening and

3 h in the morning, extending the natural photoperiod. A dramatic remission of symptoms was found and similar treatments have been effective in many other centres. Again by analogy with animal work it was assumed that short-duration melatonin created by the summer photoperiod was the effector agent. Such, however, does not appear to be the case (see Chapter 9 for further discussion).

Yet another approach to this syndrome is provided by Lewy et al. [88] who consider that the melatonin rhythm (and possibly other circadian rhythms) are phase-delayed in SAD and that a phase-advancing morning light treatment is the most appropriate (see Chapter 9). In recent studies in normal volunteers on an Antarctic base (Halley 75°S) in the winter, we have observed that 1 h of bright light (>2500 lux) in the early morning and in the late afternoon clearly produced a 2 h phase advance in the melatonin rhythm (Figure 10.5) but had no effect on mood, sleep, temperature or various performance rhythms [37]. Evidently our subjects were robust healthy young males rather than the preponderance of females with SAD. Nevertheless this study suggests that a phase advance of the melatonin rhythm is not necessarily associated with a change in mood.

Another area of interest in psychiatry is that of manic-depressive disease. Such patients are supersensitive to light as assessed by suppression of melatonin production at night [101]. If this phenomenon proves to be a trait marker, it may well be of help in diagnosis as well as in elucidating some of the causative factors of the disease.

Mechanism of action of melatonin

Undoubtedly the most important question concerning melatonin at present is how and where does it act to modify seasonal and circadian cycles. Most work and discussion in this field is directed towards the effects of melatonin within the brain, and specifically on central rhythm-generating systems. A brain site of action for melatonin has been identified in rodents [102,103]. Much research directed to identifying melatonin receptors using tritiated melatonin as a ligand has proved either fruitless or controversial so far. New tools are, however, becoming available: high specific activity iodinated melatonin appears to have high-affinity specific binding sites within the brain [67] and the retina [104]. Brain binding sites (suprachiasmatic nucleus and median eminence) suggest a direct effect of melatonin on central rhythm-generating systems situated in these areas. A major problem in the dissection of physiological responses to melatonin is the slow time course of observable effects, and, without identifying target areas, it is difficult to know what to look for, in the short term. A multitude of neurotransmitters and neuromodulators are likely to be involved.

What is important? The next few years should be very fruitful in this respect. Not only are investigations proceeding within the central nervous system, but also in the periphery. The lipophilic nature of melatonin and its rapid distribution throughout body tissues and fluids suggest to me, at least, that it is ideally constructed for a general coordinating role in physiological rhythms.

Acknowledgements

This review was written during the tenure of project grants from the MRC, the AFRC, and The Wellcome Trust to whom the author is most grateful. It was originally written for *Clinical Endocrinology* and is reproduced here, with permission, with extra illustrative material, and with excision of sections and references held to be irrelevant to this book.

References

1. Lerner, A.B., Case, J.D., Takahashi, Y., Lee, T.H. and Mori, N. Isolation of melatonin, pineal factor that lightens melanocytes. *J. Amer. Chem. Soc.*, **80**, 2587 (1958)
2. Collin, J.P. Differentiation and regression of the cells of the sensory line in the epiphysis cerebri. In *The Pineal Gland* (eds G.E.W. Wolstenholme and J. Knight), Churchill Livingstone, Edinburgh and London, pp. 79–125 (1971)
3. Vollrath, L. *The Pineal Organ*, Springer-Verlag, Berlin, Heidelberg, New York (1981)
4. Krstic, R. Pineal calcification: Its mechanism and significance. *J. Neural Transm.*, (suppl.) **21**, 415–432 (1986)
5. Kappers, J.A. Innervation of the epiphysis cerebri in the albino rat. *Anat. Rec.*, **136**, 220–221 (1960)
6. Axelrod, J. The pineal gland: a neurochemical transducer. *Science*, **184**, 1341–1348 (1974)
7. Klein, D.C. Circadian rhythms in the pineal gland. In *Endocrine Rhythms* (ed. D.T. Krieger), Raven Press, New York, pp. 203–223 (1979)
8. Vakkuri, O., Rintamaki, H. and Leppaluoto, J. Presence of immunoreactive melatonin in different tissues of the pigeon (*Columba Livia*). *Gen. Comp. Endocrinol.*, **58**, 69–75 (1985)
9. Pang, S.F., Brown, G.M., Grota, L.J., Chambers, J.W. and Rodman, R.L. Determination of N-acetyl serotonin and melatonin activities in the pineal gland, retina, Harderian gland, brain and serum of rats and chickens. *Neuroendocrinology*, **23**, 1–13 (1977)
10. Arendt, J. Mammalian pineal rhythms. *Pineal Res. Rev.*, **3**, 161–213 (1985)
11. Raikhlin, N.T., Kvetnoy, I.M. and Tolkachev, V.N. Melatonin may be synthesised in enterochromaffin cells. *Nature (London)*, **219**, 344 (1975)
12. Rollag, M.D., Morgan, R.J. and Niswender, G.D. Route of melatonin secretion in sheep. *Endocrinology*, **102**, 1–8 (1978)
13. Illnerova, H., Backstrom, M., Saapf, J., Wetterberg, L. and Vancbo, B. Melatonin in rat pineal gland and serum, rapid parallel decline after light exposure at night. *Neurosci. Lett.*, **9**, 189–193 (1978)
14. Kopin, I.J., Pare, C.M.B., Axelrod, J. and Weissbach, H. The fate of melatonin in animals. *J. Biol. Chem.*, **236**, 3072–3075 (1961)
15. Jones, R.L., McGeer, P.L. and Greiner, A.C. Metabolism of exogenous melatonin in schizophrenic and non-schizophrenic volunteers. *Clin. Chim. Acta*, **26**, 281–285 (1969)
16. Bojkowski, C.J., Arendt, J., Shih, M.C. and Markey, S.P. Melatonin secretion in humans assessed by measuring its metabolite 6-sulphatoxymelatonin. *Clin. Chem.*, **33**, 1343–1348 (1987)
17. Klein, D.C. Photoneural regulation of the mammalian pineal gland. In *Ciba Foundation Symposium 17. Photoperiodism, Melatonin and the Pineal* (eds D. Evered and S. Clark), Pitman, London, pp. 38–56 (1985)
18. O'Brien, I.A.D., Lewin, I.G., O'Hare, J.P., Arendt, J. and Corall, R.J. Abnormal circadian rhythm of melatonin in diabetic autonomic neuropathy. *Clin. Endocrinol.*, **24**, 359–364 (1986)
19. Cowen, P.J., Fraser, S., Sammons, R. and Green, A.R. Atenolol reduces plasma melatonin concentrations in man. *Brit. J. Clin. Pharmacol.*, **15**, 579–581 (1983)
20. Checkley, S.A., Palazidou, E., Bearn, J., Winton, F., Franey, C. and Arendt, J. Effects of antidepressant drugs upon melatonin secretion in man. In *Melatonin: Clinical Perspectives* (eds A. Miles, D.R.S. Philbrick and C. Thompson), Oxford University Press, Oxford, pp. 190–204 (1988)
21. Romero, J.A. and Axelrod, J. Pineal β-adrenergic receptor: diurnal variations in sensitivity. *Science*, **184**, 1091–1092 (1974)
22. Lewy, A.J., Sack, R.L. and Singer, C.M. Assessment and treatment of chronobiologic disorders using plasma melatonin levels and bright light exposure, the clock-gate model and the phase response curve. *Psychopharmacol. Bull.*, **20**, 561–565 (1984)

23. Grasby, P.M. and Cowen, P.J. Clonidine fails to suppress plasma melatonin in man. Abstracts - British Pharmacological Society, Cambridge. *Brit. J. Pharmacol.*, no. 36 (1987)
24. Wever, R.A. Characteristics of circadian rhythms in human functions. In *Melatonin in Humans* (eds R.J. Wurtman and F. Waldhauser). *J. Neural Transm.*, (suppl.) **21**, 323–374 (1986)
25. Lewy, A.J., Wehr, T.A., Goodwin, F.K., Newsome, D.A. and Markey, S.P. Light suppresses melatonin secretion in humans. *Science*, **210**, 1267–1269 (1980)
26. Reiter, R.J. Action spectra, dose–response relationships and temporal aspects of light's effects on the pineal gland. *Ann. N. Y. Acad. Sci.*, **453**, 215–230 (1985)
27. Arendt, J. Role of the pineal gland and melatonin in seasonal reproductive function in mammals. *Oxford Rev. Reprod. Biol.*, **8**, 266–320 (1986)
28. Tamarkin, L., Baird, C.J. and Almeida, O.F.X. Melatonin: a coordinating signal for mammalian reproduction. *Science*, **227**, 714–72) (1985)
29. Herbert, J. The pineal gland and photoperiodic control of the ferret's reproductive cycle. In *Biological Clocks in Seasonal Reproductive Cycles* (eds B.K. Follett and D.E. Follett), Wright, Bristol, pp. 261–276 (1981)
30. Parkes, A.S. *Patterns of Sexuality and Reproduction*, Oxford University Press, Oxford (1976)
31. Kennaway, D.J., Dunstan, E.A. and Staples, L.D. Photoperiodic control of the onset of breeding activity and fecundity in ewes. *J. Reprod. Fertil.*, (suppl.) **34**, 187–199 (1987)
32. Martinet, L. and Allain, D. Role of the pineal gland in the photoperiodic control of reproductive and non-reproductive functions in mink (Mustela vison). In *Ciba Foundation Symposium 117. Photoperiodism, Melatonin and the Pineal.* (eds D. Evered, and S. Clark), Pitman, London, pp. 170–187 (1985)
33. Duncan, M.J. and Goldman, B.D. Hormonal regulation of the annual pelage color cycle in the Djungarian hamster, *Phodopus sungorus*. II. Role of prolactin. *J. Exp. Zool.*, **230**, 97–103 (1984)
34. Carter, D.S. and Goldman, B.D. Antigonadal effects of timed melatonin infusion in pinealecto-mised male Djungarian hamsters (*Phodopus sungorus sungorus*): Duration is the critical parameter. *Endocrinology*, **113**, 1261–1267 (1983)
35. Bittman, E.L. The role of rhythms in the response to melatonin. *Ciba Foundation Symposium 117. Photoperiodism, Melatonin and the Pineal Gland* (eds D. Evered and S. Clark), Pitman, London, pp. 149–169 (1985)
36. Illnerova, H., Zvolsky, P. and Vanecek, J. The circadian rhythm in plasma melatonin concentration of the urbanised man, the effect of summer and winter time. *Brain Res.*, **328**, 186–189 (1985)
37. Broadway, J., Folkard, S. and Arendt, J. Bright light phase shifts the human melatonin rhythm in Antarctica. *Neurosci. Lett.*, **79**, 185–189 (1987)
38. Foster, D.L. Mechanism for delay of first ovulation in lambs born in the wrong season (fall). *Biol. Reprod.*, **25**, 85–92 (1981)
39. Sizonenko, P.C., Lang, U., Rivest, R.W. and Aubert, M.L. The pineal and pubertal development. In *Ciba Foundation Symposium 117. Photoperiodism, Melatonin and the Pineal* (eds D. Evered and S. Clark), Pitman, London, pp. 208–230 (1985)
40. Kitay, J.I. and Altschule, M.D. *The Pineal Gland*, Harvard University Press, Cambridge, MA, pp. 79–95 (1954)
41. Waldhauser, F., Frisch, H., Waldhauser, M., Weiszenbacher, G., Zeitlhuber, V. and Wurtman, R.J. Fall in nocturnal serum melatonin during prepuberty and pubescence. *Lancet*, **i**, 362–365 (1984)
42. Young, I.M., Francis, P.L., Leone, A.M., Stovell, P. and Silman, R.E. Night/day urinary 6-hydroxy melatonin production as a function of age, body mass and urinary creatinine levels: a population study in 110 subjects aged 3–80. *J. Endocrinol.*, **111**, suppl. abstr. no. 32 (1986)
43. Iguchi, H., Kato, K. and Ibayashi, H. Age dependent reduction in serum melatonin concentration in healthy human subjects. *J. Clin. Endocrinol. Metab.*, **55**, 27–29 (1982)
44. Lewy, A.J. and Newsome, D.A. Different types of melatonin circadian secretory rhythms in some blind subjects. *J. Clin. Endocrinol. Metab.*, **56**, 1103–1107 (1983)
45. Reiter, R.J. The pineal and its hormones in the control of reproduction in mammals. *Endocrine Res.*, **1**, 109–131 (1980)
46. Wetterberg, L., Arendt, J., Paunier, L., Sizonenko, P.C., Van Donselaar, W. and Heyden, T.

Human serum melatonin changes during the menstrual cycle. *J. Clin. Endocrinol. Metab.*, **42**, 185–188 (1976)

47. Ozaki, Y., Wurtman, R.J., Alonso, R. and Lynch, H.J. Melatonin secretion decreases during the proestrous stage in the rat estrous cycle. *Proc. Natl Acad. Sci. USA*, **75**, 531–534 (1978)

48. Webley, G.E. and Leidenberger, F. The circadian pattern of melatonin and its positive relationship with progesterone in women. *J. Clin. Endocrinol. Metab.*, **63**, 323–328 (1986)

49. Hariharasubramanian, N. and Nair, N.P.V. Circadian rhythm of plasma melatonin and cortisol during the menstrual cycle. In *The Pineal Gland, Endocrine Aspects* (eds G.M. Brown and S. Wainwright), Pergamon Press, Toronto, Vol. 1, pp. 31–35 (1984)

50. Walker, R.F., McCamant, S. and Timiras, P.S. Melatonin and the influence of the pineal gland on timing of the LH surge in rats. *Neuroendocrinology*, **39**, 37–42 (1982)

51. Brzezinski, A., Lynch, H.J., Wurtman, R.J. and Siebel, M.M. Possible contribution of melatonin to the timing of the luteinizing hormone surge. *New Engl. J. Med.*, **316**, 1550–1551 (1987)

52. Testart, J., Frydman, R. and Roger, M. Seasonal influence of diurnal rhythms in the onset of the plasma luteinising hormone surge in women. *J. Clin. Endocrinol. Metab.*, **55**, 374–377 (1982)

53. Berga, S.L., Mortola, J.F. and Yen, S.S.C. Amplification of nocturnal melatonin secretion in women with functional hypothalamic amenorrhea. *J. Clin. Endocrinol. Metab.*, **66**, 242–244 (1988)

54. Vaughan, G.M. Melatonin in humans. *Pineal Res. Rev.*, **2**, 141–201 (1984)

55. Wetterberg, L., Aperia, B., Beck-Friis, J., Kjellman, B.F., Ljunggren, J-G., Nilsonne, A., Petterson, U., Tham, A. and Umden, F. Melatonin and cortisol levels in psychiatric illness. *Lancet*, **88**, 100 (1982)

56. Murakami, N., Hayafuji, C., Sasaki, Y., Yamazaki, J. and Takahashi, K. Melatonin accelerates the re-entrainment of the circadian adrenocortical rhythm in inverted illumination cycle. *Neuroendocrinology*, **36**, 385–391 (1983)

57. Arendt, J., Aldhous, M., Marks, M., Folkard, S., English, J., Marks, V. and Arendt, J. Some effects of jet-lag and its treatment by melatonin. *Ergonomics*, **30**, 1379–1393 (1987)

58. Fevre-Montange, M., van Cauter, E., Refetoff, S., Desir, D., Tourniaire J. and Copinschi, G. Effects of "Jet Lag" on hormonal patterns. II. Adaptation of melatonin circadian periodicity. *J. Clin. Endocrinol. Metab.*, **52**, 642–649 (1981)

59. Wright, J., Aldhous, M., Franey, C., English, J. and Arendt, J. The effects of exogenous melatonin on endocrine function in man. *Clin. Endocrinol.*, **24**, 375–382 (1986)

60. Waldhauser, F., Steger, H. and Vorkapic, P. Melatonin secretion in man and the influence of exogenous melatonin on some physiological and behavioural variables. *Adv. Pineal Res.*, **2**, 207–223 (1987)

61. Vriend, J. Evidence for pineal gland modulation of the neuroendocrine–thyroid axis. *Neuroendocrinology*, **36**, 68–78 (1983)

62. Arendt, J. Assay of melatonin and its metabolites: results in normal and unusual environments. In *Melatonin in Humans* (eds R.J. Wurtman and F. Waldhauser), *J. Neural Trans.*, (suppl.) **21**, 11–33 (1986)

63. Arendt, J., Bojkowski, C., Folkard, S., Franey, C., Minors, D., Waterhouse, J.M., Wever, R.A., Wildgruber, C. and Wright, J. Some effects of melatonin and the control of its secretion in man. In *Ciba Foundation Symposium 117. Photoperiodism, Melatonin and the Pineal* (eds D. Evered and S. Clark), Pitman, London, pp. 266–283 (1985)

64. Menaker, M., Hudson, D.J. and Takahashi, J.S. Neural and endocrine components of circadian clocks in birds. In *Biological Clocks in Seasonal Reproductive Cycles* (eds B.K. Follett and D.E. Follett), Wright, Bristol, pp. 171–183 (1981)

65. Underwood, H. Circadian organisation in lizards: the role of the pineal organ. *Science*, **195**, 587–589 (1977)

66. Takahashi, J.S. Circadian oscillators at cellular levels. *Proceedings of the 18th International Conference on Chronobiology*, Pergamon, Oxford (in press)

67. Vanecek, J., Pavlik, A. and Illnerova, H. Hypothalamic melatonin receptor sites revealed by autoradiography. *Brain Res.*, **435**, 359–362 (1987)

68. Armstrong, S.M. and Redman, J. Melatonin administration: effects on rodent circadian rhythms. In *Ciba Foundation Symposium 117. Photoperiodism, Melatonin and the Pineal* (eds D. Evered and S. Clark), Pitman, London, pp. 188–207 (1985)

69. Redman, J., Armstrong, S. and Ng, K.T. Free-running activity rhythms in the rat: entrainment by melatonin. *Science*, **219**, 1089–1091 (1983)
70. Wever, R.A. *The Circadian System of Man*, Springer, Berlin, Heidelberg, New York (1979)
71. Arendt, J., Aldhous, M. and Wright, J. Synchronisation of a disturbed sleep–wake cycle in a blind man by melatonin treatment. *Lancet*, **i**, 772–773 (1988)
72. Moore-Ede, M.C., Czeisler, C.A. and Richardson, G.S. Circadian time-keeping in health and disease. Part 2. Clinical implications of circadian rhythmicity. *New Engl. J. Med.*, **309**, 530–536 (1983)
73. Minors, D.S. and Waterhouse, J.M. *Circadian Rhythms and the Human*, Wright, Bristol, pp. 143–148 (1981)
74. Arendt, J. and Marks, V. Physiological changes underlying jet-lag. *Brit. Med. J.*, **284**, 144–146 (1982)
75. Armstrong, S.M., Cassone, V.M., Chesworth, M.J., Redman, J.R. and Short, R.V. Synchronization of mammalian circadian rhythms by melatonin. *J. Neural Transm.*, (suppl.) **21**, 375–398 (1986)
76. Arendt, J., Aldhous, M. and Marks, V. Alleviation of jet-lag by melatonin: preliminary results of controlled double-blind trial. *Brit. Med. J.*, **292**, 1170 (1986)
77. Arendt, J., Borbely, A.A., Franey, C. and Wright, J. The effect of chronic, small doses of melatonin given in the late afternoon on fatigue in man: a preliminary study. *Neurosci. Lett.*, **45**, 317–321 (1984)
78. Cramer, H., Rudolph, J. and Consbruch, V. On the effects of melatonin on sleep and behaviour in man. *Adv. Biochem. Psychopharmacol.*, **11**, 187–191 (1974)
79. Vollrath, L., Semm, P. and Gammel, G. Sleep induction by intranasal application of melatonin. *Adv. Biosci.*, **29**, 327–329 (1981)
80. Lerner, A.B. and Nordlund, J.J. Melatonin: clinical pharmacology. *J. Neural Transm.*, (suppl.) **13**, 339–347 (1978)
81. Smythe, G.A. and Lazarus, L. Growth hormone responses to melatonin in man. *Science*, **134**, 1373–1374 (1974)
82. Lieberman, H.R., Waldhauser, F., Garfield, G., Lynch, H.J. and Wurtman, R.J. Effects of melatonin on human mood and performance. *Brain Res.*, **323**, 201–207 (1984)
83. Sugden, D. Psychopharmacological effects of melatonin in mouse and rat. *J. Pharmacol. Exp. Therap.*, **227**, 587–591 (1983)
84. Carman, J.S., Post, R.M., Buswell, R. and Goodwin, F.K. Negative effects of melatonin on depression. *Am. J. Psychiat.*, **133**, 1181–1186 (1976)
85. Bojkowski, C.J., Aldhous, M.E., English, J., Franey, C., Poulton, A.L., Skene, D.J. and Arendt, J. Suppression of nocturnal plasma melatonin by bright and dim light in man. *Horm. Metab. Res.*, **19**, 437–440 (1987)
86. Wever, R.A., Polasek, J. and Wildgruber, C.M. Bright light affects human circadian rhythms. *Pflügers Arch.*, **396**, 85–87 (1983)
87. Czeisler, C.A., Allan, J.S., Strogatz, S.H., Ronda, J.M., Sanchez, R., Rios, C.D., Freitag, W.O., Richardson, G.S. and Kronauer, R.E. Bright light resets the human circadian pacemaker independent of the timing of the sleep–wake cycle. *Science*, **233**, 667–671 (1986)
88. Lewy, A.J., Sack, R.L., Miller, L.S. and Hoban, T.M. Anti-depressant and circadian phase-shifting effects of light. *Science*, **235**, 352–354 (1987)
89. Lewy, A.J., Sack, R.L. and Singer, C.M. Assessment and treatment of chronobiologic disorders using plasma melatonin levels and bright light exposure, the clock-gate model and the phase response curve. *Psychopharmacol. Bull.*, **20**, 561–565 (1984)
90. Elliot, J.A. Circadian rhythms, entrainment and photoperiodism in the Syrian hamster. In *Biological Clocks in Seasonal Reproductive Cycles* (eds B.K. Follett and D.E. Follett), Scientechnica, Bristol, pp. 203–218 (1981)
91. Grasby, P.M. and Cowen, P.J. The pineal and psychiatry: still fumbling in the dark. *Psychol. Med.*, **17**, 817–820 (1987)
92. Thompson, C., Franey, C., Arendt, J. and Checkley, S.A. A comparison of melatonin secretion in depressed patients and normal subjects. *Brit. J. Psychiatr.*, **152**, 260–5 (1988)
93. Lewy, A.J., Wehr, T.A., Gold, P.W. and Goodwin, F.K. Plasma melatonin in manic depressive

illness. In *Catecholamines: Basic and Clinical Frontiers*. Volume II (eds E. Usdin, I.J. Kopin and J. Barechas), Pergamon Press, Oxford and New York, pp. 1173–1175 (1978)

94. Ferrier, I.N., Arendt, J., Johnstone, E.C. and Crow, T.J. Reduced nocturnal melatonin secretion in chronic schizophrenia: Relationship to body weight. *Clin. Endocrinol.*, **17**, 181–187 (1982)

95. Franey, C., Aldhous, A., Burton, S., Checkley, S. and Arendt, J. Acute treatment with desipramine stimulates melatonin and 6-sulphatoxymelatonin in man. *Brit. J. Clin. Pharmacol.*, **22**, 73–79 (1986)

96. Demisch, K., Demisch, L., Bodinik, H.J., Nickelson, T., Althoff, P.H., Schoffling, K. and Rieth, R. Melatonin and cortisol increase after fluvoxamine. *Brit. J. Clin. Pharmacol.*, **22**, 620–622 (1986)

97. Namboodiri, M.A., Sugden, D., Klein, D.C. and Mefford, I.N. 5-Hydroxytryptophan elevates serum melatonin. *Science*, **221**, 659–661 (1983)

98. Rosenthal, N.E., Sack, D.A., Gillin, J.C., Lewy, A.J., Goodwin, F.K., Davenport, Y., Mueller, P.S., Newsome, D.A. and Wehr, T.A. Seasonal affective disorder. A description of the syndrome and preliminary findings with light therapy. *Arch. Gen. Psychiat.*, **41**, 72–79 (1984)

99. Lewy, A.J., Kern, H.E., Rosenthal, N.E. and Wehr, T.A. Bright artificial light treatment of a manic depressive patient with seasonal mood cycle. *Amer. J. Psychiat.*, **139**, 1496–1498 (1982)

100. Bojkowski, C.J. and Arendt, J. Annual changes in 6-sulphatoxymelatonin excretion in man. *Acta Endocrinol.*, **117**, 470–476 (1988)

101. Lewy, A.J., Wehr, T.A., Goodwin, F.K., Newsome, D.A. and Rosenthal, N.E. Manic depressive patients may be supersensitive to light. *Lancet*, **i**, 383–384 (1981)

102. Hastings, M.H., Roberts, A.C. and Herbert, J. Neurotoxic lesions of the anterior hypothalamic disrupt the photoperiodic but not the circadian system of the Syrian hamster. *Neuroendocrinology*, **40**, 316–322 (1985)

103. Glass, J.D. and Knotts, L.K. A brain site for the anti-gonadal action of melatonin in the white-footed mouse *Peromyscus leucopus*: Involvement of the immunoreactive GnRH neuronal system. *Neuroendocrinology*, **46**, 48–55 (1987)

104. Dubocovich, M.L. and Takahashi, J.S. Use of 2-[^{125}I]iodomelatonin to characterise melatonin binding sites in chicken retina. *Proc. Natl Acad. Sci. USA*, **84**, 3916–3920 (1987)

Chapter 11

Circadian rhythms in general practice and occupational health

D.S. Minors and J.M. Waterhouse

It is not only in the hospital but also in general practice and the industrial environment that a knowledge of circadian rhythms can be useful. Patients can present themselves complaining of insomnia or chronic indigestion, with fatigue or even with no more than the sense of being 'run down'. In some cases, abnormal or inappropriate circadian rhythms might be to blame, particularly in susceptible individuals and in those with 'unusual' (that is, not 9-till-5) hours of work or lifestyles.

In this chapter are considered, first, those cases where circadian rhythms are abnormal – due to a biological or environmental cause – and, second, the problems that arise when the normal sleep/wake schedule is altered. Such alterations occur after a time-zone transition and during night work. A major concern in these circumstances is the possibility of deterioration in mental performance and the increased chance of making errors or even having an accident that this might cause. Accordingly, circadian rhythms in performance and effects upon these that arise from sleep loss will be considered also. In each section we will attempt to consider the cause of a problem together with advice on how to ameliorate it.

Abnormal entrainment and environments

Failure in entrainment mechanisms

'Monday morning blues' – the difficulty in getting back into a work routine after weekend rest days – is experienced by all of us to some extent. A component of this is the advance of circadian rhythms that is required on a Monday after a weekend during which the rhythms have become phase-delayed. This phase delay has occurred as a result of late nights and staying in bed in the morning longer than usual over the weekend. For most people the readjustment of their rhythms to a working routine is rapid and begins on the Monday morning. The morning alarm wakes them 'early' (compared with the weekend) and their body might take a little longer than usual to wake up fully; but these difficulties are restricted to one day only as exposure to a normal routine soon re-establishes the appropriate phase of their internal clock. However, some individuals seem to be unable to advance their internal clock so that they cannot readily adjust after the phase delay caused by their lifestyle at the weekend. Another symptom of their abnormality is that they naturally tend to retire and rise much later than the population as a whole; as a result they become sleep-deprived if their employment requires them to work conventional hours. This form of insomnia is called Delayed Sleep Phase Syndrome (DSPS) [1]. Both the insomnia and the inability to advance delayed circadian rhythms can be treated as follows (the treatment is based upon the fact that the rhythm can both be phase-delayed and entrained to a 24-h day).

1. The patients are first adjusted to a normal day by delaying their sleep/wake routines about 3 h per day until their rhythms and ability to sleep are phased normally.
2. The patients are then advised to maintain a rigorous 24-h schedule thereafter.

Why such patients cannot advance their rhythms in response to an advance in zeitgebers is not known. Possibilities are: they possess clocks with longer inherent periods than normal; the pathways by which zeitgebers influence them are less well developed; the interaction between the zeitgebers and clock is abnormal.

Cases have been described in which sleep hours are abnormally advanced and delays, rather than advances, of phase are difficult to achieve. In such cases, a progressive advance of bedtime until it is correctly phased, and a rigorously regular routine thereafter, is helpful [2]. These cases are rarer than those of DSPS. This is presumably because they are caused by an internal clock with an inherent period that is less than 24 h, and so further from the population mean [3] than are cases of DSPS.

A condition that has occasionally been reported is one in which an individual experiences difficulties in remaining synchronized to the 24-h day and his circadian rhythms appear to free-run even though he is living in a normal society [4]. In some way, normal zeitgebers (and social zeitgebers – awareness of rhythmic activity in the rest of society – might be particularly important in such cases) appear to be inadequate for entraining the internal clock to a period of 24 h. Sometimes, the individuals appear (or are forced) to choose a lifestyle in which non-conformity with the rest of society need not be a disadvantage [5]; in other cases, they find regular employment and social habits impossible to undertake.

Blind people also tend to show considerable abnormalities in their circadian rhythms including free-running rhythms not synchronized to a normal lifestyle [6–8]. Almost certainly the inability of light to act as a zeitgeber is a contributory factor but the fact that blind subjects do not show such regularity of lifestyle as do sighted individuals is no doubt important also. Stressing a regular lifestyle for blind individuals can do something to increase the stability and amplitude of their circadian rhythms.

Abnormal environments

The above cases illustrate the problems that can arise if the individual has some abnormality of the internal clock or does not respond to conventional zeitgebers. By contrast, there are some environments where the individuals do not suffer from these abnormalities but where conventional zeitgebers are weak or even absent. One example is the situation of those living away from the equator and working in artificially illuminated buildings who, during the winter, may never see natural daylight. There is evidence that artificial levels of lighting normally encountered are inadequate to suppress pineal secretion in humans [9]. As a result, it is possible that not only the phasing of plasma melatonin but also that of other rhythms – including fatigue and sleep which might be linked with the melatonin rhythm (see

Chapter 10) – will be abnormal; in effect, as with blind people, environmental lighting would be an inadequate zeitgeber. Other environments where these considerations apply are self-contained ones under the ground or the sea. Although studies of the responses to these environments are scarce, anecdotal evidence suggests that they can be associated with a sense of disorientation and confusion, and that this can lead to a decrease in work output, to depression and low morale.

Whether it is the inadequacy of the zeitgebers or rather the low level of the artificial illumination that causes such problems is not clear. However, the lack of zeitgebers can often be a marked feature in some hospital environments in which continuous care is necessary. Examples would be intensive care units (ICU) and premature baby units. In ICU, studies have found that the incidence of psychological disturbances amongst patients is high and the term 'intensive care delirium' has been coined [10]. Such unpleasant behavioural symptoms are undesirable, of course, but there is other evidence that they might act against a successful outcome. Links have been found between the patient's general mood, his 'will to live' and his chance of survival. The advantage to patients of an ICU with windows was investigated in one study which compared two ICUs, one with and one without natural daylight [11]. Patients who had stayed in the windowless unit had poorer memories of their stay, a greater sense of disorientation as to the passage of time, more sleep and visual disturbances and a greater incidence of hallucinations. Specific studies of rhythmicity in ICU patients are very few. However, in a preliminary survey [12], the circadian rhythms of axillary temperature in five patients on intensive care were abnormal. In addition, nursing staff find work in the ICU particularly stressful and they are reported to have higher sickness rates than nurses on general wards. Many factors will contribute to this, of course, but impoverished zeitgebers might be one.

In infants, there is some evidence that the development of circadian rhythms during infancy is delayed in the absence of a daily routine [13].

Advice

As far as members of the work force are concerned, it would seem desirable to provide more time cues. The effect of this would enable them to appreciate the passage of time more clearly. If conditions permit, then the day could be structured more by going out into the daylight and taking walks or bouts of exercise if conditions permit. When this is not possible then a regular routine of meals, work, leisure and sleep might help. The passage of a particular shift or duty span can be appreciated more if adherence to a regular system of breaks and mealtimes is possible.

With respect to ICU patients, the advice must be rather tentative; however, there seems to be considerable room for further research based upon the hypothesis that the means to promote normal rhythmicity would improve their prognosis [14]. Some possibilities that would not interfere with treatment are: (1) levels of the sedation used to facilitate intermittent positive pressure ventilation could be adjusted according to the time of day, i.e. deepened at night and lightened during daylight hours, thereby imparting an element of rhythmicity to the patient's level of consciousness; (2) patterns of feeding, parenteral or enteral, could be adjusted to mimic more closely the normal day/night pattern of food intake; (3) insistence on a regular lights on/lights off policy at specified times, particularly in windowless units, and efforts by the staff to keep noise at night to an absolute minimum (compared with normal noise and activity levels during the day) may all go some way towards giving the patient a sense of environmental rhythmicity. However, it should be noted that this advice is to some extent incompatible with that given to night workers (see later) to help them adjust to night work.

In nurseries for newborn babies there is also some evidence that the strengthening of zeitgebers can improve development. For example, the introduction of day/night differences into a nursery (light/dark, noise/quiet) increased the rate of general development of a group of preterm babies when compared with matched controls who stayed in a similar nursery but with less marked day/night differences. These differences in development persisted when both groups of babies were transferred into their home environments [15].

The concept of using light/dark cycles to strengthen zeitgebers and so adjust the phase of the internal clock has been promoted for some depressed patients (see Chapter 9) [16].

Time-zone transitions

Industrial man sometimes works at night and many of us, by virtue of business or pleasure, fly from one time zone to another. These actions alter the normal relationship between environmental rhythms and internal clocks (see Chapter 1). The problems that stem from such abnormal circadian rhythmicities can be regarded, in a general sense, as occupational hazards.

Jet lag

Rapid movement from one time-zone to another results in a temporary malaise known as jet lag. Individuals might feel tired during the daytime in the new time zone and yet might have difficulty in sleeping at the new night time. In addition, they might lose their appetite, suffer gastrointestinal disorders, feel irritable, suffer headaches and generally feel 'below par' [17]. The severity of these symptoms tends to increase with the number of time zones crossed and is generally worse after a flight to the east than after one to the west [18].

Many of these symptoms might reasonably be attributed to the excitement or stress of a long journey, together with the loss of sleep and change in food and customs that will be encountered. Against this view is the observation that these symptoms are as pronounced when one returns home and so could not be due to 'culture shock'. Also, jet lag is less troublesome and persistent after a north–south flight of comparable length and inconvenience. In other words, in some way these symptoms are due to the time-zone transition itself. It is now clear that many of these problems are in some way due to the slow adjustment to the new time zone of the internal clock and the dissociation between the clock and environment that is associated with this. Adjustment of the internal clock occurs after several days; it is brought about by zeitgebers in the new time zone.

As might be expected, the advice to travellers on how to deal with the problems of a time-zone transition depends upon whether they plan to stay in the new time zone for a short or longer period of time [19].

Advice to travellers during short stays

If a short stay is envisaged then adjustment cannot occur. In such cases the traveller is advised:

1. To take a nap as soon as possible after the journey in order to recuperate from any loss of sleep;
2. To arrange meetings to coincide with daytime on the old time where possible. This entails meetings later in the day on new local times after an eastward flight and as early as possible in the morning after a flight to the west. Morning meetings on local time after an eastward flight (or in the evening after a westward flight) are to be avoided since they coincide with night on old time.

Advice to travellers during long stays

By contrast, if the stay is to be longer, then it is advisable to try to adjust circadian rhythms to the new time zone as rapidly as possible by the suitable timing of zeitgebers [20]. Several means have been suggested. Not surprisingly, links exist between some of them and the techniques used in some forms of depression (Chapter 9) and in dealing with environments with impoverished zeitgebers (above).

By making use of the zeitgebers in the new time zone
The traveller should ensure as full exposure to these as possible. Thus, he should attempt to adopt a strict regimen with regard to sleep and activity that is in phase with the new local time. He should also aim for strong social contacts in the new time zone. For example, one group of volunteers whose social life was restricted to that in a hotel room after a time-zone transition adjusted less quickly than did another group who were allowed full access to the social life [21]. Another technique which has been suggested is the appropriate timing of very bright light [22]. With this method bright light given early in the activity span is postulated to advance circadian rhythms and, given late in the activity span, to delay them. In practice this generally argues again for an 'outdoor life' in the new time zone so that exposure to the natural light/dark cycle is achieved.

A regular and appropriate timing of meals can be part of the highly structured lifestyle which makes an individual more fully aware of his new local time; but it is believed that a suitable choice of food can influence the body clock in a further way [23]. It is argued that results of the hormonal changes associated with eating, the relative amounts of protein and carbohydrate ingested and the intake of theophylline derivatives, in coffee for instance, can produce changes in brain function via changes in activity of its neurotransmitters. For example, arousal is mediated by adrenergic mechanisms and so is promoted by a high-protein intake (which promotes the brain uptake of tyrosine, the precursor of adrenaline and noradrenaline). By contrast, sleep is mediated by serotoninergic mechanisms and the uptake into the brain of the precursor of this transmitter (tryptophan) is promoted by high-carbohydrate diets. Accordingly, high-protein breakfasts with coffee and high-carbohydrate dinners without coffee are recommended. However, in one study of military personnel [23] the efficacy of these dietary modifications in promoting adjustment to time-zone transitions appeared to be slight and so the exact role of meals is uncertain at the present time. A critical evaluation of dietary influence on some rhythms is presented in Chapter 8.

Use of drugs

Hypnotics and stimulants might be used at appropriate times in the new time zone, but this does not seem to have been investigated in detail, at least for civilian personnel. However, there has been a search for a drug that could promote adjustment of the internal clock, a chronobiotic [24]. A variety of substances have been tried but none has shown a substantial effect under strictly controlled circumstances. Since we are unclear as to the exact site and nature of the internal clock, as well as the means by which zeitgebers affect it, the discovery of an appropriate drug is likely to be fortuitous. There has been a recent report that administration of melatonin at a suitable time (i.e. just before bedtime on new local time) reduces the severity of symptoms of jet lag [25] but the exact mechanisms by which the effect is produced is not known at the present time. The most important effect of melatonin was undoubtedly to improve sleep. A more detailed account of this study is given in Chapter 10.

Apart from a strengthening of natural zeitgebers, no artificial method of speeding up the process of adjustment of the internal clock has yet been found that is reliable, easy to administer and has been tested thoroughly.

If possible, a preadjustment of sleep/activity schedules is best, since the traveller is fully adjusted to the new time zone immediately on arrival. He could adjust his times of rising, meals and retiring before the journey by about 2 h per day in the appropriate direction, that is 2 h earlier each day for 4 days if flying eastwards through eight time zones. The problem is that other commitments would make it impossible to live such an abnormal schedule on home time in the days before the flight. It also raises another problem, namely that it would require individuals to live at variance with the rest of society, and it is precisely this problem that exists for those who work at night.

Problems associated with night work

About 25% of the working population are involved in some form of shift system and this often requires work to be performed at night. The night worker is required to alter his lifestyle not only by working at night but also by sleeping during the daytime. In some ways, this change in timing of habits is rather similar to that experienced by the traveller after a time-zone transition and similar symptoms arise – fatigue, difficulty in sleeping at 'bedtime' and gastrointestinal disorders [26,27].

Difficulties associated with shift work

Fatigue during night work is not unexpected, being a reflection of working during the 'troughs' of circadian rhythms in mood, performance (see later), adrenaline level and deep body temperature [28]. Fatigue also during the daytime is observed and this results from a cumulative loss of sleep. External noise plays a part in reducing daytime sleep, particularly in inner city areas with more traffic and poorer housing which is smaller and less well insulated against noise. However, this lack of sleep is not wholly due to the difficulties of sleeping in a daytime environment. Subjects studied in the sound-proofed conditions of a sleep laboratory have greater difficulty in getting to sleep and staying asleep in the daytime than during the night and their sleep tends to be more fragmented than in the daytime [29]. This is because sleep is being attempted when body temperature and the sympathetic nervous system are preparing the body for a new spell of activity; even if sleep is achieved, a full bladder is likely to curtail it as urine production rises. In other words, many of the night workers' problems arise because of a mismatching between his lifestyle and his internal clock [30].

Accepting this, then it can be argued that the gastrointestinal disturbances result from eating food at 'wrong' times with abnormal patterns of gut motility and gastric acid secretion being likely [31,32]. No doubt this is a factor, but other possibilities include: the lack of provision of hot food at night so that there is a reliance on sandwiches, etc.; the tendency to nibble rather than take full meals; the higher intake of carbohydrate, caffeine and alcohol; and the higher consumption of tobacco. All of these changes have been observed in night workers and might play some role in increasing the prevalence of gastrointestinal disorder [33].

Even though the traveller suffering from jet lag and the night worker share some symptoms and the causes for them, the plight of the night worker is far worse than that of the traveller. First, the changes can continue throughout the individual's working life since, every time the shift changes, another change of routine and a temporary mismatching between routine and internal clock will occur. Second, there will always be social pressures to adjust to a 'normal' existence during holidays and rest days and even during work days. That is, unless the individual is a social 'loner' or part of an isolated community in which night work is the norm, there will be conflicting social zeitgebers [34]. Therefore, the observation that circadian rhythms adjust slowly and only partially to night work is not surprising. By contrast, during days of rest, when a normal routine is adopted, *all* zeitgebers will constrain to adjust rhythms to a normal pattern of nocturnal sleep and diurnal activity. In summary, adjustment to night work is slow but loss of adjustment during days of rest is far more rapid [35].

Differences between night workers

Workers are not equal when the difficulties associated with night work are considered. The persistence of fatigue, the development of gastrointestinal ulcers in susceptible individuals and continuing social pressure are some of the reasons why a proportion of workers 'drop out' from night work, particularly when they reach the fifth decade of their lives [36]. Can those who might be particularly susceptible to the adverse effects of night work be identified so that they can be counselled appropriately?

There are certain groups who would be advised to think very carefully before performing night work and require careful medical advice [37].

Epileptics
Epileptics are susceptible to seizures when fatigued and so cumulative sleep loss should be avoided. It is possible that a rapid rotation of shifts is desirable, since the cumulative sleep loss will be less in this circumstance (see later).

Asthmatics and those with respiratory disorders
Allergic reactions to house dust, etc., are often worse overnight and bronchial sensitivity is greatest then; irritants in the work place will exacerbate the position.

Diabetics and others with chronic medication
A problem for all who regularly take drugs is the interpretation of instructions such as 'three times per day with meals', 'once a day on rising' etc. if their schedules are continually being changed. In particular, a diabetic's insulin regimen will be very difficult to judge accurately with irregular mealtimes and for this reason he would be advised against shift work in general. As a further example, arthritic pain is often worse in the morning, due in part to a lack of the anti-inflammatory agent, cortisol, during the previous few hours. In such cases, some other anti-inflammatory agent (e.g. indomethacin) is often taken at night, when cortisol concentrations are low, to reduce pain on waking. With a changed sleep/activity schedule, should the patient be advised to take the medication always before bedtime or try to take it instead at a time coincident with the trough of his plasma cortisol rhythms? and, if the latter advice is given, by how much will his cortisol rhythm have adjusted to the changed schedule on any particular day?

There is also evidence that the efficacy of medication may vary according to the time of day that it is administered. Even though this new field of chronopharmacology is based mainly upon work performed with animals, the results are beginning to apply to man also and the occupational physician should be aware of the possibilities (see also Chapters 2 and 12).

For most of the work force such counselling would not be relevant, of course. However, as already mentioned, some of the work force ultimately leaves night work due to the difficulties they experience with it. It would be useful to be able to identify these individuals early in their careers so that they could be forewarned. At the present time no reliable predictive tests are known, but some differences between workers who are tolerant or intolerant of night work have been described [37–42].

Age
Aging is associated with a decreased tolerance to shift work. This might reflect some change in the individual's physiology or (see later) in his perception of night work [40].

The phasing of circadian rhythms
Body temperature and other rhythms are not phased identically in all individuals. In a small proportion of the population – the 'tails' of a normal distribution – rhythms rise earlier in the morning and fall earlier in the evening. Such individuals – 'larks' or 'morning types' – are better able to go to sleep and get up early and so are more suited to the morning shift (or to an eastward flight). By contrast 'owls', or 'evening types' – with slightly delayed rhythms when compared to most of us – are better suited to night work, since they are more likely to be able to stay asleep and so get sufficient sleep after having gone to bed at about 07:00 h. They also adjust more readily to a westward flight (see, for example, ref. [39]).

Amplitude
Individuals with circadian rhythms of an amplitude that is higher than average are more tolerant of shift work [43]. The reason for this is unknown but it has been suggested that such high amplitudes might result in a day-to-day stability of the phasing of rhythms and that this is desirable. However, since any rhythm is the sum of endogenous and exogenous components, the high amplitude might result,

instead or in addition, from a *stability of habits*. This point will be taken up again later.

Psychological make-up
Studies have indicated that certain psychological characteristics – such as flexible (rather than inflexible) sleeping habits and the ability (rather than a lack of it) to overcome drowsiness – are found more frequently in those who are tolerant of night work. In practice, these differences imply that those who can sleep at 'unusual' times are advantaged and that the individual who, having been woken up during a daytime sleep, turns over and tries to go back to sleep, is at an advantage compared with another who loses his temper at having been disturbed! [38,41,42].

The role of experience
Presumably the lifestyles of experienced night workers can be expected to provide information as to how to tackle successfully the problems involved. However, there is a methodological problem. The experienced group is self-selected, since those who have suffered most adverse effects will have decided to leave night work. Therefore any better adjustment to night work that might be measured in experienced workers need not be an indication that the process of adjustment becomes easier with practice, but might indicate instead that those individuals who remain have learned how to deal with night work and that there has been a loss from the sample of those who, for whatever reason, had greater problems with adjustment. Even so, when experienced night workers are considered, a fairly common finding is that the individual puts the requirements of night work above those of a conventionally timed social life [44]. This has been called commitment or motivation. For example, in one study, those nurses who coped best with night work put their need for sleep above social considerations, whereas those who coped least well had the opposite priorities. In another study, nurses who worked three or more nights in succession adopted a regular routine of meals (including one during their night work) and took naps in the afternoon before their first night shift. By contrast, those who took night work less seriously tended to show less regular routines and appeared to skimp on regular nocturnal meals and the amount of diurnal sleep [45].

Advice on shift rotas and means to adjust to them

We have considered and explained the problems that are associated with night work together with those factors that appear to affect the ease with which an individual can adjust to it. On the basis of this we can offer advice with respect to the least troublesome types of shift schedule involving night work and the means by which a worker can best deal with his particular schedule (see, for example, ref. [46]). In many cases, the worker would be advised to make use of appropriate zeitgebers as was the case with travellers across time zones or with individuals in isolated environments (above).

Permanent night work
If night work is permanent then as much adjustment to it as possible is advised. This requires the individual to be highly motivated or committed to the work pattern. Such motivation will be manifest in a variety of ways, but in general it

will require a regular and 'abnormal' time to be set aside for sleep each day which will intrude upon conventional social hours. Facilities for uninterrupted daytime sleep – in a quiet and darkened room – should exist. If sleep immediately after night work is found to be difficult, then attempting sleep at about 14:00 h – at a time when most people feel tired temporarily – might be useful. The chronic use of hypnotics is not recommended nor is the use of alcohol as its diuretic action will cause sleep to be interrupted by a full bladder. It is also desirable to adjust one's working regimen as much as possible and have a cooked meal at 'lunch-time', that is in the middle of the night.

Such a regimen is easier to adhere to if it is practised also by colleagues or acquaintances – or at least if they accept the necessity of it. It is also beneficial if there are no strong time cues which indicate the abnormal timing of the behaviour of the individual. If conditions are such that daytime sleep is poor and so a substantial cumulative sleep loss is likely, then this should be minimized by working only a limited number of nights (say, 3–5) before having rest days [47]. Where possible, during days off between night shifts the worker should not revert fully to a 'normal' diurnal lifestyle and there is a role here for daytime naps which will maintain at least some of the sleep at the same time as during night work. There is some evidence [48] that circadian rhythms would be stabilized at a phasing appropriate for night work by the use of such an anchor sleep. Perhaps the main point is that the requirements of work should take priority over those of a conventionally timed social life.

Rotation of shifts

If shifts are rotated, then the sequence 'morning shift, evening shift, night shift' is preferable to that of 'evening shift, morning shift, night shift'. The reason is that the internal clock, with an inherent period greater than 24 h, will better adjust to hours of work becoming later than earlier, for the same reason that adjustment to a westward time-zone transition is more rapid than to an eastward journey [46,49]. There is also the general rule that days off should be taken after night work so that any cumulative sleep loss can be made up before other shifts are worked.

When the speed of rotating shifts is considered, the problems of cumulative sleep loss and social disruption are potentially most marked when a slow rotation of shifts is involved. A worker in this case will benefit greatly from colleagues, friends and a family who understand and accept the difficulties. On the other hand, a slow rotation of shifts does give the greatest opportunity for adaptation (see above), even though this is never likely to become complete.

Where a weekly rotation of shifts is practised, this does not give enough time for rhythms to adjust much but it does raise the issue of social acceptability. For many people, long stretches of night work are undesirable but weekly stretches less so. Further, the unit of social planning is often the week, with special importance being attached to the regular occurrence of weekends, 'wash days' etc. [34]. Many prefer a weekly rotation of shifts for these reasons.

At the other extreme to permanent night work are the 'Continental' or 'Metropolitan' systems by which shifts rotate frequently, every 1 or 2 days. In such circumstances, adjustment is not possible. Accordingly, the advice would be to stabilize one's rhythms to a 24-h period (and so remain *unadjusted* to night work) and to achieve this by observing a regular diurnally orientated routine whenever possible. Such a regular routine also reduces the tendency for an individual to become temporally disorientated, a problem sometimes associated with the rapid rotation of shifts (as well as work in the ICU, see above). It will be realized that, with a rapid rotation of shifts, on every occasion that night work is being performed, circadian rhythms will be phased appropriately for sleep. This might have a deleterious effect upon performance on the night shift, especially if tasks are repetitive or require prolonged concentration (see later).

The length of shifts
There has been a trend recently towards 12-h shifts; these are normally divided between night and day shifts. The 12-h night shift raises the question what are the effects of prolonged work hours? If work with considerable physical effort is involved then 12-h shifts will be particularly tiring [47]; as far as performance at mental tasks is concerned, this will be dealt with later.

The 'ideal' night worker

Even though we can reasonably assume that no night worker wishes to suffer from the effects of night work, where a choice exists, an individual's decision whether or not to undertake it is often influenced far more by the advantages of financial reward, promotion, positions of responsibility than by any physiological considerations. For most workers, there are some stages of their lives when these other factors are seen as outweighing any social and physiological disadvantages. Such a stage is liable to be reached in the early years of married life, when the home and family are being set up and extra money and status are welcome. There is even a small group of workers, often single and socially independent, who *choose* night work because of the blocks of days off associated with it and the use that can be made of these in pursuing hobbies, such as fishing, in less crowded circumstances than are available to the day worker at weekends. At other stages of one's career, such as before marriage and when the family is beginning to leave home, the social disadvantages of night work dominate. Moreover, as the worker grows older so the physiological problems tend to increase (see above) and become an ever-increasing factor in the decision whether or not to continue night work.

For those who are working at night, much of the advice can be assimilated into a model that describes a committed or motivated night worker. He or she will accept the changes in lifestyle that are involved and attempt to make use of the advantages it offers rather than be irked by the disadvantages. As has been found with experienced night workers, this will require a dedication to work rather than conventional social life, or at least require social activities to be shared with others in a similar predicament. This dedication will manifest itself also as a regular lifestyle with regard to times of sleep, mealtimes and times for chores such as shopping and appointments. These regular influences have been called 'personalized zeitgebers'. Such regularity will also act as a strong exogenous component, increasing the amplitude of the circadian rhythms and so helping to stabilize circadian rhythms to a 24-h period. The details of such a lifestyle will require experiment, of course, but will come with experience. Such a model would be of use to those who work for long spells on night work since they could phase personalized zeitgebers in such a way that they could promote adjustment to night work. In connection with this, the use of appropriately timed bright lights has recently been suggested [50]. The model could also help to stabilize to a 'normal' 24-h day the rhythms of those on rapidly rotating shift systems.

Such advice cannot remove the difficulties, but can only attempt to minimize them. Some will find ultimately that the problems are greater than any advantages, and will choose to stop night work; others will have to do so due to ill health. It is a consolation to know that those who leave night work through ill health tend to find a regression of some of their symptoms and no worsening of others.

Performance decrement

Performance can be below normal values for many reasons [51,52]. When altered sleep/wake schedules are considered, the main reasons are likely to be because an individual is working (a) during the trough of his circadian rhythms (see above), (b) when he is sleep-deprived or (c) for long duty periods. The amount of decrement will also show interindividual variation [53]. We will consider these circumstances after having described means by which performance can be assessed.

Measuring performance

Interest must necessarily be concentrated upon changes that might occur in the performance of 'real tasks' (in some industrial process, for instance) and how these changes might reflect circadian rhythmicity or the effects of fatigue (see ref. [54] Figure 10.3). Studies are rare; undoubtedly this is a reflection of the difficulty of combining work for an employer with a scientific investigation. Even if access to the work place is allowed, then considerable difficulties exist when detailed assessment of performance are investigated. For example, it can be very difficult to make quantitative assessments of performance, as can be illustrated by considering the processes of decision-taking in business, of driving a vehicle or of judging some critical stage in a complex industrial process. Furthermore, any decrements that are measured during a particular shift might be due to changes in the type of task, the workload or external circumstances rather than to changes in the ability of the individual. Some of the problems that are involved can be simply illustrated by considering interpretive difficulties that arise if a difference in the accident rate between night-time or daytime driving had been measured.

In an attempt to overcome these problems, psychologists have tried to measure performance by devising a variety of 'simple' tests [55,56]. These can be of equal difficulty, the conditions under which they are given can be standardized throughout the 24 h and how well the task is performed can be assessed objectively. The exact nature of the task that is given can be varied and with it the relative importance of reaction time, of short-term memory, vigilance, or the throughput of information that is required; the tasks can also concentrate upon different combinations of sensory or motor components or the central processing of information.

These tests have shown that, provided that the short-term memory component of the task is not high, performance tends to parallel changes in body temperature or plasma adrenaline (though this parallelism need not indicate causality [57]). Decrements of performance at night in the order of 5–15% of the 24-h mean are found in many types of test. An exception to this general finding of a parallelism between performance and temperature is that of tasks involving a high short-term memory load, such as remembering a meter reading long enough to feed it into a computer or write it on a report sheet [55,56]. In such cases better performance is associated with lower body temperature, nocturnal performance outdoing that in the daytime. The implication of this is that, while rhythms are not adjusted to night work, some tasks will be performed *better* on the night shift. There is some evidence that such memory-loaded tasks adjust rapidly to a change of sleep/activity schedule; so the 'advantage' of night work is, unfortunately, short-lived [58,59].

The extent to which performance as assessed by these tests reflects that encountered in the work place is uncertain. Several attempts have been made to decrease the differences between laboratory-based tests and 'real' tasks. Some examples are as follows (see ref. [19] for more details).

1. Technological advances that have led to miniaturization and increased portability of instruments have been used, so that a test originally devised for a laboratory environment has been applied in field conditions. For example, sets of computer-based tests can be presented on site, and the results from them stored for a later full analysis in the laboratory.
2. More complex tasks have been devised that combine several elements of the 'simple' tests described above. For example, tracking a moving target might be supposed to combine considerable sensory and motor components.
3. Groups or batteries of tasks can be required to be performed simultaneously or sequentially, often in circumstances that necessitate decisions as to how best to apportion the available time to be taken.
4. In aviation and road transport research there has been the development of highly sophisticated simulators.

In broad terms these different approaches have produced results that are similar to each other and agree with those from studies performed in the work place or with simple laboratory-based tests. In summary, even if the exact relationship performance at 'real' tasks and artificial tests is not clear, this must not blind us to the usefulness of such work which does give at least some quantitative assessment of performance in the field.

Sleep loss and the role of naps

Performance is generally poor at times coincident with the trough of the deep body temperature (see above) but sleep loss can produce further decrements. The extent of this further decrement will depend on the type of task and the psychological state of the individual. The decrement is most marked for simple repetitive tests and those that require vigilance, and often less so for complex tasks that require thought and consideration [60–63].

The deterioration in performance seems to be a function of the total amount of sleep that has been lost and so will occur whether the loss is due to the partial or complete loss of a single night's sleep or to a succession of sleeps of reduced length. This last finding is of particular significance for night workers who attempt sleep in the daytime when sleep length is decreased (see above). Subjects who have lost sleep are also more liable to show 'lapses' or 'gaps' – occasions when performance at a particular task is temporarily suspended while they appear to take a 'microsleep'. Further, the possibility of 'sleep paralysis' increases, a condition in which the individual, though awake, is unable to move or speak for some minutes [64].

The type of task and the subject's response to it affects the amount of decrement due to sleep loss; thus an individual's response to an interesting and challenging task is more robust than to one that is boring or repetitive. For this reason, decrements in performance will not inevitably follow sleep loss and this is believed to apply particularly with some 'real' tasks and in some circumstances in the field. For example, in emergencies, effects of sleep loss can be overcome but it must be remembered that, by contrast, in monotonous circumstances, early indications of a potential emergency are likely to be missed. Emotional worries (which can distract the individual) or a noisy environment are also believed to impair performance, particularly at tasks requiring vigilance. Thus a balance seems to be required between a monotonous environment and bored individual on the one hand and an overstimulating environment and distracted individual on the other [51].

Performance deteriorates also with increasing time spent at a particular task, again repetitive tasks and those requiring vigilance suffering most [60,65]. This is of particular significance when 12-h shifts are considered.

These factors are additive and so the decrement in performance of an individual who is at the trough of his circadian rhythm (about 04:00 h), has slept badly (e.g. is working night shifts), has been on duty for some time (say more than 6 h) and has performed the same repetitive task or one requiring vigilance throughout his duty span is likely to be substantial.

The advantage of being able to take short sleeps or naps when the opportunity presents itself has been mentioned already [38] and, as a means of combating sleep loss, has been stressed by some [66]. In general, short sleeps or naps considerably ameliorate the performance decrements that would arise from a combination of prolonged hours, working during the circadian trough and cumulative sleep loss [67,68]. Both laboratory and field investigations support this view but there are some other factors to bear in mind.

1. Unless sleep loss is marked, there will be some times when it is more difficult to fall asleep than others (see above).
2. It is possible that naps taken at different times during the 24 h and in different circumstances (amount of noise, for example) are not equally effective in decreasing an individual's sensation of fatigue and his performance decrement [67,69].
3. Immediately after waking from a nap, performance might be *poorer* than before the nap (sleep inertia) and even *worsen* for some minutes before showing the improvement indicated above [69]. The size of such effects might depend upon the sleep stage from which an individual has been woken but this temporary decrement is over by about 12 min after waking. In practice, therefore, the time it takes to dress is ample for any deleterious effects of a nap to have worn off, but there might be a problem in the circumstance when a worker naps 'on site'.

In summary, naps seem to be useful for recuperation after a long work span, a valuable means to 'top up' daytime sleep and so guard against the effects of cumulative sleep loss and a method for stabilizing or adjusting circadian rhythms. Not surprisingly, therefore, there has been considerable interest in the possibility that hypnotics could be used to facilitate sleep at unconventional times [70]. Several problems are associated with this use. One is that many hypnotics have an initial rate of uptake that is too slow or that their metabolites have too long a half-life, so that performance is depressed the next day. Conversely, a metabolic rate that is too rapid is unsuitable for maintaining sleep. Other difficulties are that some hypnotics appear to be more effective with subjects of certain ages or when given in the night rather than in the daytime. Also, residual effects after naps rather than longer sleeps have not yet been fully investigated and whether the long-term use of hypnotics for night workers should be encouraged is a separate issue, of course. Alcohol is unsuitable, since its effects last too long, it is addictive and there are undesirable side and cumulative effects. Even so there is anecdotal evidence that it is widely used by night workers to initiate sleep.

However, a few words of caution. When the subject of performance decrement is considered it must be realized that the exact relationship between decrements in performance such as have just been described and accidents or gross errors of judgement is not clear [71]. For example, when the occurrence of aircraft and industrial accidents is considered it is clear that many factors other than circadian rhythms and fatigue must be involved [72,73]. Nevertheless, the potential difficulties associated with a decrease in performance should be understood together with the stress that an individual might suffer when attempting to perform effectively under circumstances when a decrement would be predicted. In addition, it is obviously important that individuals should not fall asleep whilst on duty. In connection with this, recent interest has been shown in the possibility of assessing when an individual appears to be entering into sleep [74]; alternatively, devices are being tested that indicate when a person has fallen asleep (see ref. [75] for example).

References

1. Richardson, G.S., Coleman, R.M., Zimmerman, J.C., Moore-Ede, M.C., Derwent, W.C. and Weitzman, D. Chronotherapy: Resetting the circadian clocks of patients with delayed sleep phase insomnia. *Sleep*, **4**, 1–21 (1981)
2. Moldofsky, H., Musisi, S. and Phillipson, E.A. Treatment of a case of advanced sleep phase syndrome by phase advanced chronotherapy. *Sleep*, **9**, 61–65 (1986)
3. Wever, R.A. *The Circadian System of Man: Results of Experiments under Temporal Isolation*, Springer-Verlag, New York (1979)
4. Chiba, Y. A school-refuser: his rest activity rhythm involved multiple circadian components. *Chronobiologia*, **11**, 21–27 (1984)
5. Wirz-Justice, A. Light and dark as a "drug". In *Progress in Drug Research* (ed. U.A. Mever), Birhaeuser Verlag, Basel, pp. 1–46 (1987)
6. Lewy, A.J. and Newsome, D.A. Different types of melatonin circadian secretory rhythms in some blind subjects. *J. Clin. Endocrinol. Metab.*, **56**, 1103–1107 (1983)
7. Tokura, H. and Hirose, F. Circadian rhythm of rectal temperature in the blind. *J. Interdiscipl. Cycle Res.*, **16**, 187–191 (1985)
8. Moog, R., Endlich, H., Hildebrandt, G. and Martens, H. Circadian rhythms in blind persons. In *Chronobiology and Chronomedicine* (eds G. Hildebrandt, R. Moog and F. Raschke), Peter Lang, Frankfurt, pp. 439–441 (1987)
9. Lewy, A.J., Wehr, T.A., Goodwin, F.K., Newsome, D.A. and Markey, S.P. Light suppresses melatonin secretion in humans. *Science*, **210**, 1267–1269 (1980)
10. Keep, P.J. Stimulus deprivation in windowless rooms. *Anaesthesia*, **32**, 598–600 (1977)
11. Keep, P., James, J. and Inman, M. Windows in the intensive therapy unit. *Anaesthesia*, **35**, 257–262 (1980)
12. Campbell, I.T., Bell, C.F., Minors, D.S. and Waterhouse, J.M. A preliminary study of body temperature rhythms on intensive care. *Chronobiologia*, **10**, 114 (1983)
13. Minors, D.S. and Waterhouse, J.M. Development of circadian rhythms in infancy. In *Scientific Foundations of Paediatrics* (eds J. Davis and J. Dobbing), Heinemann, London, pp. 980–997 (1981)
14. Campbell, I.T., Minors, D.S. and Waterhouse, J.M. Are circadian rhythms important in intensive care? *Intensive Care Nursing*, **1**, 144–150 (1986)

15. Mann, N.P., Haddow, R., Stokes, L., Goodley, S. and Rutter, N. Effect of night and day on preterm infants in a newborn nursery: randomised trial. *Brit. Med. J.*, **293**, 1265–1267 (1986)
16. Lewy, A.J., Sack, R.L., Miller, L.S. and Hoban, T.M. Antidepressant and circadian phase-shifting effects of light. *Science*, **235**, 352–354 (1987)
17. Arendt, J. and Marks, V. Physiological changes underlying jet lag. *Brit. Med. J.*, **284**, 144–146 (1982)
18. Wegmann, H.M. and Klein, K.E. Jet-lag and aircrew scheduling. In *Hours of Work. Temporal Factors in Work-Scheduling* (eds S. Folkard and T.H. Monk), Wiley, Chichester, pp. 263–276 (1985)
19. Minors, D.S. and Waterhouse, J.M. Circadian rhythms and aviation. *Aviat. Med. Q.*, **1**, 9–26 (1987)
20. Folkard, S. Our diurnal nature. *Brit. Med. J.*, **293**, 1257–1258 (1986)
21. Klein, K.E. and Wegmann, H.M. *Significance of Circadian Rhythms in Aerospace Operations*, AGARDograph no. 247, NATO-AGARD Neuilly-sur-Seine (1980)
22. Daan, S. and Lewy, A.J. Scheduled exposure to daylight: a potential strategy to reduce "jet-lag" following transmeridian flight. *Psychopharmacology Bull.*, **20**, 566–568 (1984)
23. Graeber, R.C., Sing, H.C. and Cuthbert, B.N. The impact of transmeridian flight on deploying soldiers. In *Biological Rhythms, Sleep and Shift Work* (eds L.C. Johnson, D.I. Tepas, W.P. Colquhoun and M.J. Colligan), MTP Press, Lancaster, pp. 513–553 (1981)
24. Reinberg, A., Smolensky, M. and Labreque, G. The hunting of a wonder pill for resetting all biological clocks. *Annu. Rev. Chronopharmacol.*, **4**, 171–208 (1988)
25. Arendt, J., Aldhous, M. and Marks, V. Alleviation of jet lag by melatonin: preliminary results of controlled double blind trial. *Brit. Med. J.*, **292**, 1170 (1986)
26. Moore-Ede, M.C. and Richardson, G.S. Medical implications of shift-work. *Annu. Rev. Med.*, **36**, 607–617 (1985)
27. Rutenfranz, J., Haider, M. and Koller, M. Occupational health measures for nightworkers and shiftworkers. In *Hours of Work. Temporal Factors in Work-scheduling* (eds S. Folkard and T.H. Monk), Wiley, Chichester, pp. 199–210 (1985)
28. Akerstedt, T. Adjustment of physiological circadian rhythms and the sleep–wake cycle to shiftwork. In *Hours of Work. Temporal Factors in Work-scheduling* (eds S. Folkard and T.H. Monk), Wiley, Chichester, pp. 185–198 (1985)
29. Akerstedt, T. and Gillberg, M. The circadian variation of experimentally displaced sleep. *Sleep*, **4**, 159–169 (1981)
30. Waterhouse, J.M., Minors, D.S. and Scott, A.R. Circadian rhythms, intercontinental travel and shiftwork. In *Current Approaches to Occupational Health 3* (ed. A. Ward Gardner), Wright, Bristol, pp. 101–118 (1987)
31. Kumar, D., Wingate, D. and Ruckebusch, Y. Circadian variation in the propagation velocity of the migrating motor complex. *Gastroenterology*, **91**, 926–930 (1986)
32. Lenzi, R., Cecchettin, M., Galvan, P., Poggini, G., Cariddi, A., Benvenuti, M. and Tarquini, B. Serum gastrin and pepsinogen (PGI) in foundry shiftworkers. *Chronobiologia*, **21**, 255–256 (1985)
33. Folkard, S., Minors, D.S. and Waterhouse, J.M. Chronobiology and shiftwork: Current issues and trends. *Chronobiologia*, **12**, 31–54 (1985)
34. Walker, J. Social problems of shiftwork. In *Hours of Work. Temporal Factors in Work-scheduling* (eds S. Folkard and T.H. Monk), Wiley, Chichester, pp. 211–226 (1985)
35. Knauth, P., Rutenfranz, J., Herrmann, G. and Poeppl, S.J. Re-entrainment of body temperature in experimental shift-work studies. *Ergonomics*, **21**, 775–784 (1978)
36. Frese, M. and Semmer, N. Shiftwork, stress, and psychosomatic complaints: a comparison between workers in different shiftwork schedules, non-shiftworkers, and former shiftworkers. *Ergonomics*, **29**, 99–114 (1986)
37. Minors, D.S., Scott, A.R. and Waterhouse, J.M. Circadian arrhythmia: shiftwork, travel and health. *J. Soc. Occup. Med.*, **36**, 39–44 (1986)
38. Folkard, S., Monk, T.H. and Lobban, M.C. Towards a predictive test of adjustment to shiftwork. *Ergonomics*, **22**, 79–91 (1979)
39. Hildebrandt, G. Survey of current concepts relative to rhythms and shift work. In *Chronobiology:*

Principles and Application to Shifts in Schedules (eds L. Scheving and F. Halberg), Sijthoff and Noordhoff, Alpen aande Rijn, Netherlands, pp. 261–275 (1980)

40. Kerkhof, G. Individual differences in circadian rhythms. In *Hours of Work. Temporal Factors in Work-scheduling* (eds S. Folkard and T.H. Monk), Wiley, Chichester, pp. 29–36 (1985)

41. Monk, T.H. and Folkard, S. (eds) Individual differences in shiftwork adjustment. In *Hours of Work. Temporal Factors in Work-scheduling*, Wiley, Chichester, pp. 227–237 (1985)

42. Moog, R., Hauke, P. and Kittler, H. Interindividual differences in tolerance to shift work related to morningness/eveningness. In *Biological Adaptation* (eds G. Hildebrandt and H. Hensel), Georg Thieme Verlag, Stuttgart, pp. 95–103 (1982)

43. Reinberg, A., Andlauer, P., DePrins, J., Malbecq, W., Vieux, N. and Bourdeleau, P. Desynchronization of the oral temperature circadian rhythm and intolerance to shiftwork. *Nature (London)*, **29**, 185–196 (1984)

44. Adams, J., Folkard, S. and Young, M. Coping strategies used by nurses on night duty. *Ergonomics*, **29**, 185–196 (1985)

45. Minors, D.S. and Waterhouse, J.M. Circadian rhythms in deep body temperature, urinary excretion and alertness in nurses on nightwork. *Ergonomics*, **28**, 1523–1530 (1985)

46. Rutenfranz, J. Occupational health measures for night- and shift-workers. *J. Human Ergol.*, **11**, (suppl.) 67–86 (1982)

47. Andlauer, P., Rutenfranz, J., Kogi, K., Thierry, H., Vieux, N. and Duverneuil, G. Organization of night shifts in industries where public safety is at stake. *Int. Arch. Occup. Environ. Hlth*, **49**, 353–355 (1981)

48. Minors, D.S. and Waterhouse, J.M. Anchor sleep as a synchronizer of rhythms in abnormal routines. *Int. J. Chronobiol.*, **7**, 165–188 (1980)

49. Czeisler, C.A., Moore-Ede, M.C. and Coleman, R.M. Rotating shiftwork schedules that disrupt sleep are improved by applying circadian principles. *Science*, **21**, 460–463 (1982)

50. Eastman, C.I. Bright light in work–sleep schedules for shiftworkers: application of circadian rhythm principles. In *Temporal Disorder in Human Oscillatory Systems* (eds L. Rensing, U. an der Heiden and M.C. Mackey), Springer-Verlag, New York, pp. 176–185 (1987)

51. Craig, A. Field studies of human inspection: the application of vigilance research. In *Hours of Work. Temporal Factors in Work-scheduling* (eds S. Folkard and T.H. Monk), Wiley, Chichester, pp. 199–210 (1985)

52. Davies, D.R. Individual and group differences in sustained attention. In *Hours of Work. Temporal Factors in Work-scheduling* (eds S. Folkard and T.H. Monk), Wiley, Chichester, pp. 123–132 (1985)

53. Monk, T.H. and Leng, V.C. Interactions between inter-individual and inter-task differences in the diurnal variation of human performance. *Chronobiol. Int.*, **3**, 171–177 (1986)

54. Minors, D.S. and Waterhouse, J.M. *Circadian Rhythms and the Human*, Wright, Bristol (1981)

55. Folkard, S. and Monk, T.H. (eds) Circadian performance rhythms. In *Hours of Work. Temporal Factors in Work-scheduling*, Wiley, Chichester, pp. 37–52 (1985)

56. Monk, T.H. The arousal model of time of day effects in human performance efficiency. *Chronobiologia*, **9**, 49–54 (1982)

57. Wilkinson, R.T. The relationship between body temperature and performance across circadian phase shifts. In *Rhythmic Aspects of Behaviour* (eds F.M. Brown and R.C. Graeber), Lawrence Erlbaum Associates, Hillsdale, NJ, pp. 213–240 (1982)

58. Monk, T.H. and Folkard, S. (eds) Shiftwork and performance. In *Hours of Work. Temporal Factors in Work-scheduling*, Wiley, Chichester, pp. 239–252 (1985)

59. Monk, T.H., Knauth, P., Folkard, S. and Rutenfranx, J. Memory based performance measures in studies of shiftwork. *Ergonomics*, **21**, 819–826 (1978)

60. Borland, R.G., Rogers, A.S., Nicholson, A.N., Pasco, P.A. and Spencer, M.B. Performance overnight in shiftworkers operating a day–night schedule. *Aviat. Space Environ. Med.*, **57**, 241–249 (1986)

61. Colquhoun, W.P. (ed.) *Biological Rhythms and Performance*, Academic Press, London (1971)

62. Froberg, J.E. Sleep deprivation and prolonged work hours. In *Hours of Work. Temporal Factors in Work-scheduling* (eds S. Folkard and T.H. Monk), Wiley, Chichester, pp. 67–75 (1985)

63. Webb, W.B. and Levy, C.M. Effects of spaced and repeated total sleep deprivation. *Ergonomics*, **27**, 45–58 (1984)
64. Folkard, S., Condon, R. and Herbert, M. Night shift paralysis. *Experientia*, **40**, 510–512 (1984)
65. Minors, D.S., Nicholson, A.N., Spencer, M.B., Stone, B.M. and Waterhouse, J.M. Irregularity of rest and activity: studies on circadian rhythmicity in man. *J. Physiol.*, **381**, 279–295 (1986)
66. Nicholson, A.N. Sleep and wakefulness of the airline pilot. *Aviat. Space Environ. Med.*, **58**, 395–401 (1987)
67. Naitoh, P. Circadian cycles and restorative power of naps. In *Biological Rhythms, Sleep and Shiftwork* (eds L.C. Johnson, D.I. Tepas, W.P. Colquhoun and M.J. Colligan), MTP Press, Lancaster, pp. 553–580 (1981)
68. Nicholson, A.N., Pascoe, P.A., Roehrs, T., Roth, T., Spencer, M.B., Stone, B.M. and Zorick, F. Sustained performance with short evening and morning sleeps. *Aviat. Space Environ. Med.*, **56**, 105–114 (1985)
69. Dinges, D.F., Orne, E.C., Evans, F.J. and Orne, M.T. Performance after naps in sleep-conducive and alerting environments. In *Biological Rhythms, Sleep and Shiftwork* (eds L.C. Johnson, D.I. Tepas, W.P. Colquhoun and M.J. Colliagn), MTP Press, Lancaster, pp. 539–552 (1981)
70. Nicholson, A.N., Roth, T. and Stone, B.M. Hypnotics and aircrew. *Aviat. Space Environ. Med.*, **56**, 299–303 (1985)
71. Green, R.G. Stress and accidents. *Aviat. Space Environ. Med.*, **56**, 638–641 (1985)
72. Gerbert, K. and Kemmler, R. The causes of causes: determinants and background variables of human factor incidents and accidents. *Ergonomics*, **29**, 1439–1453 (1986)
73. Wojtczak-Jaroszowa, J. and Jarosz, D. Chronohygienic and chronosocial aspects of industrial accidents. In *Advances in Chronobiology, Part B. Progress in Clinical and Biological Research* (eds J.E. Pauly and L.E. Scheving), Alan R. Liss, New York, Vol. 227B, pp. 415–426 (1987)
74. Akerstedt, T., Torsvall, L. and Gillberg, M. Sleepiness in shiftwork. A review with emphasis on continuous monitoring of EEG and EOG. *Chronobiol. Int.*, **4**, 129–140 (1987)
75. Gardner-Medwin, A.R. Device to prevent vehicle drivers falling asleep. *J. Physiol.*, **371**, 22P (1985)

Chapter 12

Preclinical and clinical cancer chronotherapy

W.J.M. Hrushesky, R.v. Roemeling and R.B. Sothern

Introduction

For more than 5000 years, traditional Chinese medicine has recognized that the concept of dose cannot possibly be isolated from the concept of timing. Thus the treatment modality or dose for the same ailment or disease may differ, depending upon the time of day, day within the week, the menstrual cycle stage or the season. Western physicians first met to consider time-dependent differences in physiology and therapy in 1937 at Ronneby, Sweden. Properties of rhythms have been repeatedly addressed in animals beginning several decades ago [1–4]. Although timing of a therapeutic intervention may profoundly affect a patient's outcome, it has not generally been effectively approached in clinical situations.

The most frequently used xenobiotic anticancer drugs are either substantially less toxic or more effective at certain circadian stages. In most instances, such drugs are both less toxic and more effective at a given circadian stage. In the near future, genetically engineered biological response modifiers and growth factors may play a primary role in the treatment of the most frequently occurring solid tumours. These new therapeutic tools may prove to be severalfold more circadian-stage dependent than the most highly time-dependent xenobiotics in terms of toxicity and anticancer activity resulting from systemic administration [5]. Proper circadian timing will therefore be of growing, rather than diminishing, importance as we learn to use these agents. An entirely independent, yet related, literature extensively documents the sequence and interval dependence of both xenobiotic (especially antimetabolite) and biological therapies. As we use an increased number of agents and more complex drug combinations, optimal drug timing will depend, in part, upon sophisticated drug administration systems. Chronotherapy delivered by this advanced technology may result in profound changes in the practice of medicine [6–8].

The search for therapeutic selectivity is most critical when life-threatening diseases are treated and when the drugs used have life-threatening toxicities [9]. This problem of narrow therapeutic index occurs in every field of medicine. However, it is nowhere more prominent than in cancer treatment. Anticancer agents affect all tissues, whether or not they are malignant. A balance between excessive toxicity in the host and for the cancer must be preserved when administering cytostatic treatments. For most drugs, dose–response curves have been established for the susceptibilities of both tumour cells and rapidly renewed cells of normal host tissues, yet limited host tolerance remains a major cause of treatment failure, intensive and frequent administration of chemotherapeutic agents (which could be accomplished by continuous infusion) may be necessary to increase tumour cell cure and to minimize the probability of drug-resistant cell clones. Furthermore, small increases (5–10%) in dose intensity (amount of drug delivered per unit of time) have been clearly shown to result in disproportionately larger increases in cure rate or degree of cancer control for Hodgkin's Disease, ovarian cancer, breast and colon cancer [10–13].

It is known that complex metabolic processes, including those involved in cellular proliferation of both healthy and tumour tissues and the malignant transformation of cells, are characterized by biological rhythms along daily, monthly, annual or other time scales [14]. These rhythms affect the cellular susceptibility to cytotoxic agents and their pharmacokinetics, metabolism and excretion [15] (for further discussion see also Chapters 2 and 13). Rhythmic variations in observable end points will result from interaction of many component rhythms, including cell cycles and endocrine and immunological rhythms. In the example given in Figure 12.1, the circadian time of best and worst drug tolerance differs between host and tumour, whereas the quantitative difference between peak and trough, and the rhythm frequency is the same. Such differences between normal and malignant cells could be used to increase the differential cell kill by drug timing.

Preclinical chronotoxicological studies have investigated whether mice or rats tolerate the same dose of the same anticancer agent differently depending upon

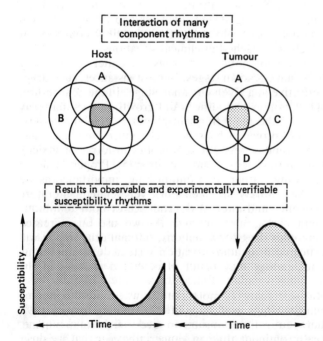

Figure 12.1 The anatomy of susceptibility rhythms observed in circadian studies may be dissected into several components, noted by the four spheres, each of which influences the frequency and amplitude of overall response. A desirable goal is to dissociate host and tumour susceptibility rhythms, as shown, in order to maximize desired therapeutic effect and minimize undesired toxicity. A, Cell cycle rhythm; B, drug absorption activation, cellular uptake, metabolism and excretion; C, overlying hormonal rhythm affecting drug toxicity; D, immunological rhythms

when it is given during a 24-h span. Survival rate and mean survival time were the most widely used end points to evaluate the effect of dosing time upon chronotolerance. Organ-specific measures of lethal and sublethal toxicity have also been thoroughly investigated for many agents.

Initial clinical chronotherapy trials have focused upon time-related differences in drug toxicity in cancer patients and were modelled from preclinical studies. The purpose of these clinical studies in patients with metastatic bladder or ovarian cancer was to reduce treatment-related toxicity and complication rates by optimal circadian timing, allowing high-dose intensity treatment to be administered safely and effectively.

To date, the toxicity and antitumour activity of some most commonly used chemotherapeutic agents (doxorubicin, cisdiamminedichloroplatinum, 5-fluoro-2-deoxyuridine (FUDR), 5-fluorouracil (5-FU] have now been documented as circadian-stage dependent in human beings [16–18]. The following sections summarize preclinical and clinical trials in Minnesota, initially with a combination of doxorubicin and cisplatin, followed by studies with FUDR.

Preclinical animal results

Doxorubicin (adriamycin) and cisplatin

The following studies were performed to investigate whether optimal circadian timing of a commonly used and highly active two-drug combination (doxorubicin and cisplatin) could reduce drug toxicity and increase treatment efficacy of a solid tumour model.

In a series of six chronotoxicity experiments with doxorubicin performed between September 1973 and May 1975, it was found that deaths of male CD_2F and BD_2F mice occurred in a time-dependent circadian rhythmic pattern following a potentially lethal overdose at one of six 4-hourly test times around the clock (Figure 12.2) [19]. When survival rate was summarized at 50% overall mortality, there were most survivors in the group given doxorubicin in the middle of the daily 12-h light (rest) span and fewest in the group treated in the middle of the daily 12-h dark (activity) span.

Initial chronotherapeutic studies performed in 1974 revealed that the rate of tumour shrinkage following doxorubicin treatment of a transplanted plasmacytoma of rats was circadian-stage dependent. When animals housed in LD12:12 were treated with doxorubicin in the middle of their daily light (resting) span, fastest shrinkage occurred [20–22]. Time-dependent synergistic effects of doxorubicin and cisplatin were then demonstrated, with the reduction of both tumour size and the rate of renal excretion of the tumour marker, Bence-Jones protein [23]. In these preliminary studies, however, the drugs were tested concomitantly in rats at one of only two circadian stages (late-light and late-dark). Animals treated with cisplatin alone or in combination with doxorubicin died more quickly than untreated animals or those treated with doxorubicin alone, indicating that the dose of cisplatin (6 mg/kg) used was too high. Despite the dosing problem, time-dependent differential toxicity was clearly observed. Animals treated in late-light tolerated the drug treatment far better than those injected in late-dark. The primary cause of death in these studies was bone marrow toxicity of the anthracycline.

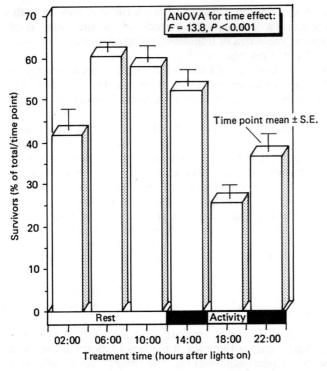

Figure 12.2 Circadian rhythm in toxicological effect of doxorubicin delivered to more than 800 male and female CD_2F_1 and BD_2F_1 mice at six different circadian stages (>130 mice/test time) in six separate studies. At 50% overall mortality, most mice were alive following treatment in the middle of their daily light (resting) span and fewest were alive if treated in the middle of their daily dark (activity) span

Two additional studies followed up on these earlier investigations, using lower doses of doxorubicin and cisplatin to test drug effects upon the host and tumour at six (rather than two) different circadian stages. The purpose of these experiments was to investigate whether circadian drug timing optimized the ability of the doxorubicin–cisplatin combination to cure cancer in a murine model. Study 1 was primarily designed to test the effect of doxorubicin as a single agent at each of six different circadian stages. By contrast, Study 2 was designed to test the effect of doxorubicin administered only at its best circadian time in combination with cisplatin at one of six different circadian stages, in order to find the most effective circadian-timed combination of these drugs. These studies are described in detail to increase awareness of the extent of control necessary for experimental chronobiological research.

Study 1
On March 21, 1977, 188 inbred LOU rats of both sexes, ranging in age from 5 to 30 weeks (median age = 17 weeks) received a subcutaneous inoculation of 0.1 cc of plasmacytoma tumour on their shaved back right flank. The plasmacytoma was selected because its tumour cell proliferation is associated with the urinary excretion of light chains which exhibit a circadian rhythm both in LOU rats and

in human beings with multiple myeloma [24,25]. Forty-eight inbred LOU rats in the same age range served as placebo-inoculated controls. All rats were singly housed in two separate sound-dampened windowless rooms that contained equal numbers of rats with temperature maintained at $24 \pm 1\,°C$, relative humidity at ~50%, and food and water available *ad libitum*. Fluorescent lights were on for 12 h and off for 12 h daily. All rats were conceived, born and raised under these standardized environmental conditions, assuring rigid synchronization of body rhythms to the light/dark schedule.

Seventeen days after tumour or placebo inoculation (when all tumours of the tumour-inoculated rats were palpable), six subgroups of rats stratified by age, weight, sex and tumour size were randomly assigned to order of treatment. A single dose of doxorubicin only (5 mg/kg, i.p.) was given at one of six circadian stages (02:00, 06:00, 10:00, 14:00, 18:00 and 22:00 *H*ours *A*fter *L*ights-*O*n, HALO). Weight, tumour size (length × width, measured by a vernier caliper) and rectal temperature (using a Yellow Springs probe) were recorded immediately prior to drug injection. These weekly measurements on each rat were repeated at precisely the same circadian times to assess drug-induced tumour and whole-body weight responses and to investigate the quality of continued group circadian synchronization to the light/dark regimen.

Three weeks after initial treatment with doxorubicin, the treatment time point associated with optimal doxorubicin-induced tumour shrinkage was determined (10 HALO). Of the surviving 147 tumour-bearing rats, 106 were then redistributed across the six test times, with each test time receiving equal representation from the previous six subgroupings. Cisplatin (2 mg/kg, i.p.) was then administered to these newly stratified subgroups of rats at one of six equi-spaced time points. Four days later, doxorubicin (3 mg/kg, i.p.) was given at 10 HALO, the circadian stage identified as most effective in shrinking tumours. After 2 weeks, a second combination cisplatin–doxorubicin treatment course identical to the first was given. Cisplatin administration time was always the same for any individual animal. In addition to the combination cisplatin–doxorubicin treatment groups, 20 tumour-bearers received doxorubicin only (without cisplatin) and 21 tumour-bearers received cisplatin only (without doxorubicin). Twenty-six tumour-bearing rats were untreated to establish reference limits of survival time and tumour growth rate, while 24 rats received neither tumour nor drug to serve as healthy untreated controls for body weight and temperature measurements.

Study 2
On May 19, 1978, 282 inbred LOU rats of both sexes, ranging in age from 3 to 44 weeks (median age = 22 weeks) were housed, stratified and randomized under conditions identical to Study 1, except that only one periodicity room was used. The lighting regimen provided a daily 8-h light span (rather than 12 h) and 16 h of dark (D) during each 24-h span, starting on the day of tumour inoculation. This LD8:16 schedule was selected in order to more closely mimic the spans of rest and activity for human beings. Other studies have shown that both LD12:12 and LD8:16 light/dark schedules yield similarly timed circadian rhythms in numerous variables, when light onset is used as time reference [26]. Tumour inoculation occurred at the identical circadian stage, i.e. from 8 to 10 HALO for both studies. Of the Study 2 rats 215 were inoculated with tumour. Rats were divided among four planned treatment groups 12 days after inoculation, when all animals displayed a palpable tumour. One group (*n* = 41) was given only cisplatin (2 mg/

kg), a second group ($n = 10$) received only doxorubicin (4 mg/kg), a third group ($n = 148$) received both cisplatin and doxorubicin, while the fourth group was not treated ($n = 16$). Five tumour-free rats served as treatment-only controls and received doxorubicin only, while two groups of 25 tumour-free rats received either cisplatin only or in combination with doxorubicin. In this study, cisplatin was given at one of six circadian stages, whereas doxorubicin was restricted to only 10 HALO. The same treatment regimen was repeated in each group, 2 weeks after the first treatment course.

Analyses

All rats were checked daily for mortality in both studies. Measurements of tumour size, body weight and body temperature continued at weekly intervals around the clock until the end of the study. Numerical data were analysed by classical statistical procedures of analysis of variance (ANOVA) and chi square. Survival duration and duration of remission were evaluated by Kruskal-Wallis life table methods. Chronobiological analyses involving the least-squares fit of a 24-h cosine were also performed to estimate the characteristics of circadian rhythms (Chapter 14) [27].

Results

In Study 1, plasmacytoma-bearing male and female LOU rats responded most favourably to the first treatment with doxorubicin when it was administered at 10 HALO on an LD12:12 schedule. Maximal tumour reduction and minimal weight

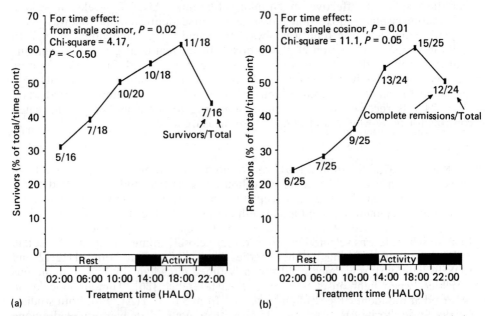

Figure 12.3 Circadian-stage dependence of immunocytoma response to cisplatin when doxorubicin is administered at an optimal time (10 HALO), gauged by survival rate (Study 1; a) and by complete remissions (Study 2; b) in LOU rats

loss were observed in these animals compared to other groups treated at five other circadian stages 4 h apart. The addition of cisplatin resulted in a statistically significant prolongation of life compared to those animals treated with doxorubicin or cisplatin only at optimal circadian stages. More rats survived longer if they were treated with doxorubicin at 10 HALO in combination with cisplatin at 18 HALO (mid-dark) (Figure 12.3a).

Study 2 was performed using lower total doses of both agents. Results corroborated Study 1 findings with detection of a statistically significant circadian rhythm in rate of complete remissions. The therapeutic index was greatest if doxorubicin was given at 10 HALO and cisplatin at 18 HALO (Figure 12.3b).

The relative contribution of drug sequence and the span between administration of these two agents to the schedule-dependent differences in therapeutic index was considered to some degree in these two studies. The pattern of therapeutic advantage across the day was very similar in both studies. However, the sequence of agents, the span between agents and the number of courses were different. Regardless of these schedule differences, the same doses of drug were substantially less toxic to the host and more effective in controlling the cancer when doxorubicin was given late in the daily light span (i.e. just prior to usual awakening) in combination with cisplatin given in mid to late activity (i.e. during the daily dark span for nocturnally active rodents).

The critical importance of timing chemotherapy according to circadian stage to improve desired therapeutic effects and minimize undesired and life-threatening side effects was documented in these studies on over 500 LOU rats. Each chemotherapeutic agent tested, while exhibiting degrees of anticancer activity, had uniquely timed optimal intervals dependent upon circadian stage.

For clinical applications, these preclinical data suggested that administration of doxorubicin and cisplatin be disparate in time by 8–12 h, with doxorubicin given near awakening (i.e. in the early morning at 06:00 h) and cisplatin given 12 h removed (i.e. at 18:00 h for a patient on a usual diurnal schedule, sleeping from 22:00 to 06:00 h). It is critical to emphasize that this suggested timing of doxorubicin and cisplatin is by circadian stage rather than sequence and interval or clock hour [28]. Thus a person on an unusual sleeping schedule (e.g. sleep from 08:00 to 16:00 h if a night worker) would receive these drugs at a different clock hour (e.g. doxorubicin upon awakening at 16:00 h and cisplatin 12 h later at 04:00 h for previous example). Although sleep/wake times can serve as reference time for this chronotherapy, an appropriate marker rhythm (e.g. temperature, urinary potassium) should be monitored before, during and after chemotherapy to confirm sleep/wake synchronization to a given schedule and, thereby, proper circadian-stage timing of the therapy [29,30].

Underlying mechanisms: additional studies

Heart muscle toxicity related to doxorubicin is thought to be secondary to its activation into a free radical intermediate. The availability of the main free radical scavenger, reduced glutathione (GSH), is circadian-stage dependent with peak levels at the time of lowest drug toxicity [15,31]. Tumour response, however, occurs secondary to drug binding to DNA intercalation, and single strand breaks. Circadian changes in cell cytokinetics (e.g. rate of cells in S-phase DNA), as well as tissue-specific differences between tumour and normal organ, may have determined the observed circadian differences in doxorubicin therapeutic index.

Furthermore, circadian changes in drug pharmacokinetics may have influenced the toxicity rhythm.

Not only is normal kidney function circadian-stage dependent (see Chapter 6), but cisplatin pharmacokinetics display this phenomenon as well [32,33]. Pronounced circadian rhythmicity in lethal toxicity from cisplatin was demonstrated in each of a series of eleven studies over a course of about 1 year. Each study entailed injection of six groups of rats with a toxic dose (11 mg/kg) of cisplatin at different circadian stages of an LD12:12 lighting regimen. Animals were subsequently observed for mortality. Cisplatin tolerance was much greater when administered late in the animals' active (daily dark) phase [34]. In addition, mortality resulted from nephrotoxicity, proven by monitoring blood urea nitrogen (BUN) and microscopic section of the severely damaged kidneys. Most extensive kidney damage was in the proximal convoluted tubules. A brush border lysosomal enzyme, N-acetyl-β-glucosaminidase (NAG), was found to be released into the urine in proportion to the degree of renal dysfunction induced by cisplatin. This enzyme was present in urine in normal animals, and its baseline concentration was found to display a high-amplitude circadian rhythm. When cisplatin was given at the time of most toxicity, the circadian rhythm in urinary NAG was maintained, but the mean peak levels increased 5-fold in direct proportion to the subsequent rise in BUN. If cisplatin was given at a favourable circadian stage, NAG did not rise significantly and little renal damage occurred with only a small rise in BUN. In another series of three studies, an intraperitoneal saline load of 3% body weight was given to or withheld from animals with cisplatin concurrently administered at six separate circadian stages [35]. The amount of kidney protection achieved by the fluid load revealed a marked circadian rhythm. A high degree of protection was found when cisplatin or cisplatin plus saline was given to the animals late in their activity span. However, when the hydration and cisplatin treatments were given to the animals at the circadian stages associated with early activity (early dark), less protection was gained from the hydration regimen. These data indicated quite clearly not only that the lethal nephrotoxicity of cisplatin was circadian-stage dependent, but also that the standard method of renal protection (hydration) was circadian-stage dependent in its ability to decrease cisplatin nephrotoxicity.

FUDR

To devise a chronobiologically based infusion schedule for clinical applications, a series of murine experiments was begun in August 1984 to explore whether FUDR toxicity and efficacy were circadian-stage dependent. The purpose was to reduce toxicity of infusional FUDR, allowing increased dose intensity and improved anticancer activity.

In an initial series of three experiments, single-bolus FUDR injections (using doses between 1000 and 2000 mg/kg) were given at either one of three (Study 1) or six equally spaced (Studies 2 and 3) circadian stages to a total of 300 female CD_2F_1 mice standardized to an LD12:12 schedule. Temperature (24 ± 1 °C) and relative humidity (~50%) were held constant in soundproofed windowless rooms with food and water provided *ad libitum*. Animals were followed for survival every 4 h around the clock. Survival varied predictably by more than 50%, depending upon the circadian stage of injection. Treatment during mid-to-late activity (18–20 HALO) was consistently associated with best drug tolerance in all studies [36].

Figure 12.4 shows the differences in long-term survival among six groups of 15

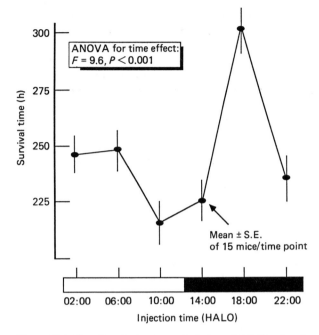

ANOVA for time effect:
$F = 9.6, P < 0.001$

Mean ± S.E.
of 15 mice/time point

Injection time (HALO)

Figure 12.4 Circadian rhythm in survival time of CD_2F_1 mice after a single injection of a lethal dose of FUDR at one of six circadian test times

animals each, treated with 2000 mg/kg FUDR i.v. at one of six circadian stages in Study 3. Probable causes of death were identified in animals by autopsy, careful macroscopic inspections and light microscopy of slides prepared from liver, small bowel, colon and bone marrow. Pathological changes were found in both small and large bowel, explaining diarrhoea and dehydration prior to death. Diffuse necrosis in the liver and bone marrow aplasia were also present. These murine studies clearly indicated that the lethal toxicity of single-bolus FUDR injection is circadian-stage dependent. However, this series of experiments did not address the question whether the same observation could be made after repeated injections at lower doses or after continuous infusion of the drug over prolonged time spans [37].

The toxicity pattern following continuous infusion might be qualitatively and quantitatively different from that of bolus injection. For rapid bolus injection, bone marrow suppression is dose limiting. If given as continuous infusion, less haematotoxicity but more diarrhoea, stomatitis and skin alterations are observed in patients. Nausea and vomiting are common for both administration modes. The longer the duration of the FUDR infusion, the lower the daily dose must be to prevent life-threatening bowel dysfunction. To simulate more closely the clinical situation, where FUDR is continuously infused over prolonged time spans, continuous infusion patterns in 3-month-old female F344 Fischer rats (average weight 195 g) were studied under the same environmental conditions as described for the mice. Continuous infusion was achieved by cannulation of the tail vein with a catheter, using the method described by Danhauser *et al.* [38], so that the rats could tolerate the catheter for at least 1 week without major compromise in their daily activity. Constant-rate (flat) infusion at 1000 mg/kg per 48 h was compared to sinusoidal infusion patterns (two 24-h cycles). The peak of these sinusoidal curves was set at six different circadian stages with 68% of the total daily dose automatically delivered over a 6-h span by programmable Intelliject pump (Intelligent Medicine, Englewood, CO, USA). Rats receiving FUDR either as a sinusoidal infusion with the peak at 4 HALO (maximum rate of infusion between 22 and 4 HALO, during late activity and early rest for nocturnally active animals) or as a constant-rate infusion, lived significantly longer than rats receiving differently timed sinusoidal patterns (Kruskal-Wallis life table analysis: $w = 11.2$; $P < 0.025$). Cosinor circadian rhythm analysis confirmed the early rest phase as the least toxic circadian treatment time ($P < 0.05$; see Figure 12.5). The centre time of best infusional FUDR tolerance was 5–7 h later than in the mouse studies. However, the peak 6-h infusion began in the second half of activity, a time associated with longest survival in the mouse. This time shift may reflect the alteration in the toxicity pattern with less bone marrow and more intestinal toxicity.

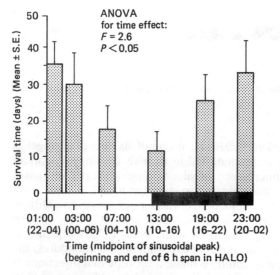

Figure 12.5 Circadian variation observed in survival time of female Fischer rats following 48 h of equal-dose (1000 mg/kg per 48 h) sinusoidal FUDR infusions with the peak infusion rate placed at different circadian stages

The effects of flat FUDR or saline infusion (control) and four equal-dose FUDR sinusoidal infusion patterns (700 mg/kg per 48 h) were also studied on Fischer rats with a transplanted NF 13762 mammary adenocarcinoma tumour. The most active schedule was identical with the least toxic sinusoidal infusion, with peak beginning near the end of activity (22 HALO) and ending in the resting span (4 HALO) (as defined by tumour response rate and overall growth retardation, see Figure 12.6). This series of experiments confirmed that circadian-stage-dependent differences in drug tolerance and efficacy for infusional FUDR depend upon timing of the infusion peak. The toxicity of the best-tolerated sinusoidally shaped infusion with a peak around 4 HALO was not significantly different from that observed after

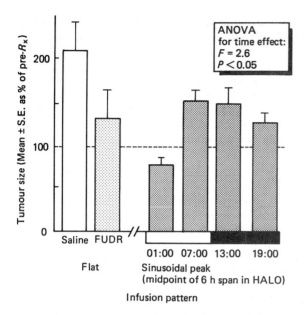

Figure 12.6 Tumour response in female Fischer rats following 48 h of equal-dose (700 mg/kg per 48 h) flat or sinusoidal FUDR infusion with the peak infusion rate placed at different circadian stages

equal-dose constant-rate infusion. However, the antitumour activity for the sinusoidal infusion curve was greater than that for the equally toxic flat infusion. Our studies showed that a variable-rate continuous i.v. FUDR infusion is substantially less toxic and most effective when it is given to rats late in their daily activity span and early in their daily sleep span. Clinical extrapolations from these observations can only be cautiously drawn, in part because the 48-h infusion duration may have been suboptimally brief.

Clinical studies

Doxorubicin and cisplatin for ovarian or bladder cancer

The preclinical results were to serve in the design of a randomized clinical trial of chronochemotherapy in human beings suffering from metastatic ovarian or bladder cancer. The most active drugs for treatment of human cancers are doxorubicin and cisplatin. This drug combination shows an advantage over single-agent therapy for response rate and survival, while dose intensity, at least in part, determines tumour control [39]. However, only about a third of patients with advanced ovarian cancer [defined as metastatic in the abdomen without liver involvement (FIGO* Stage III) or distant metastases and/or liver involvement (Stage IV)] will attain a complete clinical tumour response, while an additional third achieves partial response. Most patients relapse and have median survival times between 10 and 36 months only [40]. These disappointing treatment results render any possible improvement of therapy very urgent.

*International Federation of Gynecologic Oncology

Metastatic bladder cancer is even more difficult to treat effectively than ovarian cancer. However, chemotherapy combinations (including doxorubicin/cisplatin) and schedules have recently emerged that can result in long-lasting complete responses in some patients. Response rates, response durations and survival patterns of the entire patient population have, however, remained unsatisfactory. Higher dosages are associated with better response rates, but also result in substantially increased toxicity. As demonstrated in adjuvant studies, the extent of disease-free survival is improved for chemotherapy-treated patients when compared to those observed following operation without treatment [41].

Chronotherapy with crossover design

The first clinical study tested two different circadian schedules of the same combination of doxorubicin and cisplatin with equal doses, drug sequence and interval for possible pharmacokinetics and toxicity differences in the same patients. More than 100 monthly treatment courses of doxorubicin at $60 \, \text{mg/m}^2$ and cisplatin at $60 \, \text{mg/m}^2$ were studied in 23 patients. This first protocol randomized initial doxorubicin treatment time between 06:00 and 18:00 h for these patients, who maintained a usual sleep/wake schedule with sleep from 22:00 to 06:00 h. Cisplatin followed each doxorubicin infusion by 12 h, with each drug infused for 30 min. A standard vigorous hydration protocol using a total of 4100 cc of normal saline (with 20 meq of KCl per litre) preceded and followed each cisplatin infusion. Antiemetics and diuretics were not used. After initial treatment, the timing of doxorubicin for each subsequent monthly treatment course was alternated between 06:00 and 18:00 h. Thus, the sequence of drugs was crossed over throughout the study. Two patients refused further therapy after the initial treatment. Each of the remaining 21 patients had advanced malignancy, 12 with Stage III and IV ovarian cancer and 9 with metastatic D2 transitional cell cancer of the bladder.

Cisplatin excretion
Pharmacokinetics were studied using an HPLC method for the quantitative identification of urinary cisplatin. The pattern of urinary excretion of cisplatin was examined after 51 courses of $60 \, \text{mg/m}^2$ of this agent. Urine samples were obtained immediately prior to and every 30 min after cisplatin infusion for 4.5 h. It was found that urinary cisplatin kinetics (peak concentration, time to peak, area under the curve) were predictably different depending upon when the drug was infused. Significantly higher concentrations following morning administration were discovered [42,43]. In these same patients, a statistically greater per course drop in creatinine clearance followed morning cisplatin administration compared to evening administration. This difference was most striking following the first course and then diminished as treatment time was alternated. There was either no creatinine clearance decline or a permanent 30% fall following the first dose of cisplatin.

Acute drug toxicity
When doxorubicin was given at 06:00 and cisplatin at 18:00 h, there was less neutropenia and thrombocytopenia compared to doxorubicin given at 18:00 h followed by cisplatin at 06:00 h. The morning doxorubicin schedule resulted in statistically significantly less depressed nadir blood cell counts and in full recovery of all counts to pretreatment levels, usually within 21 days of treatment. The

evening doxorubicin schedule led to less than full recovery, even 28 days after therapy. For the entire group of patients after a total of 50 courses on each circadian schedule, all counts had rebounded to more than 100% of pretreatment value following morning doxorubicin 1 month after treatment, but had not fully recovered after evening treatment. The clinical relevance of these findings is demonstrated by the fact that morning doxorubicin treatment resulted in statistically significantly fewer dose reductions and fewer treatment delays than the opposite circadian drug schedule.

Cisplatin treatment is usually discontinued because the patient refuses to permit further therapy. Severe nausea, vomiting and anorexia are caused in nearly all cases by cisplatin and no antiemetic regimen is available to eliminate this often dose-limiting toxicity totally. Nausea and vomiting were studied quantitatively in 101 courses of combination doxorubicin and cisplatin chemotherapy administered without antiemetics. Cisplatin given at 06:00 h resulted in more vomiting episodes ($P<0.01$), which tended to begin sooner and last longer [9]. In addition, nephrotoxicity, chronic anaemia and transfusion episodes were each statistically significantly different, supporting the schedule of morning doxorubicin and evening cisplatin [41].

Chronotherapy with randomized non-crossover design

In the subsequent protocol, patients were randomized to receive each of the nine planned doxorubicin–cisplatin treatments at fixed times always beginning at 06:00 (morning) or 18:00 h (evening). Circadian Schedule A consisted of morning doxorubicin followed by evening cisplatin, and Schedule B consisted of evening doxorubicin followed by morning cisplatin. This fixed assignment of circadian treatment stage allowed analysis of the effect of drug timing upon all acute and cumulative drug toxicities, as well as the quality of tumour response (partial versus complete response rate), time to response, response duration, patient survival and cure rates.

Cumulative drug toxicity
Complete evaluation of the bone marrow toxicity of the first 37 patients receiving all of nine planned treatments revealed that the circadian stage of chemotherapy administration determines whether or not this combination of drugs induces cumulative bone marrow toxicity. Most patients treated on Schedule B received doxorubicin doses reduced by greater than 33% and many of them experienced treatment delays of more than 2 weeks because of leukopenia, compared to patients on Schedule A. Assessment by linear regression analysis of individual white blood cell decrease and recovery (on days 1, 7, 14 and 28) after treatment revealed more cumulative bone marrow toxicity for the majority of patients treated on circadian Schedule B, despite substantial dose reductions, than for Schedule A [16].

Effect of cancer on circadian time structure
Patients with cancer or another serious illness may not display precisely synchronized circadian rhythms important for determining the extent of drug toxicity. To investigate this premise more thoroughly, circadian rhythm characteristics of body temperature, neutrophil count, lymphocyte count, heart rate, blood

pressure and urinary volume, sodium, potassium and cortisol excretion were studied. These variables were studied in 43 patients prior to 295 separate treatment courses. Creatinine clearance reduction after each treatment was then compared. Least nephrotoxicity was seen when cisplatin was given at 18:00 h as compared to 06:00 h. Urine was collected every 2 h and rate of potassium excretion was determined for 24–48 h prior to each treatment. The circadian rhythm in urinary potassium excretion (expressed as meq per h) was calculated for each course for each individual. The amount of subsequent renal damage was represented by the creatinine clearance determination prior to the next course of treatment. Creatinine clearance results were assigned to a time corresponding to how far removed from the daily potassium peak excretion that patient had, in fact, received cisplatin. Creatinine clearance results were analysed on the basis of when cisplatin was received (0–6 h or 6–12 h before or after the daily peak in potassium excretion). This procedure compared treatment times as gauged by a measure of internal, rather than external, time. Patients treated within 3 h on either side of the span during which their rate of potassium excretion was highest suffered no subsequent loss of renal function. Those patients receiving cisplatin farthest away from the time of highest potassium excretion had an average loss of 8 ml/min in creatinine clearance per treatment course. Inappropriate timing of repeated cisplatin administration resulted in a substantial and preventable loss of kidney function of more than 50%, since the standard treatment course of cisplatin for this group of patients was nine courses of therapy.

Overall toxicity comparison
Toxicity evaluation following each of the 247 treatment courses that could be evaluated consisted of weekly sampling of haemoglobin, total and differential white blood cell count, platelet count and creatinine clearance at 08:00 h. These weekly laboratory values guided dose and schedule modifications, in addition to a monthly interim history and physical examination. Doxorubicin dose modifications or schedule delays were necessitated by three events, namely (1) a recovery (day 28) absolute granulocyte count below 1500 cells/mm^3 or (2) a recovery platelet count under 100 000 cells/m^3 or (3) interim infection or bleeding. If any of these conditions were present, a 25% doxorubicin dose reduction or 1-week treatment delay with subsequent re-evaluation was instituted. Doxorubicin doses were more often reduced if an infection or bleeding complication supravened, and treatment delays were more frequent with a poor recovery of blood cell counts.

Treatment complications were defined as: (1) interim clinical infections requiring oral or parenteral antibiotics; (2) interim bleeding episodes of any kind (whether or not platelet transfusions were administered); and (3) anaemia requiring a transfusion episode (Hb < 8.0 g/dl, or Hct (haematocrit) < 25%, or symptoms related to anaemia). Each transfusion episode usually required administration of two or three units of packed red blood cells. Dose or schedule modifications were not instituted on the basis of nadir counts. Cisplatin was given at full dose unless creatinine clearance fell below 30 ml/min, in which case it was discontinued. The rates of chemotherapy-related toxicity following either treatment schedule were calculated by patient group and treatment course. Rates and kinds of modifications and complications are displayed in Figures 12.7 and 12.8.

Effect of drug timing upon tumour response and patient survival
To test whether drug timing affected tumour control, 63 consecutively diagnosed women (median age 60, range 29–87) with FIGO Stage III (n=46) and IV (n=17)

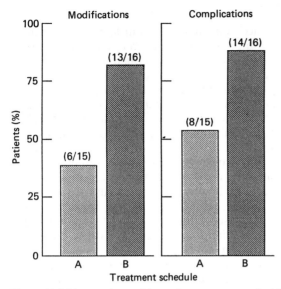

Figure 12.7 More patients with ovarian cancer treated with cisplatin and doxorubicin on Schedule B had to have both dose reductions and treatment delays (6/15 versus 13/16; $\chi^2 = 4.0$, $P<0.05$). Even though more patients on Schedule B had dose and schedule modifications, episodes of infection, bleeding and transfusions each occurred more commonly in patients receiving Schedule B than in those on Schedule A (8/15 versus 14/16; $\chi^2 = 2.9$, $0.10>P>0.05$)

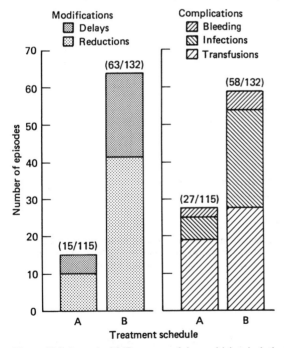

Figure 12.8 A total of 247 courses of doxorubicin–cisplatin therapy were administered to patients with ovarian cancer: 115 on Schedule A and 132 on Schedule B. Dose reductions were three times more frequent when the drugs were given on Schedule B (31% vs 9%, $\chi^2 = 17.4$. $P<0.01$). Despite Schedule B dose reductions and treatment delays, 44% of Schedule B treatments were associated with bleeding, infection, or transfusion requirement, while only 23% of treatment given on Schedule A were associated with these complications ($\chi^2 = 10.5$, $P<0.01$)

epithelial ovarian cancer were treated according to one of four temporal schedules of the same two-drug protocol (60 mg/m² of both doxorubicin and cisplatin every 28 days for 9 months). Of the 63 women, 15 had optimal debulking operations and 48 had bulky disease with residual masses (massive disease of >10 cm masses in 40 patients). The four treatment groups were comparable in terms of patient age, FIGO stage, histological grade of cancer and quality of debulking surgery. Sixteen women had received prior chemotherapy and nine had abdominal pelvic irradiation. The four different treatment schedules were defined as follows: U, doxorubicin and cisplatin administered at unspecified times of day with no consistent sequence or interval between drugs; A, doxorubicin administered at 06:00 h followed 12 h later by cisplatin; B, doxorubicin administered at 18:00 h, followed 12 h later by cisplatin; A/B, monthly alternation of A and B (crossover regimen).

Circadian scheduling significantly increased clinical complete response (CR) rates ($\chi^2 = 38.8$, $P < 0.001$) and survival. Median follow-up of all patients exceeded 67 months (16–105 months). Pathological complete response (PR) rates were also higher with chronobiological administration. All patients treated without drug timing (Schedule U) died within 3 years. Patients receiving Schedule A had a 5-year survival of 50%, exceeded by patients treated with the crossover timing regimen (Schedule A/B). Patients treated on Schedule B had a 5-year survival of 25% (Figure 12.9).

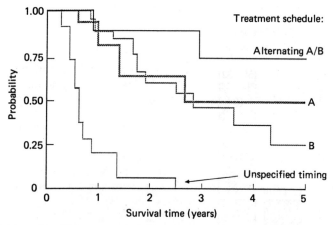

Figure 12.9 Five-year survival time of ovarian cancer patients varied depending on the circadian timing of doxorubicin/cisplatin treatment. This was only in part due to variations in dose intensity. No patient receiving treatment 'as usual' (timing and drug interval unspecified) survived longer than 2.5 years

Treatment-time-dependent differences in dose intensity
Differences in average dose intensity clearly accounted for part of the schedule-dependent difference in patient survival. Mean dose intensity (as % of planned dose) was statistically significantly lower for each agent in Schedule B (80% for doxorubicin and 82% for cisplatin) as compared to Schedule A (94% for doxorubicin and 95% for cisplatin) and the crossover regimen A/B (89% for

doxorubicin and 90% for cisplatin). Patients on Schedule U failed very rapidly, although they received the drugs at the same or higher dose intensity (94% for doxorubicin and 103% for cisplatin) as patients treated with Schedule A or A/B. At first glance, a difference of 10–15% in dose intensity may not appear important. However, the relationship between decrease in dose intensity and decrease in disease control and cure rate is not linear. The work of Hryniuk and others [9,10] demonstrates that a decrease of 10% in dose intensity may result in as much as a 50% decrease in the ability of that regimen to control cancer. Therefore, this statistically significant drop in dose intensity is undoubtedly important to these findings that timing of doxorubicin–cisplatin administration markedly affects patient survival. The observation that unspecified treatment timing results in relatively high dose intensity but poor disease control also requires additional clarification. The dose intensity formula does not consider the possibility of early treatment failure. It is clear from reviewing the mean number of courses for patients receiving unspecified treatment time that early failures occurred far more frequently, as compared to those receiving time-specified treatment. In fact, the mean number of treatment courses in this group is only slightly more than three, whereas eight to nine treatment courses were given using all time-specified treatment regimens. The other conclusion to be drawn about dose intensity and circadian timing is that although dose intensity is important in determining the success of a combination of treatment for controlling cancer, there may also be effects of timing that are separate from and additive to dose intensity effects. In summary, it is clear that dose intensity can be maximized by appropriate circadian treatment timing, resulting in prolongation of patient survival in advanced ovarian cancer.

Chronotherapy of metastatic bladder cancer
The same two-drug combination of doxorubicin and cisplatin was given to patients with transitional cell carcinoma of the bladder (TCCB). Patients were randomized to receive the drugs at a dose of 60 mg/m^2 each in monthly courses according to Schedule A or Schedule B as described previously. Forty-three consecutively diagnosed patients with widely metastatic cancer received up to nine monthly courses of the two-drug combination followed by cyclophosphamide and 5-fluorouracil concurrently with cisplatin as maintenance for up to 2 years. Of the 35 patients that could be evaluated, 57% responded objectively and 23% displayed complete clinical response. Median survival from the first treatment for complete responders was more than 2 years and for partial responders was 1 year. Of the complete responders, three were alive without evidence of cancer more than 2 years after cessation of all therapy.

   This chronotherapeutic approach allowed safe application of high-dose intensity treatment. The stipulations covering the order of the drugs, interval between them and the circadian time may have been favourable factors for this treatment's success, which compares very favourably to other chemotherapy regimens currently reported. The fact that three patients with biopsy-proven metastatic TCCB were removed from all therapy without disease recurrence may augur the eventual chemotherapeutic curability of this disease, which has not been previously possible. Unfortunately, the numbers of patients per treatment group did not permit interpretation of schedule-dependent differences in drug efficacy. However, Schedule A was superior to Schedule B, resulting in lower toxicity despite higher dose intensity.

Adjuvant bladder cancer chronotherapy
Finally, the same two-drug combination was given to 16 patients with TCCB who received chronotherapy monthly either on Schedule A or Schedule B immediately after radical cystectomy. Cancer had penetrated through the serosa of the bladder wall into the perivesical fat (stage C) in five patients and had metastasized further to other pelvic organs and pelvic lymph nodes (stage D1) in 11 patients. Of these 16 patients, 11 showed no recurrence of the disease after a median follow-up time of 3.5 years (range: 1–>5.5 years). Of the five patients who ultimately failed, two had local tumour recurrence that developed much later than usual (at 37 and 42 months). The circadian-timed drug regimen (given as adjuvant treatment in full doses for nine courses) delayed and possibly prevented local and distant recurrence of the stage C and D1 bladder cancer, expected in more than 90% of patients within 2 years of the surgery [44]. Similar differences in schedule-dependent toxicity were observed, but again the number of patients per treatment was too low to test properly for differences in antitumour activity. To enhance testing, accrual continues in clinical studies involving metastatic ovarian cancer and transitional cell cancer of the bladder.

FUDR: programmable automatic pumps

Therapeutic index may be improved if certain drugs are given by long-term infusion. Automatic drug-delivery systems are required to facilitate this infusional therapy. Programmable pumps may automatically vary the flow rate over time and allow chronotherapy with a maximum and minimum drug flow during specified time periods. We have recently discovered that infusional intravenous FUDR is an effective treatment for progressive metastatic renal cell carcinoma [45]. FUDR has mainly been used via hepatic arterial infusion. This treatment is clinically indicated in cases in which the primary or metastatic disease is confined to the liver. The following studies aimed to define optimally safe and effective schedules of infusional intravenous FUDR in order to make this therapy more widely available to patients with kidney cancer.

After the implantable Medtronic pump (Medtronic Inc., Minneapolis, MN, USA) became available in 1985, the application of time-modified treatment

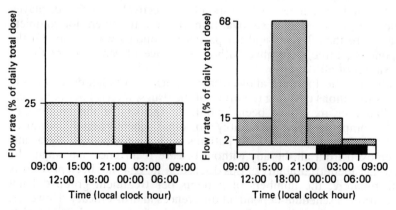

Figure 12.10 Scheme of flat (a) vs sinusoidal (b) continuous FUDR infusional patterns. Note that the AUC for each pattern is equivalent

schedules to cancer patients could be started on an outpatient basis. Serial 14-day courses of FUDR followed by 14 days of rest were given to 100 patients with metastatic adenocarcinomas (28 colorectal, 48 kidney, 7 pancreatic, 17 other) either by constant-rate infusion or by continuous time-modified infusion.

When malignancy was confined to the liver, hepatic arterial infusion (HAI) was given; all other cases received intravenous infusion, with either constant flat-rate (CI) or sinusoidal (SI) patterns and with 68% of the daily dose given between 15:00 and 21:00 h (Figure 12.10). This choice of a daily 6-h dose division was an arbitrary estimation of the best way to divide the dose which corresponded precisely to what had been done in the preclinical rat studies.

Toxicity and dose intensity
Constant-rate hepatic arterial infusion resulted in significantly more severe toxicity for both routes as compared to sinusoidal infusion. Following HAI in 38 patients (19 flat vs 17 time-modified), the incidence of chemical cholestasis was 66 vs 31% and jaundice was observed in 24 vs 0%. Gastrointestinal toxicity was likewise more frequent and more severe after flat infusion (nausea 63 vs 18%; vomiting 47 vs 12%; diarrhoea 26 vs 0%; toxicity-related hospital admissions 16 vs 6%) and cholangitis occurred earlier (after 3.8 vs 6.0 months, on average). In those patients receiving flat-rate HAI, the mean dose intensity had to be markedly reduced in patients due to toxicity, but was maintained for those patients receiving time-modified infusion (see Figure 12.11).

Toxicity following i.v. infusion in 30 patients was virtually an all-or-none phenomenon, depending upon the infusion pattern. At equal dose intensity, the rates of nausea and vomiting were 50 vs 19% and diarrhoea 43 vs 6% for flat ($n=14$) vs sinusoidal ($n=16$) infusion. Because of toxicity 21 vs 0% of the patients had to be hospitalized. Time-modified sinusoidal infusion permitted higher FUDR dose intensity. For i.v. FUDR infusion, the mean dose intensity could be increased

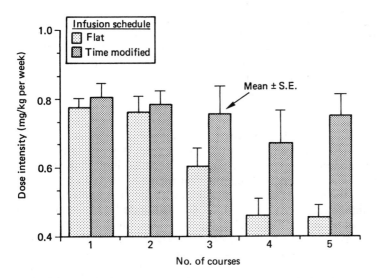

Figure 12.11 Flat vs time-modified continuous intra-arterial (IA) FUDR: Mean dose intensity per course

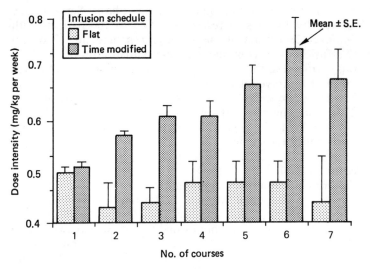

Figure 12.12 Flat vs time-modified intravenous (i.v.) FUDR: Mean dose intensity per course

substantially on the time-modified schedule, but had to be reduced due to toxicity for constant flat-rate infusion (see Figure 12.12).

In a subgroup of 28 patients with colon cancer metastatic to the liver, objective tumour responses [determined by computer tomography and substantiated by reduction in carcinoembryonic antigen (CEA) levels] were observed in 50% of both patient groups receiving flat-rate intra-arterial (i.a.) FUDR or time-modified i.a. FUDR. A complete response was seen in a single case (flat-rate infusion). More patients need to be studied, and the median observation time must be extended to compare flat- and variable-rate infusion for tumour response duration and survival.

Among the patients treated with infusional FUDR, there were 48 cases with proven progressive measurable metastatic renal cell cancer (RCC) (7 females, 41 males, ages 36–73), 38% of whom had received previous systemic therapy. Forty-two patients received programmable Medtronic pumps for automatic drug delivery and six patients received Infusaid pumps. Forty-two patients had i.v. infusion. Because RCC was limited to the liver in six cases, these patients were given hepatic i.a. therapy. FUDR was continuously infused for 14 days at monthly intervals at starting doses of 0.15 mg/kg per day i.v. or 0.25 mg/kg per day i.a., which were escalated and de-escalated in increments of 0.025 mg/kg per day as permitted by toxicity. As expected, abdominal pain, diarrhoea and mucositis limited the i.v. CI, whereas malaise, anorexia and hepatic function abnormalities limited i.a. CI.

Time modification of the infusion shape (sinusoidal with the peak centred around 18:00 h) virtually eliminated toxicity of i.v. CI. Mean tolerated dose intensity of time-modified i.v. infusion was 0.55 ± 0.02 mg/kg per week, which is twice that of constant-rate infusion, as found in a previous study and described by others [46,47]. In 47 patients evaluated for response who had had at least two courses, five complete, seven partial and five minor responses were observed. Only nine of the 47 patients had objective tumour progression (none of the responders). Objective responses have been durable; one complete response has lasted longer than 1 year

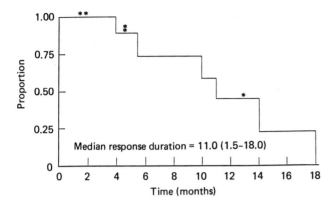

Figure 12.13 Objective response duration for patients with metastatic renal cell carcinoma receiving sinusoidal continuous FUDR infusion. Since all patients did not enter the protocol on the same date, asterisks represent patients who have survived up to the point indicated (in months) without a relapse and are still being followed

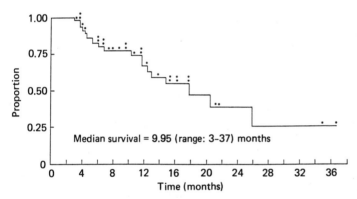

Figure 12.14 Survival duration for patients with metastatic renal cell carcinoma receiving sinusoidal continuous FUDR infusion. Since, as in Figure 12.13, all patients did not enter the protocol on the same date, asterisks represent patients who have survived up to the point indicated (in months) and are still being followed. Thus 29 patients were still alive at the months indicated on the time scale

(6 months off therapy) (see Figure 12.13). Twenty-four (50%) of the 48 patients are alive at the 16-month median follow-up span (see Figure 12.14). Further chronobiological optimization of the treatment schedule might result in a truly effective chemotherapy regimen for this usually chemotherapy-refractory disease [48].

Discussion

The ability to detect and quantify meaningful biological rhythms is a precondition to the improvement of therapeutic index by optimal circadian drug timing [49].

Rhythmic changes in normal organ function relating to drug susceptibility have been studied extensively in murine models. DNA synthesis, RNA synthesis, RNA translational activity, mitotic index, weight, glycogen content and the activity of numerous enzymes in the mouse and rat liver have all been shown to be circadian rhythmic [50]. The liver's detoxification potential of various drugs, including para-oxon, nicotine, antimycin A, phenobarbital, hexobarbital and cytosine arabinoside [51–53], has also revealed substantial circadian-stage dependence.

Rhythmic changes at the cellular and subcellular level will certainly affect drug pharmacokinetics and, indeed, circadian rhythmicity in drug pharmacokinetics has been described for 5-fluorouracil, cisdiamminedichloroplatinum (cisplatin), oxali-platin, methotrexate, 6-mercaptopurine and doxorubicin [42,43,53–55] (R.v. Roemeling, unpublished results). At the whole organ level, it has also been shown that kidney function exhibits circadian rhythmicity, which determines renal toxicity and the excretion pattern of certain drugs [7] (see also Chapters 2 and 6). At the cellular level, we have shown that the reduced glutathione (GSH) content of murine heart muscle cells, determining the redox potential and salvage from free oxygen radicals, maintained significant circadian rhythmicity [31]. At the subcellular level, circadian rhythmicity has also been demonstrated for mitotic index and DNA synthesis of rat and mouse stomach, duodenum, rectum and bone marrow [56,57]. It is known that some of these rhythms can be predictably shifted, but not eliminated, by changing the lighting regimen or feeding pattern of the animals [58–60]. In addition, hepatic regeneration in rats after partial hepatectomy showed a rhythmic circadian pattern which could be shifted by altering the lighting schedule [61].

Another focus of attention has been whether or not tumour cells proliferate rhythmically. Many transplantable tumours and some spontaneously arising ones in the laboratory rodents have been studied around the clock for mitotic index and/or DNA synthesis. Data on a rapidly or slowly growing hepatoma have shown that tumour cell division exhibits a more or less strong circadian organization, depending upon the stage of tumour growth, with earlier-stage tumours (prior to the development of necrosis) more tightly tied to host circadian time structure than later-stage malignancies [62]. Results with other experimental tumours support the hypothesis that well-differentiated slow-growing tumours may retain a circadian time structure, whereas poorly differentiated, fast-growing tumours tend to lose this rhythmicity. Such a loss of circadian rhythmicity may also be acquired along the course of tumour growth [63].

Data on rhythms of proliferation in normal and human neoplastic cells are documented, but are relatively scarce, primarily because of ethical problems involved in frequent tissue sampling in human beings. However, rhythmic activity of most normal organ functions can be indirectly concluded from almost all laboratory tests, which express more or less strong circadian rhythmicity [64,65]. This rhythmic activity has also been directly documented in many normal human tissues and cells, and such rhythms may have a significant impact on drug pharmacodynamics [66–78].

Mitotic index, DNA synthesis and temperature measurements in cancerous lesions and normal tissues have been measured frequently and periodicities determined. Large interindividual differences, as well as inter- and intra-tumour differences in circadian organization and resultant chronopharmacological effect may be present in malignant tissues. These differences are related to tumour stage and grade, and performance status of the host [15].

Haus et al. [79] reported in 1972 that chemotherapy schedules adjusted to circadian rhythms result in better drug tolerance and greater efficacy for arabinosylcytosine in leukaemic mice. Experimental evidence documenting and extending the critical importance of circadian timing of cytotoxic treatment has been steadily and rapidly accumulating for three decades [80]. At certain circadian stages, the most common anticancer drugs have been proven to be substantially less toxic or more effective, or both, at certain circadian stages. Optimal timing may differ from drug to drug, which has been shown even when two drugs differ by a few atoms or by arrangement of precisely the same molecular structure [22,81].

More recently, genetically engineered biological response modifiers and growth factors have entered clinical trials. They provide a broader basis for hope in the fight against solid tumours most commonly afflicting human beings. Chronobiological studies initially revealed that these new therapeutic tools are several times more dramatically circadian-stage dependent in terms of toxicity and anticancer activity [5].

Careful extrapolation from extensive preclinical investigations has allowed design of time-qualified clinical treatment schedules using FUDR and the combination of doxorubicin and cisplatin. Such optimal drug timing resulted in less toxicity, higher dose intensity, improved tumour control and increased patient survival. Similar clinical studies performed elsewhere confirm and emphasize the importance of circadian drug timing [82].

Since the extent of host tolerance for each anticancer agent tested in human beings differed markedly as a function of its dosing time, the extension of circadian-timed therapy is logical [83]. Circadian monitoring of marker variables must be considered and developed because interindividual differences may determine host chronotolerance and to some extent tumour susceptibility [34,35,84,85].

Complex drug timing schedules are only feasible if automatic programmable delivery systems are available. Devices with one or multiple reservoirs (each reservoir independently complexly programmable, with many steps completely coordinated by the program) can now be used for optimized chronotherapy [86,87]. Closed-loop systems may eventually become available in which delivery of each drug or hormone is determined by an array of physiological signals sensed by the device and fed through algorithms determining the appropriate dose, dose timing, sequence of the agents, and span between pulses or patterns of these agents [8].

Only a few metastatic solid tumours can be cured by chemotherapy alone. Most malignancies are primarily chemotherapy-resistant or will develop resistance. This is particularly true for the more frequently occurring cancer types. The currently available tools must be rendered more powerful by careful consideration of circadian drug timing, mode, route, drug sequence and intervals to maximize dose intensity, reduce host toxicity and minimize natural and acquired drug resistance.

Numerous preclinical studies have documented that the therapeutic index of anticancer drugs can be significantly improved, if those drugs are given at optimal circadian stages. These optimal application times may differ between drugs and may also depend upon the mode of drug administration (e.g. bolus injection versus continuous infusion). Careful extrapolations from these studies have now resulted in the first clinical studies showing improved antitumour activity and reduced toxicity, even at higher dose intensity, achieved by chronotherapy. Improved cancer control is urgently needed because of the disappointing treatment results following conventional therapy approaches in the most frequently occurring metastatic human cancer types.

Chronotherapy offers an opportunity to break the vicious circle of insufficient therapeutic selectivity, tumour cell resistance and subsequent treatment failure. Advanced technology now allows the administration of chronotherapy automatically and safely.

Acknowledgements

Preclinical trials with doxorubicin–cisplatin were performed in the laboratory of Professor Franz Halberg, who is also acknowledged for his guidance and suggestions. The authors are most indebted to Mr Todd Langevin and Jeffrey Rabatin for help with the clinical data base and to Ms Terri Wurscher, who provided invaluable help in preparation of this manuscript. This work was supported by a grant NIH R02 31635 to W.J.M.H.

References

1. Halberg, F. Temporal coordination of physiologic function. *Cold Spring Harbor Symp. Quant. Biol.*, **25**, 289–310 (1960)
2. Aschoff, J. Exogenous and endogenous components in circadian rhythms. *Cold Spring Harbor Symp. Quant. Biol.*, **25**, 11–28 (1960)
3. Pittendrigh, C.S. Circadian rhythms and the circadian organization of living systems. *Cold Spring Harbor Symp. Quant. Biol.*, **25**, 159–184 (1960)
4. Hastings, J.W. Biochemical aspects of rhythms: phase-shifting by chemicals. *Cold Spring Harbor Symp. Quant. Biol.*, **25**, 131–143 (1960)
5. Langevin, T., Young, J., Walker, K., Roemeling, R., Nygaard, S. and Hrushesky, W.J.M. The toxicity of tumor necrosis factor (TNF) is reproducibly different at specific times of the day. *Proc. AACR*, **28**, 398 (1987)
6. Scheving, L.E., Halberg, F. and Ehret, C.E. *Chronobiotechnology and Chronobiological Engineering*, NATO ASI Series E: Applied Sciences No. 120, Martinus Nijhoff, Dordrecht, 453 pp. (1987)
7. Hrushesky, W.J.M. The clinical application of chronobiology to oncology. *Amer. J. Anat.*, **168**, 519–542 (1983)
8. Hrushesky, W.J.M. The rationale for non-zero-order drug delivery systems (chronotherapy). *J. Biol. Resp. Mod.*, **6**, 587–598 (1987)
9. Focan, C. Chronobiologie et marqueurs biochimiques du cancer humain. *Pathol. Biol.*, **35**, 951–959 (1987)
10. Hryniuk, W.M., Levine, M.N. and Levin, L. Analysis of dose intensity for chemotherapy in early (stage II) and advanced breast cancer. *NCI Monogr.*, **1**, 87–94 (1986)
11. Levin, L. and Hryniuk, W. The use of dose intensity (DI) to solve problems in gynecologic oncology. *Proc. ASCO*, **6**, 119 (1987)
12. Longo, D.L., Young, R.C., Wesley, M., Hubbard, S.M., Duffey, P.L., Jaffe, E.S. and DeVita, V.T. Jr. Twenty years of MOPP therapy for Hodgkin's disease. *J. Clin. Oncol.*, **4**, 1295–1306 (1986)
13. Scheving, L.E. Chronobiology of cell proliferation. In *Biological Rhythms and Medicine* (eds A. Reinberg and M. Smolensky), Springer Verlag, New York, pp. 79–130 (1983)
14. Scheving, L.E. Chronobiology of cell proliferation. In *Biological Rhythms and Medicine* (eds A. Reinberg and M. Smolensky), Springer Verlag, New York, pp. 79–130 (1983)
15. Levi, F., Halberg, F., Nesbit, M., Haus, E. and Levine, H. Chrono-oncology. In *Neoplasma – Comparative Pathology of Growth in Animals, Plants and Man* (ed. H. Kaiser), Williams and Wilkins, Baltimore, pp. 267–316 (1981)
16. Hrushesky, W.J.M. Circadian timing of cancer chemotherapy. *Science*, **228**, 73–75 (1985)

17. Roemeling, R., Mormont, M.-C., Walker, K., Olshefski, R., Langevin, T., Rabatin, J., Wick, M. and Hruschesky, W. Cancer control depends upon the circadian shape of continuous FUDR infusion. *Proc. AACR*, **28**, 1293 (1987)
18. Peters, G.J., Van Dijk, J., Nadal, J.C., Van Groeningen, C.J., Lankelma, J. and Pinedo, H.M. Diurnal variation in the therapeutic efficacy of 5-fluorouracil against murine colon cancer. *In Vivo*, **1**, 113–118 (1987)
19. Sothern, R.B., Nelson, W.L. and Halberg, F. A circadian rhythm in susceptibility of mice to the anticancer drug, adriamycin. In *Proc. XIIth Int. Conf. Int. Soc. Chronobiol.*, Washington D.C.. Il Ponte, Milano, Italy, pp. 433–438 (1977)
20. Good, R.A., Sothern, R.B., Stoney, P.J., Simpson, H.W., Halberg, E. and Halberg, F. Circadian state dependence of adriamycin-induced tumor regression and recurrence rates in immunocytoma-bearing LOU rats. *Chronobiologia*, **4**, 174 (1977)
21. Halberg, F., Gupta, B.D., Haus, E., Halberg, E., Deka, A.C., Nelson, W., Sothern, R.B., Cornelissen, G., Lee, J.K., Lakatua, D.J., Scheving, L.E. and Burns, E.R. Steps toward a cancer chronopolytherapy. In *Proc. XIVth Int. Congr. Therapeutics*, Montpellier, France, L'Expansion Scientifique Francaise, Paris, pp. 151–196 (1977)
22. Sothern, R.B., Halberg, F., Good, R.A., Simpson, H.W. and Grage, T.B. Difference in timing of circadian susceptibility rhythm in murine tolerance of chemically-related antimalignant antibiotics: adriamycin and daumomycin. In *Chronopharmacology and Chronotherapeutics* (eds C.A. Walker, C.M. Winget and K.F.A. Soliman), Florida A & M University Foundation, Tallahassee, pp. 257–268 (1981)
23. Sothern, R.B., Halberg, F., Halberg, E., Zinneman, H.H. and Kennedy, B.J. Circadian and methodologic aspects of toxicity from cis-diamminedichloroplatinum, adriamycin and methylpred-nisolone interaction in rats with immunocytoma. In *Chronopharmacology and Chronotherapeutics* (eds C.A. Walker, C.M. Winget and K.F.A. Soliman), Florida A & M University Foundation, Tallahassee, pp. 247–256 (1981)
24. Zinneman, H.H., Halberg, F., Haus, E. and Kaplan, M. Circadian rhythms in urinary light chains, serum iron and other variables of multiple myeloma patients. *Int. J. Chronobiol.*, **2**, 3–16 (1974)
25. Nelson, W., Zinneman, H., Selden, J., Schaper, K., Halberg, F. and Bazin, H. Circadian rhythm in Bence-Jones protein excretion by LOU rats bearing a transplantable immunocytoma, responsive to adriamycin treatment. *Int. J. Chronobiol.*, **2**, 359–366 (1974)
26. Sothern, R.B. and Halberg, F. Timing of circadian core temperature rhythm in rats on 5 lighting schedules with different photofractions. *Chronobiologia*, **6**, 158–159 (1974)
27. Nelson, W., Tong, Y., Lee, J.K. and Halberg, F. Methods for cosinor rhythmometry. *Chronobiologia*, **6**, 305–323 (1979)
28. Sothern, R.B., Halberg, F. and Hruschesky, W.J.M. Persistence of doxorubicin susceptibility rhythm for mice in constant light: circadian stage versus time of day. In *Biological Rhythms and Medications, Proc. 3rd Int. Conf. Chronopharmacol.*, Nice, March 14–17, p. VI-14 (1988)
29. Hruschesky, W.J.M., Haus, E., Lakatua, D.J., Halberg, F., Langevin, T. and Kennedy, B.J. Marker rhythms for cancer chrono-chemotherapy. In *Chronobiology 1981–1983* (eds E. Haus and H.F. Kabat), Karger Publishers, New York, pp. 493–499 (1985)
30. Hermida Dominguez, R.C., Sothern, R.B., Halberg, F. and Langevin, T.R. Variability of circadian acrophase of urinary potassium excretion as a potential marker for cancer chronotherapy. In *Proc. 2nd Int. Conf. Medico-Social Aspects Chronobiol.* (eds F. Halberg, L. Reale and B. Tarquini), Instituto Italiano di Medicina Sociale, Rome, pp. 313–325 (1986)
31. Hruschesky, W.J.M., Dell, I., Eaton, J. and Halberg, F. Circadian-stage-dependent effect of doxorubicin upon reduced glutathione in the murine heart. *Proc. AACR*, **23**, 12 (1982)
32. Wesson, L.F. Electrolyte excretion in relation to diurnal cycles of renal function. *Medicine*, **43**, 547–592 (1964)
33. Hecquet, B., Meynadier, J., Bonneterre, J., Adenis, L. and Demaille, A. Time dependency in plasmatic protein binding of cisplatin. *Cancer Treat. Rep.*, **69**, 79–82 (1985)
34. Levi, F.A., Hruschesky, W.J.M., Blomquist, C.H., Lakatua, D., Haus, E., Halberg, F. and Kennedy, B.J. Reduction of cis-diamminedichloroplatinum nephrotoxicity in rats by optimal circadian drug timing. *Cancer Res.*, **42**, 950–955 (1982)
35. Levi, F.A., Hruschesky, W.J.M., Halberg, F., Haus, E., Langevin, T. and Kennedy, B.J. Lethal

nephrotoxicity and hematologic toxicity of cis-diamminedichloroplatinum ameliorated by optimal circadian timing and hydration. *Eur. J. Cancer Clin. Oncol.*, **18**, 471–477 (1982)

36. Roemeling, R.v., Wick, M., Rabatin, J., Berestka, J., Langevin, T.R., Lakatua, D., Mormont, C.M., Mushiya, T. and Hrushesky, W.J.M. Circadian stage dependence of FUDR toxicity. In *Annual Review of Chronopharmacology* (eds A. Reinberg, M. Smolensky and G. Labrecque), Pergamon Press, New York, Vol. 3, pp. 191–194 (1986)

37. Bixby, L., Levi, F., Haus, E., Sackett, L., Halberg, F. and Hrushesky, W. Circaseptan aspects of cisplatin nephrotoxicity. In *Toward Chronopharmacology, Adv. Biosci. 41* (eds R. Takahashi, F. Halberg and C. Walker), Pergamon Press, Oxford, pp. 339–347 (1982)

38. Danhauser, L.L. and Rustum, Y.M. A method for continuous drug infusion in unrestrained rats: its application in evaluating the toxicity of 5-fluorouracil/thymidine combinations. *J. Lab. Clin. Med.*, **93**, 1047–1053 (1979)

39. Levin, L. and Hryniuk, W.M. Dose intensity analysis of chemotherapy regimens in ovarian cancer. *J. Clin. Oncol.*, **5**, 756–767 (1987)

40. Young, R.C., Knapp, R.C. Fuks, Z. and Disaia, P.J. Cancer of the ovary. In *Cancer, Principles and Practice of Oncology* (eds V.T. DeVita, Jr., S. Hellman and S.A. Rosenberg), J.P. Lippincott Co., Philadelphia, pp. 1083–1118 (1984)

41. Roemeling, R.v. and Hrushesky, W.J.M. Advanced transitional cell bladder cancer: a treatable disease. *Semin. Surg. Oncol.*, **2**, 76–89 (1986)

42. Levi, F., Hrushesky, W.J.M., Borch, R.F., Pleasants, M.E., Kennedy, B.J. and Halberg, F. Cisplatin urinary pharmacokinetics and nephrotoxicity: a common circadian mechanism. *Cancer Treat. Rep.*, **66**, 1933–1938 (1982)

43. Hrushesky, W.J.M., Borch, R. and Levi, F. Circadian time dependence of cisplatin urinary kinetics. *Clin. Pharmacol. Ther.*, **32**, 330–339 (1982)

44. Roemeling, R.v., Hrushesky, W.J.M. and Fraley, E. Long-term control of locally advanced transitional cell bladder cancer (TCCB) by high-dose intensity, circadian-based adjuvant chemotherapy. In *Adjuvant Treatment of Cancer V* (ed. S.E. Salmon), Grune Stratton, Orlando, pp. 571–580 (1987)

45. Roemeling, R.v., Rabatin, J.T., Fraley, E.E. and Hrushesky, W.H. Progressive metastatic renal cell carcinoma controlled by continuous 5-fluoro-2-deoxyuridine infusion. *J. Urol.*, **139**, 259–262 (1988)

46. Lokich, J.J., Sonneborn, H., Paus, S. and Zipoli, T. Phase I study of continuous venous infusion of floxuridine (5-FUDR) chemotherapy. *Cancer Treat. Rep.*, **67**, 791–793 (1983)

47. Kemeny, N. and Daly, J. Randomized study of intrahepatic versus systemic infusion of FUDR in patients with liver metastases from colorectal carcinoma. *ICRCT 85*, Giesen, Italy, p. 25 (1985)

48. Hrushesky, W.J.M., Roemeling, R.v., Rabatin, J.T. and Fraley, E. Continuous FUDR infusion is effective in progressive renal cell cancer. *Proc. ASCO*, **7**, 425 (1987)

49. Halberg, F., Haus, E., Cardoso, S.S., Scheving, L.E., Kühl, J.F.W., Shiotsuka, R., Rosene, G., Pauly, J.E., Runge, W., Spalding, J.F., Lee, J.K. and Good, R.A. Toward a chronotherapy of neoplasia: tolerance of treatment depends upon host rhythms. *Experientia*, **29**, 909–934 (1972)

50. Feuers, R.J. and Scheving, L.E. Chronobiology of hepatic enzymes. *Annu. Rev. Chronopharmacol.*, **4**, 209–256 (1988)

51. Scheving, L.E. Chronobiology of cell proliferation in mammals: implications for basic research and cancer chemotherapy. In *Cell Cycle Clocks* (ed. L.N. Edmunds), Marcel Dekker, New York, pp. 455–499 (1984)

52. Mayersbach, H.v. Die zeitstruktur des organismus. Auswirkungen auf zellulaere leistungsfaehigkeit und medikamentenempfindlichkeit. *Arznisem. Forsch./Drug Res.*, **28**, 1824–1836 (1978)

53. Kinlaw, W.B., Fish, L.H., Schwartz, H.L. and Oppenheimer, J.H. Diurnal variation in hepatic expression of the rat S14 gene is synchronized by the photoperiod. *Endocrinology*, **120**, 1563–1567 (1987)

54. Boughattas, A.N., Levi, F., Roulon, A., Mechkouri, M., Lemaigre, G., Cal, J.C., Camber, J., Reinberg, A. and Mathe, G. Similar circadian rhythm in murine host tolerance for two platinum analogs: carboplatin (CBDCA) and oxaliplatin (I-OHP). *Proc. AACR*, **28**, 1788 (1987)

55. Aherne, G.W., English, J., Burton, N., Arendt, J. and Marks, V. Chronopharmacokinetics and their relationship to toxicity and effect with reference to methotrexate, 6-mercaptopurine and morphine. *Satellite Symposia Proc. ECCO*, **4**, 40 (1987)

56. Scheving, L.E. Circadian rhythms in cell proliferation: their importance when investigating the basic mechanism of normal versus abnormal growth. In *11th Int. Congr. Anat. Biol. Rhythms Struct. Funct.*, Alan R. Liss, New York, pp. 39–79 (1981)

57. Burns, R.E. Circadian rhythmicity in DNA synthesis in untreated mice as a basis for improved chemotherapy. *Cancer Res.*, **41**, 2795–2802 (1981)

58. Walker, P.R. and Van Potter, R. Diurnal rhythms of hepatic enzymes from rats adapted to controlled feeding schedules. In *Chronobiology* (eds L.E. Scheving, F. Halberg and J.E. Pauly), Igaku Shoin Ltd., Tokyo, pp. 17–22 (1974)

59. Mayersbach, H.v. Rhythms at morphological levels. In *Chronobiology: Principles and Applications to Shifts in Schedules* (eds L.E. Scheving and F. Halberg), Sijthoff and Noordhoff, The Netherlands, pp. 95–107 (1980)

60. Nelson, W., Scheving, F. and Halberg, F. Circadian rhythms in mice fed a single daily meal at different stages of lighting regimen. *J. Nutr.*, **105**, 171–184 (1975)

61. LaBrecque, D.R., Feigenbaum, A. and Bachur, N.R. Diurnal rhythm: effects on hepatic regeneration and hepatic regenerative stimulator substance. *Science*, **199**, 1082–1084 (1978)

62. Nash, R.E. and Echave Llanos, J.M. Circadian variations in DNA synthesis of a fast-growing and a slow-growing hepatoma: DNA synthesis rhythm in hepatoma. *J. Natl. Cancer Inst.*, **47**, 1007–1012 (1971)

63. Burns, E.R., Scheving, L.E. and Tsai, T.H. Circadian rhythms in DNA synthesis and mitosis in normal mice and in mice bearing the Lewis lung carcinoma. *Eur. J. Cancer*, **15**, 233–242 (1979)

64. Haus, E., Lakatua, D.J., Swoyer, J. and Sackett-Lundeen, L. Chronobiology in hematology and immunology. *Amer. J. Anat.*, **168**, 467 (1983)

65. Swoyer, J., Haus, E., Lakatua, D., Sackett-Lundeen, L. and Thompson, M. Chronobiology in the clinical laboratory. In *Chronobiology 1982–1983* (eds E. Haus and H.F. Kabat), Karger Publishing, New York, pp. 533–543 (1984)

66. Levi, F.A., Canon, C., Blum, J.P., Mechkouri, M., Reinberg, A. and Mathe, G. Circadian and/or circahemidian rhythms in nine lymphocyte-related variables from peripheral blood of healthy subjects. *J. Immunol.*, **134**, 217–220 (1985)

67. Levi, F.A., Canon, C., Blum, J.P., Mechkouri, M., Reinberg, A. and Mathe, G. Circadian and/or circahemidian rhythms in nine lymphocyte-related variables from peripheral blood of healthy subjects. *J. Immnol.*, **134**, 217–220 (1985)

68. Gatti, G., Cavallo, R., Del Ponte, D., Sartori, M., Masera, R., Carignola, R., Carandente, F. and Angeli, A. Circadian changes of human natural killer (NK) cells and their *in vitro* susceptibility to cortisol inhibition. In *Annual Review of Chronopharmacology* (eds A. Reinberg, M. Smolensky and G. Labrecque), Pergamon Press, New York, pp. 75–78 (1986)

69. Levi, F., Canon, C., Blum, J.P., Reinberg, A. and Mathes, G. Large-amplitude circadian rhythm in helper:suppressor ratio of peripheral blood lymphocytes. *Lancet*, **2**, 462–463 (1983)

70. Ross, D.D., Pollak, A., Akman, S.A. and Bachur, N.R. Diurnal variation of circulating human myeloid progenitor cells. *Exp. Hematol.*, **8**, 954–960 (1980)

71. Verma, D.S., Fisher, R., Spitzer, G., Zander, A.R., McCredie, K.B. and Dicke, K.A. Diurnal changes in circulating myeloid progenitor cells in man. *Amer. J. Hematol.*, **9**, 185–192 (1980)

72. Killmann, S.A., Cronkite, E.P., Fliedner, T.M. and Bond, V.P. Mitotic indices of human bone marrow cells. I. Number and cytologic distribution of mitoses. *Blood*, **19**, 743–750 (1962)

73. Mauer, A.M. Diurnal variation of proliferative activity in the human bone marrow. *Blood*, **26**, 1–7 (1965)

74. Bellamy, W.T., Alberts, D.S. and Dorr, R.T. Circadian variation in non-protein sulfhydryl levels of human bone marrow. *Eur. J. Cancer Clin. Oncol.*, **29** No. 11, 1759–1762 (1988)

75. Smaaland, R., Sletvold, O., Bjerknes, R., Lote, K. and Laerum, O.D. Circadian variations of cell cycle distribution in human bone marrow. *Chronobiologia*, **14**, 239 (1987)

76. Buchi, K.N., Moore, J.G. and Rubin, N.H. Circadian cellular proliferation measurements in human rectal mucosa. *Chronobiologia*, **14**, 155–156 (1987)

77. Buchi, K.N., Hrushesky, W.J.M., Sothern, R.B., Rubin, N. and Moore, J.G. Circadian rhythm of cellular proliferation in the human rectal mucosa. *Gastroenterology* (in press)

78. Markiewicz, A., Lelek, A., Panz, B., Wagiel, J., Boldys, H., Hartleb, M. and Kaminski, M. Chronomorphology of jejunum in man. *Chronobiologia*, **14**, 202 (1987)

79. Haus, E., Halberg, F., Scheving, L.E., Cardoso, S., Kuhl, J.F.W., Sothern, R., Shiotsuka, R.N.,

Hwang, D.S. and Pauly, J.E. Increased tolerance of leukemic mice to arabinosyl cytosine with schedule adjusted to circadian system. *Science*, **177**, 80–82 (1972)

80. Scheving, L.E., Pauly, J.E. and Tsai, T.H. The importance of chronobiology in modern research and medicine. *Verh. Anat. Ges.*, **77**, 59–84 (1983)

81. Mormont, M.C., Roemeling, R.v., Sothern, R.B., Berestka, J.S., Langvin, T.R., Wick, M. and Hrushesky, W.J.M. Circadian rhythm and seasonal dependence in tolerance of mice to 4'-epi-doxorubicin. *Investigational New Drugs*, **6**, 273–283 (1988)

82. Huben, R.P., Dragone, N., Wolf, R.M. Early results of a phase II study of continuous infusion FUDR in metastatic renal cell carcinoma. *Proc. Am. Soc. Clin. Oncol.*, abstract 546, May (1989)

83. Halberg, F. Protection by timing treatment according to bodily rhythms – analogy to protection by scrubbing before surgery. In *Chronobiological Aspects of Endocrinology* (eds J. Aschoff, F. Ceresa and F. Halberg), Il Ponte, Milano, pp. 27–72 (1974)

84. Klevecz, R.R., Shymko, R.M., Blumenfeld, D. and Braly, P.S. Circadian gating of S phase in human ovarian cancer. *Cancer Res.*, **47**, 6267–6271 (1987)

85. Garcia Sainz, M. and Halberg, F. Mitotic rhythm in human cancer, reevaluated by electronic computer programs – evidence for chronopathology. *J. Natl. Cancer Inst.*, **37**, 279–292 (1966)

86. Roemeling, R. and Hrushesky, W.J.M. Circadian shaping of FUDR infusion reduces toxicity even at high-dose intensity. *Proc. ASCO*, **6**, 293 (1987)

87. Roemeling, R., Hrushesky, W.J.M., Kennedy, B.J. and Buchwald, H. Programmed automatic FUDR chronotherapy improves therapeutic index. *Surg. Forum*, **27**, 401–402 (1987)

Chapter 13

Present achievements and future prospects for clinical chronobiology

M.H. Smolensky

Introduction

The results of chronobiological research conducted during the past 30 years or so
are now realizing applications in clinical medicine. Early on, the findings of
biological rhythm research were challenged by contemporary medical scientists
since they were often inconsistent with the prevailing dogma of homoeostatic
theory purporting constancy of bioprocesses and functions. Today the situation is
different. Chronobiology is being recognized by an increasing number of clinicians
as offering a new avenue for improving the diagnosis and treatment of human
diseases as well as the research of their epidemiology and underlying mechanisms.
At the present time, the field of clinical chronobiology is just emerging. In certain
countries, particularly in Europe, advances are proceeding more rapidly than in
others. Applications of chronobiological methods and findings in medicine are
occurring at different rates in different medical specialities. The purpose of this
epilogue is to chronicle the current status of clinical chronobiology in relation to
the prospects for future applications to medicine. Although it is proper to discuss
the field of medical chronobiology in terms of the epidemiology and mechanisms
of disease, owing to a limitation of space here the clinical aspects of the field will
be emphasized primarily from two perspectives – the diagnosis and treatment of
human disease.

Chronobiology and diagnostic procedures

Diagnostic procedures are typically carried out without consideration of influences
or dependencies of biological rhythms. This is the case in spite of the fact that the
timing of certain tests can be critical [1–16]. A few examples are given in the
following sections.

Allergic response

The diagnosis of allergy in most clinics is based on the cutaneous response to
intradermal injections of allergen extracts [1–3]. Generally, such diagnostic
procedures are done in the clinic during the morning (between 07:00 and 11:00 h),
at which time the biological responses of erythema and induration in day-active
persons are minimal. When the same diagnostic procedures are done later,

between 19:00 and 23:00 h, the biological responses are much greater (see Figure 7.14). On average, cutaneous reaction to antigens in tests conducted in the morning is only one-third of that of those done in the evening [1–3]. However, there are individual differences between patients, such that the morning–evening variation in biological responses to skin testing can be as great as 7–11-fold [1,2]. The point to be made is that the time at which intradermal diagnostic tests are conducted for the purpose of determining specific allergen sensitivities can profoundly affect the clinical findings. If the procedures are done in the morning in day-active persons, the biological responses are likely to represent an underestimation of the true allergic sensitivity and, moreover, there exists the likelihood of 'false negatives'. In contrast, tests conducted in the evening are likely to result in very strong biological responses. It is unknown, at present, whether testing at night results in an overestimation of true allergen sensitivity or even 'false positives' in certain cases; this awaits further research.

Even though the importance of circadian rhythms in cutaneous reactivity was reported some 20 years ago, many practising allergists and family physicians still do not know of it today. Most clinicians are completely unaware of how the timing of intradermal skin testing with allergens can influence the results of their diagnostic evaluations. For those clinicians who do know of this chronobiological phenomenon, the manner of how best to take account of it in their clinical practices and office routines remains to be resolved. Some clinicians try to compensate for the circadian rhythm by concomitantly applying histamine controls, thereby allowing interpretation of the cutaneous reaction to antigens relative to that of histamine injected at the same clock-time. However, this approach may be flawed. The amplitude, that is the day–night variation, of the cutaneous reactivity may differ between antigens, perhaps in proportion to the severity of the specific allergen sensitivity of the patient, and also from that of histamine. Some clinicians believe that the best solution is to schedule the intradermal tests in the afternoon, since this is the span during the 24 h when the response to antigens is most likely to be indicative of the patients' average reactivity. While the latter approach seems the most sensible for now, it does not represent a perfect solution; not all patients can be scheduled for afternoon tests and not many clinicians are willing to alter their office routine to accomplish this. More work is required to bring the knowledge of circadian change in cutaneous reactivity to antigens into the clinic for practical purposes.

It is also of relevance that the diagnosis of airway hyperreactivity, as in asthma, to various chemical substances and antigens is greatly affected by the time, during the 24 h, at which procedures are scheduled [4–7]. The airways are least reactive to the inhaled aerosolized test agents, acetylcholine and histamine, and the antigen, house dust (in house-dust-sensitive asthmatic patients) during the afternoon as compared to early in the morning and overnight. On the other hand, the airways of individuals induced into bronchospasm by the hyperventilation of cold dry air are more reactive during the afternoon than overnight (Figure 13.1). Thus the time of day at which the tests are done will affect the reactivity of the airways to chemical agents and antigens and thus the physician's determination of the magnitude of sensitivity to them.

Commonly, aerosolized beta-agonist medications are used to help make the differential diagnosis between reversible and non-reversible forms of obstructive airways disease. A series of investigations have shown that the time when such agents are inhaled determined the extent of airway responsiveness, which in turn

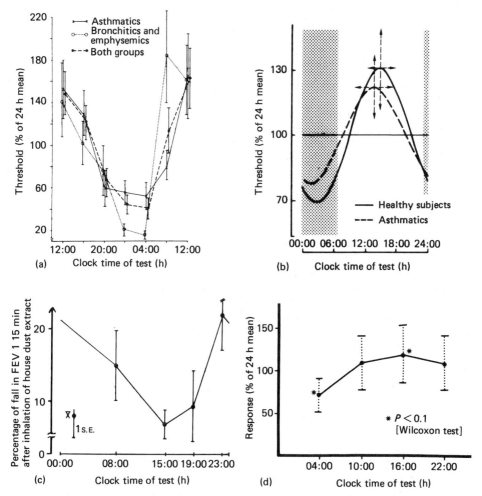

Figure 13.1 Circadian change in airway hyperreactivity to chemical challenges of histamine (a), acetylcholine (b), house dust antigen (c) and hyperventilation with cold dry air (d). For house dust and hyperventilation with cold dry air [6,7], the measured response was the change in airway patency from the respective clock-time baseline. For histamine and acetylcholine [4,5], the measured end point was the concentration required to induce a 15–20% change in airway patency at each clock time. Except for the plot of the house dust antigen, the temporal changes are plotted relative to the group 24-h mean values. The plots indicate extensive temporal variability in the response to the various diagnostic test agents. For aerosolized histamine, acetylcholine and house dust, the reactivity of the airways (bronchial constriction) was consistently greater between 00:00 and 04:00 h than at midday

may influence the diagnosis made [8–11]. Most clinicians expect the inhalation of a beta-agonist drug to induce a bronchodilatory response equal to 15–20% of the pretreatment baseline level in patients with reversible airway obstruction. Results of studies on asthmatic patients demonstrate that the increase in airway patency following inhalation of a standardized dose of a beta-agonist aerosol around midday or during the afternoon is far less than that produced early in the day or late in the evening [8,9]. It is of interest, too, that the response of healthy normal airways to beta-agonist agents also varies, although to a lesser degree than in asthmatics, according to the (biological) time at which such procedures are carried out [10,11].

Time-qualified reference values

The results of various kinds of diagnostic tests can be affected by the time at which they are conducted. In a great number of clinical situations, blood and urine samples are taken routinely to assess selected indicators of health status. It has long been recognized that certain constituents of both the blood and urine undergo moderate to profound circadian and sometimes other rhythmic changes. Haus and his colleagues [12] have established time-qualified reference values (TQRVs) to allow clinicians to interpret properly clock-time samples of those constituents that exhibit large-amplitude circadian variability.

TQRVs are generated by around-the-clock investigations on large groups of healthy persons of both sexes and various age groups. At present, TQRVs exist for most of the variables routinely analysed by clinical laboratories. They differ from conventionally derived and published reference values in that the latter represent sources of variation due to a number of factors including individual differences between healthy persons as well as those due to time of sampling, reflecting rhythmic alterations. TQRVs represent more precisely the expected range of values due to individual variability with respect to a specific time span. They are thus likely to be more sensitive than conventionally derived normal ranges which incorporate values derived from different biological times of sampling. Knowledge of the sleep/activity schedule of the patient plus the clock time of the

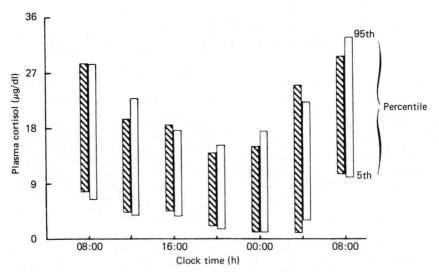

Figure 13.2 Circadian variation in the usual range of plasma cortisol concentrations based on frequent (every 4-h) blood samples of diurnally active healthy young male ▨ and female □ volunteers. Note that a plasma cortisol concentration of 5 μg/dl is considered normal if found for samples taken between 20:00 and 04:00 h, but not for a sample taken at 08:00 h. On the other hand, a concentration of 20 μg/ dl is considered normal if found for samples taken at 08:00 or 12:00 h but not for samples taken at 20:00 h or 00:00 h. (Courtesy of Erhard Haus, University of Minnesota Medical School, Department of Pathology, Minneapolis, Minnesota)

blood withdrawal or urine voiding (and, if need be, day of week, month or year) makes possible the use of TQRVs for a more precise interpretation of clinical laboratory analyses. It enables determination of whether the values are within the normal range for the comparable age and sex reference groups and in relation to the time of sampling.

For many chemical constituents of the blood and urine, the amplitude of the 24-h rhythms is small and inconsequential in terms of diagnostic relevance. However, for certain constituents of the blood (Figure 13.2) as well as of the urine, TQRVs represent an indispensable tool for the sensitive scrutiny of test results. For example, TQRVs pertaining to plasma cortisol are quite commonly utilized to diagnose hyper- or hypo-adrenocortism as well as iatrogenically induced adreno-cortical suppression [17].

Common chronic diseases

Many relevant biological parameters serve as indicator end points for the diagnosis of disease. Typically, in the clinic these end points are examined at a single clock time during the 24 h, usually during a brief daytime appointment. Many of these exhibit moderate- to high-amplitude circadian change. This is the case for blood pressure [13–16], the severity of joint stiffness, pain and inflammation in arthritis [18.19], and airway patency assessed by spirometry or other methods when asthma is suspected [20,21], for example. In the case of asthma, the measurement of airway patency by peak expiratory flow (PEF) or the forced expiratory volume in 1 s (FEV 1) is greatly affected by the time during the 24 h at which it is done [21]. Commonly, the day/night difference in airway patency amounts to 25–40% of the 24-h mean level [21,22].

Underlying biological rhythms in physiochemical processes and functions constitute the mechanisms of predictable temporal variation over the 24 h in the manifestation and intensity of the symptoms or markers of several human diseases [22–25]. Single or even repeated blood pressure readings in the clinician's office done over a restricted span of the day may be insufficient to differentiate between normotension versus hypertension if the examination is done at the wrong biological time and if the patient's blood pressure varies circadian rhythmically [13–16]. The day/night variation in diastolic or systolic blood pressure can amount to 10–20 mmHg or more as found in many studies [13–16]. In addition, the assessment of the severity of illnesses such as arthritis or asthma may be biased if the examination is done at the wrong biological time. Since the symptoms and acute exacerbations of disease [for example, the dyspnoea of asthma (Figure 13.3)] exhibit rhythmicity as well as other non-periodic temporal variability [25], the need to achieve a more careful and precise medical assessment of patients is a current urgent concern for all.

Autorhythmometry

For many years, investigative clinical chronobiologists have relied upon what they refer to as autorhythmometry to gather data over time from ambulatory human beings to detect and describe biological rhythms of various periods [26,27]. Autorhythmometry is the frequent self-monitoring of biological variables by

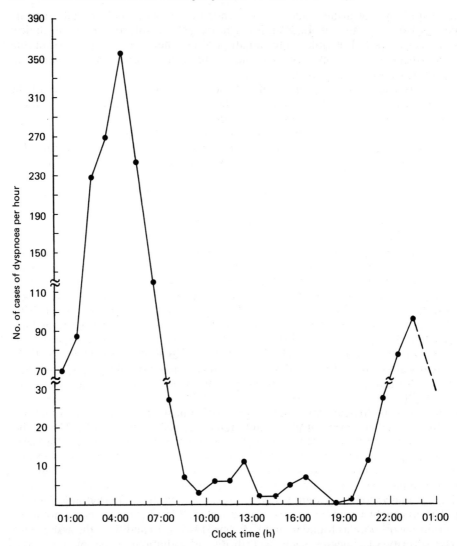

Figure 13.3 Day/night variation in the occurrence of 1631 asthma attacks in 3129 untreated patients. Most attacks take place between 02:00 and 07:00 h; very few occur during the daytime, especially between 10:00 and 19:00 h. The risk of asthma at 05:00 is nearly 70-fold that between 13:00 and 15:00 h. (Redrawn from Dethlesen and Repges [31])

persons using especially designed light-weight portable instrumentation to determine and objectively quantify the characteristics of rhythms by applying appropriate statistical methods to the collected time series data [26,27]. In order to gather sufficient data, patients are instructed to conduct their self-assessments four to five times daily, i.e. upon awakening, before midday, in the afternoon, before supper and before bedtime, to evaluate day/night and circadian variability.

The concept of self-monitoring in medicine for assessing the biological status of patients is not at all new. For generations, pre-menopausal women have monitored fertile and infertile spans of their menstrual cycles by charting their 'basal' morning oral temperatures. Diabetic patients nowadays routinely self-monitor their blood glucose levels in relation to insulin requirements or dietary modification. Autorhythmometry has proven useful for documenting numerous rhythms of various periods in healthy persons in the past. Its significance in the future lies with clinical applications. In recent years physicians have become more willing to accept the findings of self-measurements by patients, for example, blood pressure obtained several times daily at home during both the day and night using traditional or automated ambulatory blood pressure devices [14]. Data obtained in this way have been used to assess the diagnosis and severity of hypertension and also the response of patients to specific antihypertensive medications [15].

It is in pulmonary medicine that self-monitoring procedures have been most often incorporated. Physicians in many European countries routinely distribute peak flow meters to patients for self-assessment of the severity of asthma as well as the efficacy of prescribed bronchodilator medications [28.29]. In a majority of patients, airway status is poorest in the early morning and late evening [22,30,31], times when clinicians do not normally have access to their patients. Moreover, asthma itself is mainly a nocturnal disease (Figure 13.3 and Chapter 5). Since airway patency varies so greatly over the 24 h, PEF autorhythmometry is advised, especially in those patients with severe disease. PEF autorhythmometry has proven useful for the assessment of workers suspected of suffering from occupationally induced asthma, as demonstrated for chromium- and colophony-induced asthma [32,33], and as a valuable tool in the epidemiological study of the deleterious effects of air pollutants on the airways of asthmatic and other patient samples [34,35].

There are additional inexpensive, yet clinically meaningful, techniques for obtaining data throughout the day for the purpose of assessing a patient's condition other than by reliance on instrumentation. For years clinicians and researchers alike have utilized visual analogue scales (VAS) to monitor the course of various diseases in patients or for evaluating the effects of medical interventions. All too often, however, patients have been requested to perform their self-assessments only once or perhaps twice daily, sometimes only weekly. Chronobiologists have utilized VAS to determine how the symptoms or severity of medical conditions vary during the 24 h by having patients carry out their self-assessments a number (up to five) of times daily during the waking span for several consecutive days. Studies done on patients suffering from allergic asthma, rheumatoid and osteoarthritis, chronic pain and nasal rhinitis confirm that autorhythmometry utilizing VAS is an economical, sensitive and reliable means of not only characterizing the severity of a disease or set of symptoms in question over the 24 h (Figure 13.4), but also evaluating the efficacy of medications in clinical trials involving patients [19,28,31,36–39].

The content and examples presented in the preceding paragraphs represent, in part, future prospects for the application of chronobiological methods and findings for the improvement of diagnostic procedures. Earlier in this century, chronobiologists took advantage of technological advances in order to market portable and light-weight medical instrumentation for the at-home self-monitoring of selected biological variables. In this manner, circadian and other rhythms were detected and quantitatively described with the aid of computers to analyse collected data. Today, new instrumentation, along with visual analogue scales, is being utilized by clinicians of some medical specialities to diagnose more accurately the health status of patients. Additional applications are expected in the future.

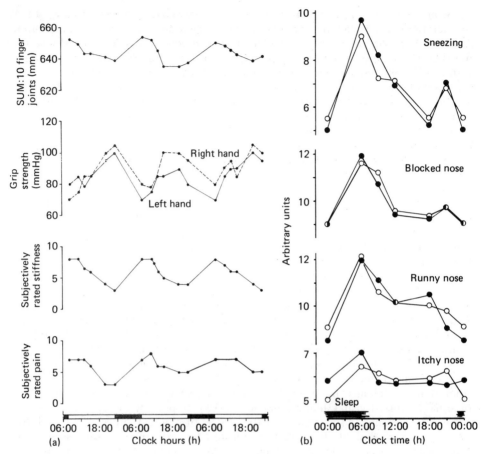

Figure 13.4 Examples of applications of self-assessment of disease status using visual analogue scales (VAS) a number of times daily for several consecutive days in individual (a) or a group (b) of patients. In (a) are shown circadian changes in the symptoms and signs of rheumatoid arthritis, and in (b) is shown the severity of hay fever symptoms in 330 men (●) and 435 women (○). The units of measurement for the VAS self-monitoring are arbitrary ones, typically, the distance in millimetres between the left-hand margin of the scale (no symptom intensity) and the placement of the mark on the scale by the patient. SUM is the circumference of 10 finger joints summed. (Adapted from graphs published in refs [25] and [46])

Chronotherapeutics

In Chapters 1 and 2, the concepts of chronopharmacology and chronotherapeutics were presented. Chronotherapy has as its goal the optimization of medications by tailoring drug administrations to biological rhythms so as to enhance their efficacy and/or reduce their toxicity [40]. In some instances, investigators have concentrated on administration-time-dependent variation in drug kinetics in order to make inferences regarding dosing schedules. Too often the findings of kinetic studies alone have been used as the basis for devising chronotherapeutic interventions. To achieve a true optimization of treatments for human disease, clinical investigations are necessary to ensure that medications are delivered at the most opportune time to avert the occurrence and exacerbation of symptoms, which themselves may vary predictably over the course of 24 h, or other time domains, with minimal or no toxicity. There is ample evidence that the severity of several chronic illnesses in many patients varies during 24 h [25]. This is the case for the symptoms of allergic rhinitis [38] and rheumatoid arthritis [18,36] which are typically at their worst in the morning; osteoarthritis [39,41] which is usually worst in the afternoon and evening; and asthma as well as Prinzmetal's variant angina [42] which tend to be at their worst overnight or very early in the morning, to mention but a few examples. Moreover, for persons who are at risk from certain pathological events, such as myocardial [25] and cerebral [43] infarction and cerebral haemorrhage [25] (Figure 13.5), which on a population basis exhibit significant 24-h patterns, the

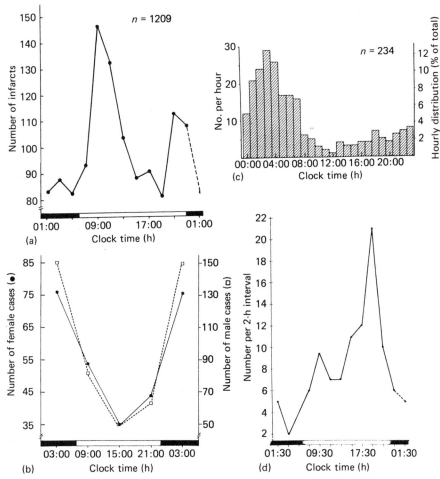

Figure 13.5 Examples of human circadian chronopathologies [25,42,43] observed with diseases of the cardiovascular system. The vulnerability of populations of human beings to the morbid events of myocardial infarction (a), cerebral infarction (b), ST-segment anomaly of Prizmetal's variant angina (c) and spontaneous intracerebral haemorrhage (d) is not random over 24 h. Instead, the temporal patterns appear to represent underlying circadian rhythms in biological processes interacting with cyclic environmental factors.

scheduling of medication must take into account identified temporal patterns of risk over this time period. For these diseases, a chronotherapeutic approach is worthy of investigation.

Apparently, the first large-scale attempt at chronotherapy was the morning alternate-day treatment schedule of orally administered methylprednisolone, a synthetic corticosteroid marketed in the United States during the 1960s and 70s [44]. The chronotherapy of methylprednisolone and other corticosteroids of this family of drugs is based primarily on the finding that the timing of moderate doses of orally administered corticosteroids in the morning, which in diurnally active persons corresponds to the peak cortisol level during the 24 h (Figure 13.2), results in slight or no adrenal suppression as a side effect. The circadian rhythm in the inhibition of the pituitary–adrenal axis due to exogenously administered synthetic corticosteroid drugs has been repeatedly confirmed [17]. Today, it is known that both the toxicity and benefit of corticosteroid medications, such as prednisolone and methylprednisolone, depend on the biological time of their administration. In the case of asthma, adrenocortical suppression can be averted, bone density maintained and airway status improved optimally when all (or most) of the daily oral dose is taken in the morning, whether or not a small supplemental dose is also taken early in the afternoon [17,28,45].

During the past 5–10 years, the concept of chronotherapeutics has rapidly gained the attention of medical researchers and officials of several pharmaceutical companies. For instance, Hrushesky in Chapter 12 has reviewed the progress of cancer chronotherapy. Significant steps have also been taken recently in the chronotherapy of several chronic diseases, such as allergic rhinitis (by H_1-receptor antagonist antihistamines), rheumatoid and osteoarthritis (by non-steroidal anti-inflammatory drugs), asthma (by theophylline, corticosteroids and beta-agonists) and ulcers (by H_2-receptor antagonists) [for example 9,17,39,41,46–51]. As the life expectancy of the population increases, the number of persons at risk from and under treatment for chronic diseases will also increase. As many of the currently available chemotherapies produce side effects and the development of new medications devoid of such side effects will require many years of work with great expense, practitioners are faced with the task of learning how better to utilize available drugs to optimize their therapeutic attributes while controlling toxicity. The field of chronotherapeutics provides a practical and economical approach to better management of many chronic diseases including cardiovascular ones [52].

In retrospect, it has not always been clear how chronotherapeutic strategies arose for some of the chronic diseases mentioned above. In some instances, they may have represented the thoughts of marketing executives of pharmaceutical companies culminating in either proven or unproven claims. A scientific approach, on the other hand, incorporates initial surveys of patients to examine temporal patterns in disease processes and symptoms and to determine the basis for a differential requirement for medication over 24 h. Thereafter, a study of candidate medications must involve evaluations in terms of their chronoeffectiveness and chronotoxicity. Drug-administration schedules to be investigated should include not only traditional ones (that is, equal-interval equal-dose) but also unequal morning–evening ones, especially if the occurrence or severity of symptoms of the disease to be treated varies quite predictably over time [40].

In clinical medicine, there appear to be certain clear indications when a chronotherapeutic approach is likely to be advantageous and these are outlined in Table 13.1.

Table 13.1 Situations indicating the prudence of a chronotherapeutic approach for the treatment of human disease

1. When the risk of symptoms or the exacerbation of disease exhibits day/night or other temporal variability
2. When the therapeutic window for a given medication is rather narrow relative to the potential for toxicity
3. When drug toxicity is the dose-limiting factor in aggressively treating patients
4. When drug kinetics and effects are known to be administration (biological)-time-dependent
5. When the goal of treatment, such as in hormonal substitution therapy, is to simulate the temporal pattern of the natural substance observed in normal persons
6. When optimal drug effect(s) can only be achieved by a time-modulated treatment mode [53]

Resetting circadian clocks

Most persons adhering to a diurnal activity/nocturnal rest cycle possess a 24-h circadian time structure synchronized by temporal patterns or stimuli of social interaction, sleep and activity, light and darkness and/or noise and quiet, among other environmental signals [54–57]. In synchronized individuals, there exists a specific precise phase relationship between the multitude of circadian processes. However, there are exceptions. Some persons exhibit free-running rhythms with periods closer to 25 h [54–56]. For brief periods, shiftworkers, when working nights, and travellers, when transported rapidly over several time zones, become desynchronized [58–60] (see Chapters 10 and 11). Finally, patients suffering from certain types of affective illness may exhibit abnormalities of the sleep/activity cycle and/or critical endogenous circadian rhythms [61–63] (see Chapter 9).

A current clinical concern is the resetting of circadian clocks and processes in subjects with disrupted or abnormal rhythms. During the past decade in particular, a clearer understanding of the mechanisms of biological time-keeping has resulted in exciting new developments in the management of individuals with these conditions. For several decades chronobiologists have been searching for chrono-biotics, i.e. physical or chemical agents capable of resetting or enhancing the rapid resetting of disrupted biological clocks [64]. Several candidates have been proposed: these include, for example, bright light exposure, melatonin administration, benzodiazepine treatment, theophylline dosing, exercise scheduling and meal timings, to mention a few [65–84] (see Chapters 9, 10 and 11).

Administration of both melatonin and the benzodiazepine, triazolam, has been evaluated in controlled laboratory animal experiments and human trials. Experiments with melatonin are treated extensively in Chapter 10. In brief, from real-time and simulated 'jet lag' studies it appears that both may serve as chronobiotics by improving attributes of sleep quality as well as possibly speeding up the resetting of circadian processes. In another investigation [73], a single acute administration of triazolam to shiftworkers was shown initially to promote sleep maintenance and quality, but the effect was not carried over to subsequent days. The effect of triazolam may not be a result of a resetting of biological clocks, but rather a direct sleep-inducing effect of the drug. Flurazepam [74] was also shown to exert a positive effect on promoting daytime sleep following a 12-h shift in the sleep/activity routine; however, use of the drug was associated with performance impairment. Additional investigations involving larger numbers of participants are yet required to evaluate fully the potential of all these agents as chronobiotics in human beings.

Bright light (2500 lux) is currently used clinically by psychiatrists to manage effectively patients who experience seasonal affective disorder (SAD) [62,63,76,77,84] (see Chapter 9). A common type of seasonal affective disorder is marked by the regular recurrence of depression during the winter, in the absence of identifiable psychosocial stress, and by the remission of symptoms in the spring, even without treatment. It appears that in some SAD patients circadian rhythms tend to be abnormally phase-delayed [62,63,77]. Since bright light has been shown to influence the melatonin rhythm [63,67,77], it was hypothesized by Lewy and colleagues that patients would be most responsive to the scheduling of bright light in the mornings [63,77]. Some studies suggest that 2 h of morning bright-light treatment is more effective in ameliorating SAD than evening treatment. It is of interest, however, that some patients respond to phototherapy when scheduled at other times than in the morning [63,77] and many reports consider that the timing of phototherapy is not critical. In relation to these findings, it has been suggested that patients be 'chronotyped' initially to determine the optimum treatment time for phototherapy for the resetting of disturbed circadian clocks and rhythms [63].

It is worthy of mention that various investigators claim to have induced alteration in circadian systems in human beings with other agents. For example, an ACTH analogue (Synchrodyn; Hoechst, Italy) proved capable of altering the staging of several circadian rhythms depending on its administration time [85]. The circadian rhythms that were shifted in phase, however, were those known to be affected by the adrenal hormones stimulated into secretion from the adrenal cortex by ACTH. Theophylline was also reported to produce slight alteration of the sleep/activity rhythm of one group of subjects [72]. Very large numbers of patients are routinely treated with theophylline for managing respiratory disease; yet, to date no reports of altered circadian time structure in such patients have been published. In reviewing the findings of the afore-mentioned studies, it appears that the particular chemical interventions exert an effect on the 'hands of the biological clocks' rather than on the clocks themselves. Thus, these agents are either suboptimal or inappropriate for correcting disturbances of biological clocks.

In summary, research on laboratory animals and human beings indicates promising prospects for the use of chronobiotics for resetting disturbed biological clocks. Thus far, the clinical experience with candidate chronobiotics, whether bright light or melatonin, has involved a relatively small number of subjects. Nonetheless, the initial findings are most promising. The results of human studies involving benzodiazepines are not as convincing. Although daytime sleep can be induced by such medications, there is little evidence as yet from studies on human beings that triazolam or flurazepam has the effect of speeding up the resetting of biological clocks. The concept of a class of medication that possesses the attribute of regulating and resetting disturbed circadian clocks and processes is indeed exciting, having direct applications to psychiatry, shiftwork management and jet lag.

Some future prospects

The field of medical chronobiology is currently benefitting from the results of investigations conducted during the past 30–40 years. A major obstacle to the large-scale adoption of chronobiological concepts and findings by clinicians is the absence of an educational foundation which would allow clinicians to comprehend them completely and apply them efficiently. In the majority of medical schools world wide, there is only a minimum amount of teaching time devoted to chronobiology. Thus most young clinicians and medical students have only a rudimentary knowledge (if any) of chronobiology. The future prospects for chronobiological applications in clinical medicine rely on the education of clinicians and medical researchers about this field as part of their basic coursework. For established practitioners, continuing education programmes focusing on medical chronobiology must be implemented if the findings and methods of chronobiology are to be widely and rapidly introduced.

Although the field of chronopharmacology is rapidly emerging as a scientific discipline in its own right, the implications of a chronobiological approach in clinical medicine transcend mere scientific considerations. In particular, the methods of chronobiology enable a more personal and sensitive approach to the diagnosis and treatment of disease in individual patients. With developing technology, inexpensive light-weight portable instrumentation has become available for the routine outpatient monitoring of various biological indicators of disease [86]. Use of such instrumentation as well as visual analogue scales to obtain relevant data several times daily (for example, upon awakening, mid-morning, midday, afternoon and at bedtime) provides a firm basis for accurately ascertaining and understanding the nature and severity of the patient's disease and his response to conventional (homoeostatically based) or non-conventional (chronotherapeutically based) treatment schedules. Obviously, the implementation of autorhythmometry in clinical practice will entail the generation of large amounts of data thereby requiring data reduction into relevant and meaningful end points, such as time series means (mesor), amplitudes (measure of the within-period variability), acrophases (index of the peak time) and prominent periodicities using computer technology and time series analytical procedures [26,27,87] (see Chapter 14). Autorhythmometry offers the clinician the opportunity to acquire specific information about the health status of patients during the hours of usual activity and even overnight or whenever the symptoms of disease break through. These data thus serve to supplement the physician's relatively brief survey of the patient in his office. Continued technological developments relating to data acquisition and analysis make the future prospects of autorhythmometry for applications to several medical specialities promising [86].

The practice of chronotherapeutics presents challenges to both the pharmaceutical industry and practitioners. The pharmaceutical industry faces the task of developing drug-delivery technologies that will enable the release of medication to target tissues at the proper biological times using a route and dosing schedule that will ensure high patient compliance. It must be recalled that early findings by chronobiologists indicating an unequal requirement for a drug during the morning and evening, for example for the treatment of the nocturnal symptoms of asthma, were not heeded. This was due to the fact that a means of formulating a drug such as theophylline as a single administration during the activity span to protect patients from asthma during sleep had not yet been developed. Today, several different formulations of sustained-release theophylline are available for the once-a-day evening administration or unequal (low-dose) morning, (high-dose) evening dosing for the management of patients who suffer from nocturnal symptoms of asthma [47]. In addition, a more efficient management of duodenal ulcers has been produced by a once-in-the evening (rather than an equal-interval equal-dose) administration of sustained-release H_2-receptor antagonist medication, a treatment schedule that has as its goal the suppression of the nocturnal surge of acid secretion [24,48,49].

Advances in chronotherapeutics and in medical chronobiology are closely linked to corresponding advances in medical technology. This has been the case in the recent past and will be true in the future. When early findings of cancer drug studies indicated a circadian difference in the toxicity of antitumour agents, oncologists and hospital pharmacists were not in a position to utilize such results. Reliance on hospital staff to deliver treatments at set times is impractical due to shortcomings in the manpower of hospitals and the dependability of personnel as well as cost. With the current availability of programmable pumps for 'clocking' medications, multicentre trials of the chronotherapeutics of cancer drugs are now possible. The emergence of new drug-delivery technologies makes the future prospect of chronotherapeutics more of a likelihood for several classes of medication. However, only through refinement of pump technology resulting in a simplification of their utilization in clinical practice will chronotherapeutics of cancer be accepted by a large number of oncologists.

The emphasis of this chapter has been future prospects for clinical chronobiology. Although biological rhythms in relation to diagnostic procedures and drug treatment have been the topics considered, other chronobiological matters have direct clinical significance. For example, most of our knowledge concerning the pathophysiology of human diseases is based on findings derived from investigations conducted during the daytime by diurnally active researchers. For those diseases with symptoms that intensify or occur only at night, the daytime study of patients may not result in the proper evaluation of the mechanisms involved. This could be the case for allergic nasal rhinitis and rheumatoid arthritis, the symptoms of which become aggravated overnight and are at their worst in the morning, and also for asthma which has been termed a nocturnal disease [22,51]. One cannot expect to understand fully the mechanisms of a disease that exhibits great day/night variability unless investigations are conducted during the night as well as during the day.

Chronobiological factors are equally important in the evaluation of medications such as in clinical drug trials. With reference to the contents of Table 13.1, there are several indications implicating the relevance of a chronotherapeutic approach for modulating drug toxicity and/or increasing efficiency. An additional indication for chronotherapy is when the goal of treatment is the resetting or correction of biological clocks and rhythms. Some steps have already been taken in optimizing the effects of several medications used in the treatment of chronic diseases, for example, theophylline [31,47,51] and non-steroidal anti-inflammatory [36,39,41], steroidal [17,28,44,45] and H_2-receptor antagonist drugs [48,49], to mention a few. Admittedly, chronotherapeutics has been researched primarily in terms of timing and scheduling of drug administration during 24 h. Although ultradian (short period) rhythms have received attention for the chronotherapy of infertility with analogues of gonadotropin-releasing hormone [88,89] and to a lesser extent circannual (one-year) rhythms for other illnesses [90,91], the potential for optimizing the effects of medications by taking into account bioperiodicities other than just the circadian one remains to be more fully explored. The importance of biological periodicities of, for example, 7 days, 1 month and 1 year, in addition to circadian ones, awaits further study. Future directives for medical chronobiologists include the study of biological time structure in paediatric [92] and geriatric [93] patients. Currently, the knowledge base for clinical chronobiology pertains mainly to college-aged persons. The challenge for medical chronobiologists of today and tomorrow will be to investigate how biological rhythms of various frequencies in all age groups affect procedures in clinical practice.

Results of chronobiological research demonstrate that disruption of circadian time-keeping is associated with certain forms of mental illness and with disturbances associated with sudden alteration of the sleep/wake schedule due to rotating shiftwork or rapid geographical displacement by air travel. Although early attempts to develop chronobiotics were unsuccessful, recent ones utilizing melatonin and bright light have proven positive. Findings of this nature are significant for several reasons. First, they support the concept that disease can arise from altered (desynchronized) biological rhythms; this represents a new perspective concerning the diagnosis and pathogenesis of illness. Second, the findings reveal that factors other than those conventionally considered in medicating patients, such as choice of drug and dose, are critical. The timing of drug administration, with reference to the staging of key biological rhythms and clocks, may constitute the difference between the success or failure of a therapeutic regimen. At the present time, the significance of an alteration in period (τ), phase (acrophase) and/or amplitude of circadian rhythms in relation to illness and its management is yet to be fully appreciated or evaluated [61,62]. This must await future study.

Scientists and industry alike are taking note of the new ideas and concepts of chronopharmacology. Acceptance of chronobiological methods by the pharmaceutical industry and medical scientists suggests a bright outlook for clinical chronobiology. The prospects for the future are enhanced also by the increasing number of investigators researching the field of medical chronobiology and the developing technology making applications feasible in clinical practice. The future for clinical chronobiology is bright and exciting. Medical chronobiologists world wide look forward to the realization of new applications arising from continuing research on biological rhythms and body clocks.

References

1. Reinberg, A., Sidi, E. and Ghata, J. Circadian rhythms of human skin to histamine or allergen and the adrenal cycle. *J. Allergy*, **36**, 273–283 (1965)
2. Lee, R.E., Smolensky, M.H., Leach, C. and McGovern, J.P. Circadian rhythms in the cutaneous sensitivity to histamine and selected antigens including phase relationship to urinary cortisol excretion. *Ann. Allergy*, **38**, 231–236 (1977)
3. McGovern, J.P., Smolensky, M.H. and Reinberg, A. Circadian and circamensual rhythmicity in cutaneous reactivity to histamine and allergenic extracts. In *Chronobiology in Allergy and Immunology* (eds J.P. McGovern, M.H. Smolensky and A. Reinberg), C.C. Thomas, Springfield, Il, pp. 117–138 (1977)
4. De Vries, G., Goei, J.T., Booy-Noord, H. and Orie, N.G. Changes during 24-hours in lung function and histamine hyperreactivity of the bronchial tree in asthmatic and bronchitic patients. *Int. Arch. Allergy*, **20**, 93–101 (1962)
5. Reinberg, A., Gervais, P., Morin, P. and Abulker, C. Rhythme circadien humain du seuil de la reponse bronchique a l'acetylcholine. *C.R. Acad. Sci.*, **272**, 1879–1881 (1971)
6. Gervais, P., Reinberg, A., Gervais, C., Smolensky, M. and De France, O. Twenty-four-hour rhythm in the bronchial hyperreactivity to house dust in asthmatics. *J. Allergy Clin. Immunol.*, **59**, 207–213 (1977)

7. Sly, P.D. and Landau, L.I. Diurnal variation in bronchial responsiveness in asthmatic children. *Pediatr. Pulmonol.*, **2**, 344–352 (1986)

8. Barnes, P.J., Fitzgerald, G.A. and Dollery, C.T. Circadian variation in adrenergic responses in asthmatic subjects. *Clin. Sci.*, **62**, 349–354 (1982)

9. Gaultier, C., Reinberg, A. and Motohashi, Y. Time of day dependent effectiveness of a β-agonist agent in asthmatic children gauged by changes of total pulmonary resistance (R). *Chronobiol. Int.*, **5**, 285–2980 (1988)

10. Gaultier, C., Reinberg, A., Gerbeaux, J. and Gerard, F. Circadian changes in lung resistance and dynamic compliance in healthy and asthmatic children. Effects of two bronchodilators. *Respir. Physiol.*, **31**, 169–182 (1975)

11. Brown, A., Smolensky, M.H., D'Alonzo, G.E., Frankoff, H., Gianotti, L. and Nilsestuen, J. Circadian chronesthesy of the airways of healthy adults to the β-agonist bronchodilator isoproterenol. *Annu. Rev. Chronopharmacol.*, **5**, 163–166 (1989)

12. Haus, E., Grazziela, Y., Lakatua, D. and Sackett-Lundeen, L. Reference values for chronopharmacology. *Annu. Rev. Chronopharmacol.*, **4**, 338–424 (1988)

13. Carandente, F. and Halberg, F. Chronobiology of blood pressure in 1985. *Chronobiologia*, **11**, 189–309 (1984)

14. Drayer, J.I.M., Weber, M.A. and Nakamura, D.K. Automated ambulatory blood pressure monitoring: a study in age-matched normotensive and hypertensive men. *Amer. Heart J.*, **109**, 1334–1338 (1985)

15. Drayer, J.I.M., Weber, M.A., De Young, J.L. and Brewer, D.D. Long-term blood pressure monitoring in the evaluation of antihypertensive therapy. *Arch. Int. Med.*, **143**, 898–901 (1983)

16. Smolensky, M.H., Tartar, S.E., Bergman, S.A., Losman, J.G., Barnard, C.N., Dacso, C.C. and Kraft, I.A. Circadian rhythmic aspects of cardiovascular function. A review by chronobiologic statistical methods. *Chronobiologia*, **3**, 337–371 (1977)

17. Reinberg, A., Smolensky, M.H., D'Alonzo, G.E. and McGovern, J.P. Chronobiology and asthma. III. Timing corticotherapy to biological rhythms to optimize treatment goals. *J. Asthma*, **25**, 219–248 (1988)

18. Harkness, J.A.L., Richter, M.B., Panayi, G.S., Van de Pette, K., Unger, A., Pownall, R. and Geddawi, M. Circadian variation in disease activity in rheumatoid arthritis. *Brit. Med. J.*, **284**, 551–554 (1982)

19. Kowanko, I.C., Knapp, M.S., Pownall, R. and Swannell, A.J. Domiciliary self-measurement in rheumatoid arthritis and the demonstration of circadian rhythmicity. *Ann. Rheum. Dis.*, **41**, 447–452 (1982)

20. Hetzel, M.R. and Clark, T.J.H. Comparison of normal and asthmatic circadian rhythms in peak expiratory flow rate. *Thorax*, **35**, 732–738 (1980)

21. Smolensky, M.H. and Halberg, F. Circadian rhythms in airways patency and lung volumes. In *Chronobiology in Allergy and Immunology* (eds J.P. McGovern, M.H. Smolensky and A. Reinberg), C.C. Thomas, Springfield, IL, pp. 117–138 (1977)

22. Smolensky, M.H., D'Alonzo, G.E., Kunkel, G. and Barnes, P.J. Day–night patterns in bronchial patency and dyspnea: basis for once-daily and unequally divided, twice daily theophylline schedules. *Chronobiol. Int.*, **4**, 303–317 (1987)

23. Labrecque, G. and Belanger, P. The chronopharmacology of the inflammatory process. *Annu. Rev. Chronopharmacol.*, **2**, 291–326 (1986)

24. Vener, K.J. and Moore, J.G. Chronobiologic properties of the alimentary canal affecting xenobiotic absorption. *Annu. Rev. Chronopharmacol.*, **4**, 259–282 (1988)

25. Smolensky, M.H. Aspects of human chronopathology. In *Biological Rhythms and Medicine* (eds A. Reinberg and M.H. Smolensky), Springer Verlag, New York, pp. 131–209 (1983)

26. Halberg, F., Tong, Y.L. and Johnson, E.A. Circadian system phase: an aspect of temporal morphology; procedure and illustrative examples. In *The Cellular Aspects of Biorhythms* (ed. H. von Mayersbach), Springer Verlag, Berlin, pp. 20–48 (1967)

27. Halberg, F., Johnson, E.A., Nelson, W., Runge, W. and Sothern, R. Autorhythmometry. Procedures for physiologic self-measurements and their analysis. *Physiol. Teacher*, **1**, 1–11 (1972)

28. Reinberg, A., Guillet, P., Gervais, P., Ghata, J., Vignaud, D. and Abulker, C. One-month

chronocorticotherapy (Dutimelan 8-15© mite). Control of the asthmatic condition without adrenal suppression and ciradian rhythm alteration. *Chronobiologia*, **4**, 295–312 (1977)

29. Bonini, S., Toccaceli, F., Dato, A. and Brostoff, J. The circadian assessment of peak expiratory flow as an additional tool for adequate treatment (and prevention) of bronchial asthma. In *Recent Advances in the Chronobiology of Allergy and Immunology* (eds M.H. Smolensky, A. Reinberg and J.P. McGovern), Pergamon Press, New York, pp. 33–40 (1980)

30. Turner-Warwick, M. Epidemiology of nocturnal asthma. *Amer. J. Med.*, **85**, (Suppl. 18), 6–8 (1988)

31. Dethlefsen, U. and Repges, R. Éin Neues Therapieprinzip bei nächtlichem Asthma. *Klin. Med.*, **80**, 44–47 (1985)

32. Gervais, P. Clinical chronobiology of asthma. Practical implications. In *Recent Advances in the Chronobiology of Allergy and Immunology* (eds M.H. Smolensky, A. Reinberg and J.P. McGovern), Pergamon Press, New York, pp. 15–24 (1980)

33. Randem, B., Smolensky, M.H., Hsi, B., Albright, D. and Burge, S. Field survey of circadian rhythm in PEF of electronics workers suffering from colophony-induced asthma. *Chronobiol. Int.*, **4**, 263–272 (1987)

34. Smolensky, M.H., Reinberg, A., Prevost, R.J., McGovern, J.P. and Gervais, P. The application of chronobiologic findings and methods to the epidemiological investigation of the health effects of air pollutants on sentinel patients. In *Recent Advances in the Chronobiology of Allergy and Immunology* (eds M.H. Smolensky, A. Reinberg and J.P. McGovern), Pergamon Press, New York, pp. 211–236 (1980)

35. Halberg, F., Reinberg, A. and Reinberg, A. Chronobiologic serial sections gauge circadian rhythm adjustments following transmeridian flight and life in a novel environment. *Waking and Sleeping*, **1**, 259–279 (1977)

36. Kowanko, I.C., Pownall, R., Knapp, M.S., Swannell, A.J. and Mahoney, P.G.C. Circadian variations in the signs and symptoms of rheumatoid arthritis and in the therapeutic effectiveness of flurbiprofen at different times of day. *Brit. J. Clin. Pharmacol.*, **11**, 477–484 (1981)

37. Folkard, S. Diurnal variation and individual differences in the perception of intractable pain. *J. Psychosom. Res.*, **20**, 289–301 (1976)

38. Reinberg, A., Gervais, P., Levi, F., Smolensky, M.H., Del Cerro, L. and Ugolini, C. Circadian and circannual rhythms of allergic rhinitis. A chronoepidemiologic study. *J. Allergy Clin. Immunol.*, **81**, 51–62 (1988)

39. Levi, F., LeLouarn, C. and Reinberg, A. Chronotherapy of osteoarthritis patients: optimization of indomethacin sustained release (ISR). *Annu. Rev. Chronopharmacol.*, **1**, 345–348 (1984)

40. Reinberg, A., Smolensky, M.H. and Labrecque, G. New aspects in chronopharmacology. *Annu. Rev. Chronopharmacol.*, **2**, 3–26 (1985)

41. Levi, F., LeLouarn, C. and Reinberg, A. Timing optimizes sustained release indomethacin treatment of osteoarthritis. *Clin. Pharmacol. Ther.*, **37**, 77–84 (1986)

42. Kuroiwa, A. Sympatomatology of variant angina. *Jpn. Circ. J.*, **42**, 459–476 (1978)

43. Marshall, J. Diurnal variation in the occurrence of strokes. *Stroke*, **8**, 230–231 (1977)

44. Harter, J.G., Reddy, W.J. and Thorn, G.W. Studies on an intermittent corticosteroid dosage regimen. *New Engl. J. Med.*, **296**, 591–595 (1963)

45. Reinberg, A., Touitou, Y., Bothol, M., Gervais, P., Gervais, A., Choauat, D., Levi, F. and Bicakova-Rocher, A. Oral morning dosing of corticosteroids in long-term treated cortico-dependent asthmatics: increased tolerance and preservation of the adrenocortical function. *Annu. Rev. Chronopharmacol.*, **5**, in press (1989)

46. Reinberg, A., Gervais, P., Ugolini, C., Del Cerro, L., Bicakova-Rocher and Nicolaï, A. A multicentric chronotherapeutic study of mequitazine in allergic rhinitis. *Annu. Rev. Chronopharmacol.*, **3**, 441–444 (1986)

47. Smolensky, M.H., D'Alonzo, G.E., Kunkel, G. and Barnes, P.J. (eds) Circadian rhythm-adapted theophylline schedules for asthma. *Chronobiol. Int.*, **4**, 301–466 (1987)

48. Humphries, T.J. and Berlin, R.G. The suppression of nocturnal secretion by H.S. famotidine therapy is sufficient to heal benign gastric ulcers. *Annu. Rev. Chronopharmacol.*, **5**, 291–294 (1989)

49. Simon, B., Dammann, H.G., Jakob, G., Miederer, S.E., Müller, P., Ottenjann, R., Paul, F., Scholtery, T., Schütz, E., Seifert, E. and Stadelmann, O. Famotidine versus ranitidine for the short-term treatment of duodenal ulcer. *Digestion*, **32** (Suppl. 1), 32–37 (1985)
50. Reinberg, A., Gervais, P., Chaursade, M., Fraboulet, G. and Duburque, B. Circadian changes in effectiveness of corticosteroids in eight patients with allergic asthma. *J. Allergy Clin. Immunol.*, **71**, 425–433 (1983)
51. McFadden, E.R., Jr. (ed.) Asthma: A nocturnal disease. *Amer. J. Med.*, **85** (Suppl. 1B), 1–70 (1988)
52. Lemmer, B. The chronopharmacology of cardiovascular medications. *Annu. Rev. Chronopharmacol.*, **2**, 199–228 (1986)
53. Smolensky, M.H. and D'Alonzo, G.E. Biologic rhythms and medicine. *Amer. J. Med.*, **85** (Suppl. 1B), 34–46 (1988)
54. Czeisler, C.A., Allan, J.S., Strogatz, S.H., Ronda, M.J., Sanchez, R., Ross, C.D., Freitag, W.O., Richardson, G.S. and Kronauer, R.E. Bright light resets the human circadian pacemaker independent of the timing of the sleep/wake cycle. *Science*, **233**, 667–670 (1986)
55. Reinberg, A. and Smolensky, M.H. *Biological Rhythms and Medicine*, Springer-Verlag, New York (1983)
56. Wever, R.A. *The Circadian System of Man*, Springer-Verlag, New York (1979)
57. Halberg, F. and Simpson, H. Circadian acrophase of 17-hydroxycorticosteroid excretion referenced to midsleep rather than midnight. *Hum. Biol.*, **39**, 405–413 (1967)
58. Reinberg, A. (ed.) Chronobiologic field studies of shiftworkers. *Chronobiologia*, **6** (Suppl. 1) (1979)
59. Halberg, F., Reinberg, Al. and Reinberg, Ag. Chronobiologic serial sections gauge circadian rhythm adjustments following transmeridian flight and life in novel environment. *Waking and Sleep*, **1**, 259–279 (1977)
60. Klein, K.E. and Wegmann, H.M. The effect of transmeridian and transequatorial air travel on psychological well-being and performance. In *Chronobiology: Principles and Applications to Shifts in Schedules* (eds L.E. Scheving and F. Halberg), Sijhoff and Nordhoff, The Netherlands, pp. 339–352 (1980)
61. von Zerssen, D. Circadian phenomena in depression: theoretical concepts and empirical findings. In *Trends in Chronobiology* (eds W.Th.J.M. Hekkens, G.A. Kerkhof and W.J. Rietveld), Pergamon Press, Oxford, pp. 357–366 (1988)
62. Wehr, T.A. Chronobiology of affective illness. In *Trends in Chronobiology* (eds W.Th.J.M. Hekkens, G.A. Kerkhof and W.J. Rietveld), Pergamon Press, Oxford, pp. 367–379 (1988)
63. Lewy, A.J. and Sack, R.L. Phase typing and bright light therapy of chronobiologic sleep and mood disorders. In *Chronobiology and Psychiatric Disorders* (ed. A. Halaris), Elsevier, New York, pp. 181–206 (1987)
64. Simpson, H.W., Bellamy, N., Bohlen, J. and Halberg, F. Double-blind trial of a possible chronobiotic: quiadon. *Int. J. Chronobiol.*, **1**, 287–311 (1973)
65. Armstrong, S.M., Cassone, V.M., Chesworth, M.J., Redman, J.R. and Short, R.V. Synchronization of mammalian circadian rhythms by melatonin. In *Melatonin in Humans. Proceedings of the First International Conference on Melatonin in Humans* (Vienna, Austria) (eds R.J. Wurtman and F. Waldhauser), *J. Neural Trans.*, (Suppl. 21), 375–396 (1986)
66. Arendt, J., Broadway, J., English, J.E., Kemp, M., Poulton, A.L. and Symons, A.M. Pineal and photoperiodicity: practical aspects. In *Trends in Chronobiology* (eds W.Th.J.M. Hekkens, G.A. Kerkhof and W.J. Rietveld), Pergamon Press, Oxford, pp. 137–148 (1988)
67. Broadway, J., Arendt, J. and Folkard, S. Bright light phase shifts the human melatonin rhythm during the Antarctic winter. *Neurosci. Lett.*, **79**, 185–189 (1987)
68. Ehret, C.F., Groh, K.H. and Meinert, J.C. Consideration of diet on alleviating jet lag. In *Chronobiology: Principles and Applications to Shifts in Schedules* (eds L.E. Scheving and F. Halberg), Sijthoff and Nordhoff, The Netherlands, pp. 393–402 (1980)
69. Ehret, C.F., Potter, V.R. and Dobra, K.W. Chronotypic action of theophylline and of pentobarbital as circadian zeitgebers in the rat. *Science*, **188**, 1212–1215 (1975)
70. Turek, F.W. and Losee-Olson, S. A benzodiazepine used in the treatment of insomnia phase-shifts the mammalian circadian clock. *Nature*, **321**, 167–168 (1986)

71. Armstrong, S.M. and Chesworth, M.J. Melatonin phase-shifts a mammalian circadian clock. *Abstracts of the Fourth Colloquium of the European Pineal Study Group* (Modena, Italy, 1987)
72. Reinberg, A., Smolensky, M.H. and Labrecque, G. The hunting of a wonder pill for resetting all biological clocks. *Annu. Rev. Chronopharmacol.*, **4**, 171–201 (1988)
73. Walsh, J.K., Muehlbach, M.J. and Sweitzer, P.K. Acute administration of triazolam for the daytime sleep of rotating shift workers. *Sleep*, **7**, 223–229 (1974)
74. Seidel, W.F., Roth, T., Roehrs, T., Zorick, F. and Dement, W.C. Treatment of a 12-hour shift of sleep schedule with benzodiazepines. *Science*, **224**, 1262–1274 (1984)
75. Daan, S. and Lewy, A.J. Scheduled exposure to day light. A potential strategy to reduce jet-lag following transmeridional flight. *Psychopharmacol. Bull.*, **20**, 566–568 (1984)
76. Kripke, D., Gillin, J.C., Mullaney, D.J., Risch, S.C. and Janowsky, D.S. Treatment of major depressive disorders by bright white light for 5 days. In *Chronobiology and Psychiatric Disorders* (ed. A. Hilaris), Elsevier, New York, pp. 207–218 (1987)
77. Lewy, A.J., Sack, R.L., Miller, L.S. and Hoban, T.M. Antidepressant and circadian phase-shifting effects of light. *Science*, **235**, 352–355 (1987)
78. Redman, J., Armstrong, S. and Ng, K.T. Free-running activity rhythms in the rat: entrainment by melatonin. *Science*, **219**, 1089–1091 (1983)
79. Mrosovsky, N. and Salmon, P.A. A behavioral method for accelerating re-entrainment of rhythms to new light–dark cycles. *Nature*, **330**, 372–373 (1987)
80. Sack, R.L. and Lewy, A.J. Melatonin advances circadian rhythms in humans. Abstract NR175, *141st Annual Meeting of the American Psychiatric Association* (Montreal, Canada, May, 1988), abstract NR175 (1988)
81. Arendt, J., Aldhous, M. and Wright, J. Synchronisation of a disturbed sleep–wake cycle in a blind man by melatonin treatment. *Lancet*, 772–773 (1988)
82. Arendt, J., Aldhous, M. and Marks, V. Alleviation of jet lag by melatonin: preliminary results of controlled double blind trial. *Brit. Med. J.*, **292**, 1170 (1986)
83. Arendt, J., Aldhous, M., English, J., Marks, V. and Arendt, J.H. Some effects of jet-lag and their alleviation by melatonin. *Ergonomics*, **30**, 1379–1393 (1987)
84. Lewy, A.J., Wehr, T.A., Goodwin, F.K., Newson, D.A. and Markey, S.P. Light suppresses melatonin secretion in humans. *Science*, **210**, 1267–1269 (1980)
85. Reinberg, A., Touitou, Y., Lévi, F. and Nicolai, A. Circadian and seasonal changes in ACTH-induced effects of healthy young men. *Eur. J. Clin. Pharmacol.*, **25**, 657–665 (1983)
86. Scheving, L.E., Halberg, F. and Ehert, C.F. (eds) *Chronobiotechnology and Chronobiological Engineering*, NATO ASI Series, Applied Sciences; No. 120; Martinus Nijhoff Publishers, Dordrecht (1987)
87. De Prins, J., Cornelissen, G. and Malbecq, W. Statistical procedures in chronobiology and chronopharmacology. *Annu. Rev. Chronopharmacol.*, **2**, 27–141 (1984)
88. Hoffman, A.R. and Crowley, W.F. Induction of puberty in men by long-term pulsatile administration of low-dose gonadotropin-releasing hormone. *New Engl. J. Med.*, **307**, 1237–1241 (1982)
89. Gompel, A., DePlunkett, T., Mandelbaum, J. and Mauvais-Jarvis, P. Induction of ovulation by a luteinizing hormone-releasing hormone pump. Principles, indications and results. *Press Med.*, **14**, 963–966 (1985)
90. Kolopp, M., Bicakova-Rocher, A., Reinberg, A., Drouin, P., Mejean, L., Levi, F. and Debry, G. Ultradian, circadian and circannual rhythms of blood glucose and injected insulins documented in six self-controlled adult diabetics. *Chronobiol. Int.*, **3**, 265–280 (1986)
91. Descorps-Déclère, A., Bonnafous, M., Reinberg, A. and Begon, C. Sex-related differences in diurnal and seasonal changes in effectiveness of pancuronium bromide in man. *Chronobiologia*, **10**, 121–122 (1983)
92. Reinberg, A., Smolensky, M.H., Labrecque, G. and Hallek, M. Aspects of chronopharmacology and chronotherapy in children. *Chronobiologia*, **14**, 303–325 (1987)
93. Smith, H.V. and Capobianco, S. (eds) *Aging and Biological Rhythms*, Plenum, London (1978)

Chapter 14

Analysis of biological time series

D.S. Minors and J.M. Waterhouse

The analysis of time series can be extremely complex as evidenced by the numerous texts devoted to the subject (see, for examples, [1–4]). Most of these texts are devoted to the analysis of time series derived from physical systems, such as in engineering, or economic series, where numerous cycles of a periodic phenomenon are frequently available with a high rate of equidistant sampling. With biological time series, particularly clinical data, we rarely meet all of these conditions – often infrequent non-equidistant sampling over one or a few samples is the norm. This considerably limits the analyses that can be performed with validity.

In the present text we will give what we hope is an easy-to-follow account of methods available for the detection and analysis of rhythms in biological systems. We will draw attention to the limitations and assumptions underlying each test and, wherever possible, will avoid mathematical symbols which often make the specialist text (for example, those cited above) unintelligible to the non-mathematician. In addition, we will exemplify the use of each test by analysing the data shown in Figure 14.1, which shows the rectal temperature, measured every 12 min, of a single subject living in a normal nychthermal environment over a period of 10 days.

Further reviews of the analysis of biological rhythms can be found [5,6].

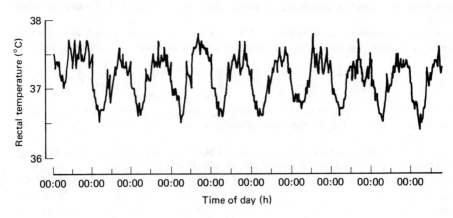

Figure 14.1 Rectal temperature measured every 12 min in a single subject over a 10-day span

Experimental design

Experiments are most frequently performed to test a particular null hypothesis and/ or estimate certain parameters, and statistics provide a means of testing the probability with which the null hypothesis can be rejected or of providing confidence limits for the parameters. (Note that statistical procedures provide a probability only – they do not tell one categorically whether a null hypothesis is correct or incorrect.) Implicit in this statement is that the experiment must be designed appropriately for the null hypothesis that is to be tested. In the case of the simple example where one is testing whether the efficacy of treatment A is better than that of treatment B, it is essential that the only variation is between treatments. Thus if different groups are used for the two treatments, they should be matched for age, sex, etc.

In chronobiological experiments a prime factor is time so that if, for example, circadian variation is sought, measurements across the day must be taken. If it is desired to know that any detected rhythm is a reflection of some internal oscillator rather than masking effects (Chapter 1), then the conditions at the different times of measurement should be identical. For example, if the peak plasma concentration of a drug is greater following ingestion of the drug during the middle of the day than at night, this might simply reflect changes in meal ingestion (and hence absorption rate of the drug) unless meals are specifically controlled. In other cases, the origin of the rhythms may be unimportant, and so control of environmental and behavioural rhythms is less important. For example, the rapid morning rise in blood pressure is associated with the processes of waking and becoming active. Nonetheless, this provides an indication of times at which care of those with cardiac disease might be more critical.

Whether or not it is desired to know the origin of any rhythm, an important feature of any chronobiological study is the frequency of sampling the variable under investigation, since this has consequences not only for assessing whether or not a rhythm is present and its parameters, but also for dealing with the statistical tests that can be performed.

Frequency of sampling

The minimum rate of sampling required for the detection of any rhythm is twice the frequency of that rhythm. In the case of a circadian rhythm, this would imply two measurements per 24 h. However, the hazards of such infrequent sampling should be evident; for example, at an extreme, no rhythm would be detected if the two times of measurement coincided with points where the rhythm crosses the mean value. Furthermore, even if a statistical difference between the two measurements can be shown, it would not indicate whether or not this is the maximum range of the oscillation nor would it enable an estimate of the true time of maximum or minimum of the rhythm to be made.

A further problem associated with a restriction in the frequency of sampling is that this considerably influences the result obtained. Consider, for example, the data shown in Figure 14.2. In Figure 14.2(a) are shown the plasma concentrations of cortisol measured at half-hourly intervals throughout a single 24-h period. If the measurements had been made at 4-hourly intervals only, Figure 14.2(b), the general shape of the rhythm (high morning values, low evening values) is still evident but the pulsatile nature of the secretion of this hormone would be missed.

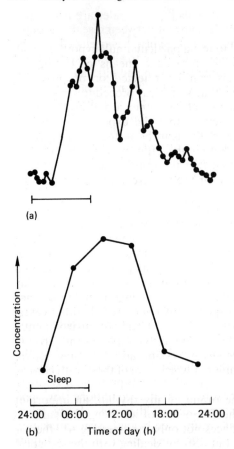

(a)

Concentration ——→

Sleep

| 24:00 | 06:00 | 12:00 | 18:00 | 24:00 |

(b)   Time of day (h)

Figure 14.2 Circadian rhythm of plasma cortisol. (a) Data plotted for half-hourly measurements. (b) Starting at 02:00 h, every 8th sample is plotted (corresponding to points if 4-hourly measurements only had been made). (After Krieger [7])

Thus, in general, a rhythm is more precisely defined the greater the frequency of sampling. However, if the sampling rate is too high, consecutive measurements are not independent and this can affect some statistical analyses. For example, if the cosinor analysis (see below) is used, although estimates of the rhythm parameters are still valid, confidence intervals for these parameters tend to be too liberal.

What is the minimum recommended sampling rate? The answer to this question often depends on the variable under investigation and the aims of the experiment. In general, if there is no prior information about the timing of the rhythm a minimum of six time points per cycle is recommended. If a high degree of characterization of the rhythm is required, more frequent sampling is advocated. If such a high rate of sampling is not possible throughout the whole cycle, perhaps due to subject intolerance or ethical considerations, then this might be resolved by more frequent measurements at a time when rapid fluctuations are expected and less frequent sampling at times when changes are smaller.

These general considerations apply also to the assessment of ultradian rhythms and, when hormone rhythms are considered, of pulses. In some aspects, however, the assessment of a pulse is slightly different. First, it is often required to know the number of secretory pulses that has occurred during a particular time interval. Algorithms exist for establishing the presence of such an event; they enable a transient rise in concentration of a hormone (a pulse) to be distinguished from random changes by the application of a set of rules [8]. The rules are necessarily arbitrary to some extent and so they will differ somewhat between research groups; as a result, some disagreement as to whether or not a pulse has occurred is to be expected. The second difference is that a pulse is unlikely to show a symmetrical concentration profile, in contrast to at least some circadian and ultradian rhythms. Thus, it is observed that often the rising phase is considerably more rapid than the declining one. This is hardly surprising since the rate of rise is a function of the secretion of the hormone (and can be very rapid), but the rate of decline is due to its metabolism. The implication of this is that the frequency of sampling that is required to define the time course of a pulse will require careful consideration.

Although a high frequency of sampling is required for detailed characterization of a rhythm, a rhythm can often be *detected* with a lower sampling rate. Indeed, several recent papers have been devoted to resolving how infrequent sampling and missing data affect the assessment of rhythm parameters (see, for example, [9–11] and Chapter 3).

Single subjects versus groups

In chronobiological studies it is always preferable to study a single subject longitudinally over time. Such a study avoids the problem of variability between subjects (see below) which can be a problem if different groups contribute to the measurements at different time points. However, the disadvantage of the longitudinal study is that the subject chosen may be unrepresentative of the population at large. Therefore, such studies should be repeated on several individuals and the mean rhythm parameters from all subjects presented. In doing so, however, care must be taken to ensure that the conditions for, and synchronization of, all subjects are identical, precautions that must also be taken when time points are derived from different groups (see below). Synchronization can be achieved by exposing the individuals to the same zeitgebers (see Chapter 1). Failure to achieve such synchrony will tend to broaden the timing of any peaks and troughs and reduce the amplitude of the mean rhythm. In a completely desynchronized population, the combined output could be arrhythmic in spite of the individual components showing marked rhythms. To check for synchrony it is often best to measure in each individual some marker rhythm, for example body temperature, which reflects the timing of the endogenous component of the circadian system.

A second problem with grouping data from several individuals is that the variable under consideration must show the same 24-h mean value and amplitude in the different individuals. In many cases, differences between individuals may be corrected for by 'standardizing' results from them. This often consists of expressing the results in terms of the percentage of the 24-h mean, which corrects for different mean values in the raw data. However, there is a statistical implication in doing this insofar as some tests should not be used with ratios (see under 'General methods of rhythm detection').

In spite of the desirability of studying a rhythm in a single subject, it is not always possible to make measurements at the desired frequency within a single cycle. For example, ethical or technical considerations may limit the samples taken to one or a few each day. In such a case measurements can be made at different time points on different cycles. Thus, for example, if 2-hourly time points are required but sampling within any one cycle is limited to four time points per cycle, then on the first day these samples could be taken at 00:00, 06:00, 12:00 and 18:00 h; on the second day at 02:00, 08:00, 14:00 and 20:00 h; and on the third at 04:00, 10:00, 16:00 and 22:00 h. The measurements can then be combined and represented as coming from a single cycle. Again, however, precautions must be taken to ensure that conditions are identical on the different days of measurement.

Occasionally it may be necessary to derive different time points from different groups of subjects. Indeed, there is an advantage to such a design insofar as random differences between individuals or between time points cancel each other out. However, care must be taken to ensure that the different individuals constituting the group are in synchrony with one another, otherwise the problems described above will arise. Again, such synchrony can be checked by measuring a marker rhythm in each individual.

Smoothing data

It must be remembered that when a variable is measured over time, one is not only measuring some rhythmic variation, but also biological noise – random fluctuations. If it is suspected that there is a considerable degree of such noise in the data, then some form of 'smoothing' should be performed. Often this takes the form of averaging adjacent time points. In the 'moving average' technique, 'weighted' or 'unweighted' means of different numbers of adjacent points may be taken. For example, an unweighted three-point moving average would require calculation of a value at time t_i which was the mean of values at times t_{i-1}, t_i and t_{i+1}. An unweighted five-point moving average would use values obtained at times t_{i-2}, t_{i-1}, t_i, t_{i+1} and t_{i+2}. When a 'weighted' three-point moving average is calculated, the central value of each set of three is weighted; a ratio 1:2:1 is common. With a five-point moving average, the weightings might be 1:2:3:2:1. Note that any moving average technique decreases the number of points, since the first and last times of the original data span cannot have moving averages calculated for them. Further, as the number of adjacent points that is averaged increases so too does the amount of smoothing; this is because the proportion of data that is being used for each assessment is increasing.

Smoothing the data in this way is not the same as decreasing the sampling frequency. Rather, smoothing the data gives an averaged result that better describes a general trend at the expense of fluctuations, whether these are caused by secretory pulses, ultradian oscillations or random fluctuations. By contrast, less frequent sampling of point data does not change the value that is measured at any time; what it changes is the confidence with which a peak or trough can be identified and the likelihood of missing such events.

Although a 'smoothing' technique can enable general trends to be distinguished from background noise and thus enable a more representative value of a variable at a particular time to be found, it can raise another potential problem. Under some circumstances it can introduce spurious periods into the data (and so can be disadvantageous if the period is being sought). A simple explanation of this is that the smoothing process has divided each result between adjacent time points. If, for example, two random fluctuations that both have high values are separated by some time interval, then the effect of using a five-point moving average is to distribute such high values over *two sets of five points* rather than the original pair; therefore, contrary to the original intention, smoothing in this case *accentuates* fluctuations in the raw data.

Detection of a rhythm and parameter estimation

The start of any rhythm analysis is to plot on rectangular coordinates values of the variable being measured at the different time points, as in Figure 14.1. Such a simple step is essential, for its gives some indication of the shape of the rhythm, an important point since some analyses (see under 'General methods of rhythm detection') assume a particular waveform. When a rhythm has been measured over several cycles in the same individual, the average waveform, termed the form estimate, can be calculated. The advantage of doing this is that it reduces random variation in the time series data (in effect, one has 'smoothed' data between cycles). This form estimate is calculated by averaging equivalent data points from successive cycles and can be best be visualized by constructing a Buys-Ballott table of the form shown in Table 14.1. Note that this method requires the period of the rhythm to be known (though see under 'Modern periodogram analysis' if it is unknown).

Table 14.1 Constructing a Buys-Ballot Table to derive the form estimate

Cycle no.	Time			
1	X_1	X_2	X_3	... X_P
2	X_{P+1}	X_{P+2}	X_{P+3}	... X_{2P}
3	X_{2P+1}	X_{2P+2}	X_{2P+3}	... X_{3P}
Last cycle	X_{N-P+1}	X_{N-P+2}	X_{N-P+3}	... X_N
Average	C_1	C_2	C_3	... C_P

The table is constructed for N data points (X_i) obtained at hourly intervals for a period P.

Though plotting the values of a variable against time is an essential step, it is usual to require some objective test to assess whether a rhythmic component is present in the data rather than any variation being due to random fluctuations. In the following sections we will describe the statistical tests that may be used to detect a rhythm and assess estimates of the rhythm parameters.

General methods of rhythm detection

A change in the value of a variable with time may, at its simplest, be detected by comparing means from two time points by Student's t test. Of course, such a comparison will require several measurements at each of the time points. If the same group of individuals is measured at each time point a paired test can be used; otherwise it should be unpaired.

There are many pitfalls with this technique, however. First, if the maximum and minimum values are chosen there is the danger that 'aberrant' values (outliers) have been used and no true rhythm exists. Second, this simple test will only give a probability of a difference existing at the two chosen time points – it takes no account of the whole time series. The Student's t test should not be used repeatedly to test for a difference between means at several time points. The reason for this is that if, for example, eight sets of measurements are made over a single cycle, there are 28 possible combinations of pairs of means; it can be calculated from the binomial distribution that, even if the means are drawn from the same population (and so not significantly different), on about three out of four occasions on which all these comparisons are made, one or more of the pairs will appear to be significantly different at the $P<0.05$ level.

If it is desired to test whether there is significant variation between several time points, the correct analysis is the analysis of variance (ANOVA). Usually the one-factor (time-of-day) ANOVA is used. This assesses whether the variation between time points is significantly greater than the random variation within them. The analysis requires several readings to be taken at each of a group of times within a cycle but the times of assessment do not have to be evenly spaced. The statistical tests are more likely to establish the presence of a time-of-day effect (that is, for a null hypothesis not to be accepted falsely) as the number of groups (time points) and number of values within each group increases. A powerful design is when the *same* individual is assessed at different times of day since the matched data are reducing interindividual variations.

As well as for tests for parametric data, ANOVA tests are available for non-parametric measurements (the Kruskal–Wallis and Friedman tests). The criteria for use of parametric or non-parametric statistical tests are those that are normally applied. It will be noted that data that have been 'standardized' by expressing them as a percentage of the 24-h mean (see under 'Single subjects versus groups') should, in the strictest sense, be assessed by non-parametric tests.

The strength of ANOVA methods is that the shape of the rhythm does not affect the statistical outcome. Furthermore, provided that the period is known *a priori*, data with any period can be analysed. In the case of the detection of a circadian rhythm where the period is not exactly 24 h, this will require sampling which, on real (24-h) time, is at equivalent points in each cycle of the rhythm. Thus if a 25-h period is assumed and one of the measurements is made at 06:00 h (real time) on the first cycle then on the second and third cycles equivalent points would occur at 07:00 and 08:00 h real time respectively.

The shortcoming of the ANOVA tests is that, even if they establish that rhythmicity exists, they do not give information as to its characteristics, for example, amplitude or phase. Furthermore, as implied above, this method cannot be used to detect the period of the rhythm when this is unknown.

Rhythm assessment when the period is known – cosinor analysis

Probably the most frequently used (and misused) method of rhythm analysis is the single cosinor analysis, described by Halberg *et al.* [12] and fully documented by Nelson *et al.* [13]. This method involves representing the data span by the best-fitting cosine function. The method assumes that the variable y_i can be represented by:

$$y_i = M + A\cos(\omega t_i + \phi) + e_i \qquad (14.1)$$

where y_i = value of the ith point in the data span, t_i = time when this point was measured, M = the mean level (termed mesor) of the cosine curve, A = the amplitude of the curve, ω = angular frequency of the curve = $2\pi/\tau$ (τ = period), ϕ = phase angle of the maximum value (termed acrophase) of the curve and e_i = residual error of the ith point, assumed to be independent random normal deviates with a mean value of zero when all time points are considered.

Equation 14.1 may be expressed in the linear form:

$$y_i = M + \beta x_i + \gamma z_i + e_i \qquad (14.2)$$

where $x_i = \cos\omega t_i$, $z_i = \sin\omega t_i$, $\beta = A\cos\phi$ and $\gamma = -A\sin\phi$.

When the period (and hence ω) is known or can be assumed, this equation is linear and the parameters β and γ can be estimated by conventional methods of linear least squares regression analysis, minimizing the residual sum of squares (RSS). This can be accomplished by solving the three least squares simultaneous equations:

$$\Sigma y_i = Mn + \beta\Sigma x_i + \gamma\Sigma z_i$$

$$\Sigma x_i y_i = M\Sigma x_i + \beta\Sigma x_i^2 + \gamma\Sigma x_i z_i$$

$$\Sigma z_i y_i = M\Sigma z_i + \beta\Sigma x_i z_i + \gamma\Sigma z_i^2$$

for the time points $i = 1 \ldots n$

These equations may be solved by calculating the following:

$$\Sigma x_i^2 - \frac{1}{n}(\Sigma x_i)^2 = P$$

$$\Sigma x_i z_i - \frac{1}{n}(\Sigma x_i)(\Sigma z_i) = Q$$

$$\Sigma z_i^2 - \frac{1}{n}(\Sigma z_i)^2 = R$$

$$\Sigma x_i y_i - \frac{1}{n}(\Sigma x_i)(\Sigma y_i) = S$$

$$\Sigma z_i y_i - \frac{1}{n}(\Sigma z_i)(\Sigma y_i) = T$$

If we let $D = PR - Q^2$

Then

$$\beta = \frac{RS - QT}{D} \; ; \gamma = \frac{PT - QS}{D}$$

and $M = (\Sigma y_i - \beta\Sigma x_i - \gamma\Sigma z_i)/n$

This is the corrected equation ↓

$$M = (\Sigma y_i - \beta \cdot \Sigma x_i - \gamma \cdot \Sigma z_i)/n$$

The computations can be greatly simplified if the measurements, y_i, are taken at equidistant times over an integral number of cycles. In this special case:

$$M = \frac{\Sigma y_i}{n} \; ; \beta = \frac{2}{n}\Sigma x_i y_i \text{ and } \gamma = \frac{2}{n}\Sigma z_i y_i$$

Having estimated β and γ, the amplitude (A) and acrophase (ϕ) may be derived:

$$A = (\beta^2 + \gamma^2)^{\frac{1}{2}} \tag{14.3}$$

$$\phi = K + s\,[\arctan(\gamma/\beta)] \tag{14.4}$$

where K and s depend on the sign of β and γ and may be derived from the following table:

Sign of β	Sign of γ	K	s
+	+	0	−1
+	−	−2π	+1
−	+	−π	+1
−	−	−π	−1

The significance of the fitted curve may then be tested against the null hypothesis that the amplitude, A, equals zero (this has been termed the zero amplitude test). To do this a variance ratio (F) statistic is used. The F ratio is computed from:

the total sum of squares about the mean (TSS) $= \Sigma(y_i - \bar{y})^2$

and the residual sum of squares (RSS) $= \Sigma[y_i - (M + \beta x_i + \gamma z_i)]^2$

The sum of squares due to the regression, that is, the amount of the total variability accounted for by the fitted curve $=$ TSS $-$ RSS. Then

$$F = \frac{(\text{TSS} - \text{RSS})2}{\text{RSS}(n - 3)} \tag{14.5}$$

This value can then be compared with tables of $F_{1-\alpha}$, that is the $(1 - \alpha)$ percentile of an F distribution, with $(2, n-3)$ degrees of freedom. A value for F greater than that derived from F tables allows the null hypothesis to be rejected at the chosen level of probability (α). In addition, this F-statistic can be used to calculate a confidence region for (β, γ) from which confidence limits for the amplitude and acrophase can be derived. Readers are referred to Nelson et al. [13] for the necessary calculations. Figure 14.3 shows the data plotted in Figure 14.1 with the best-fitting cosine curve with period of 24 h superimposed (this period was assumed since the subject was entrained to the solar day). The parameters for this curve are: mesor $= 37.16$; amplitude $= 0.34$; acrophase $= 17{:}12$ (clock time).

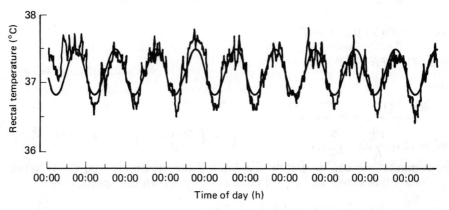

Figure 14.3 Data of Figure 14.1 shown with best-fitting cosine curve, derived from cosinor analysis, superimposed

The cosinor analysis is a very powerful technique since it can deal with irregular as well as regular sampling times. Further, as well as dealing with discrete point data (e.g. body temperature or plasma concentration of a substance), by integration of Equation 14.2 it can also deal with time-averaged data (e.g. urine samples) [14]. In addition to the single cosinor which deals with data from a single time series, cosinor methods that describe groups or a population of individuals over several cycles exist [13]. Thus, to calculate the rhythm parameters for a population, estimate of the regression coefficients β and γ are derived for each individual by the single cosinor method and the means $\bar{\beta}$ and $\bar{\gamma}$ are calculated.

From these means, by substitution in Equations 14.3 and 14.4 the population amplitude and acrophase can be determined.

Computer programs to perform the single cosinor analysis have been published [15] or can be obtained [16–17].

Because of its versatility, simplicity and availability of documentation, the cosinor analysis is the method that has been most frequently used to assess biological rhythms. However, the method does make several assumptions, often ignored by its users, so that it is also frequently misused. These assumptions are discussed below.

1. The cosinor involves fitting a cosine curve to the data and thus assumes that the time series is approximated by a cosine curve. Therefore, the method should always be used in conjunction with inspection of the raw data. Even if the raw data are only approximately a cosine curve the rhythm parameters derived by the analysis often provide objective assessments. However, if the raw data are far from cosinusoidal or the peak and trough not separated by half the period, the estimates of the rhythm parameters may be erroneous.

In this context it must be mentioned that the *F*-test described above (Equation 14.5), assesses whether the amplitude of the fitted cosine curve is significantly different from zero. In other words, the zero amplitude test gives a probability of the data being better described by a straight line than by a cosine curve. The test does not indicate that the data *are* cosinusoidal in shape. By analogy, the more familiar situation of fitting a regression line through a set of data investigates whether a straight line fits the data better than a circle and whether the slope of this line differs significantly from the vertical or horizontal. The demonstration that the coefficient of correlation between two variables is significantly different from zero does not mean that a straight line fits the data perfectly (unless $r = \pm 1$), nor does it necessarily mean that the basic assumption – of a linear relationship between the two variables throughout their ranges – is correct.

Even if a 'significant' fit of a cosine curve to the data span is obtained by cosinor analysis, it is often informative to assess how well the curve fits the data by a different method. One method is to assess the percentage of variability in the data that is accounted for by the fitted curve; this is the percentage rhythm. To calculate this, a direct comparison is made between the variability of the fitted curve about the mean (the sum of squares accounted for by the regression) and the total variability present (summed squared deviations about the mean – the total sum of squares). The percentage rhythm can be calculated as:

$$\text{Percentage rhythm} = 100 \times \left(\frac{\text{TSS} - \text{RSS}}{\text{TSS}} \right)$$

where TSS = total sum of squares about the mean, RSS = residual sum of square about the curve and thus TSS − RSS = sum of squares accounted for by the regression.

A perfect fit would give a value of 100% since RSS would equal zero. It is sometimes found that even though the cosine curve is 'significant', nevertheless it accounts for only a small percentage rhythm (say, under 30%). This kind of result is sometimes found if the data are 'noisy' and if large numbers of data points have been collected (particularly if there are serial correlations in the residuals – see below). By analogy, with sufficient data, correlation coefficients that are only slightly different from zero – and hence of little use in predicting values of Y from known values of X – are statistically significant. In all such cases, the biological, as opposed to statistical, value of the significance should be questioned.

If it is desired to investigate whether the cosine curve described the data span adequately (and here one is stressing the *shape* of the data), then this can be investigated by a statistical test such as the Sinusoidality Test [13]. However, if such a test indicates that the cosine curve is an inadequate description, the problem of then how best to describe the data remains. Several solutions have been suggested and will be discussed later (see under 'Some alterantives to the single cosinor').

2. Equation 14.2 is linear in its parameters (and hence the equation solved by a linear least squares regression) only if the period is known or can be assumed *a priori*. In the case of human circadian rhythms, if an individual is living in a normal environment exposed to all the zeitgebers associated with the solar day, it can usually be assumed that the period of the individual's rhythms will be 24 h. However, if the individual is denied such zeitgebers or is insensitive to them, no such assumption can be made. Under these circumstances the period of the rhythm should be determined by techniques such as those described under 'Assessing the period of a rhythm when it is unknown'. As will be described, these techniques often require data collected frequently and over a long period of time. If such data cannot be obtained for the variable under investigation, a marker rhythm, such as body temperature, which can be measured frequently, may be used to derive the rhythm's period. Once the period has been determined then this can be used in Equation 14.1 and the other rhythm parameters determined by cosinor analysis. An alternative method is to solve Equation 14.1 using a non-linear regression analysis using estimates of the period, mesor, amplitude and acrophase (for example, [18]).

3. In a linear regression analysis it is assumed that the residual errors are independent normally distributed deviations with zero mean and common variance. The normal distribution of the errors may be tested by the Kolmogorov–Smirnov test and the independence of successive errors tested for serial correlation by a test such as the Runs Test. In this respect it is to be noted that often the successive values of a biological variable are not independent, particularly if sampled at a high frequency. In view of this, methods have recently been developed that use autoregressive and moving average filtering (ARMA) of the data and so are not subject to this problem [19].

Although one may not be able to show the residuals are independent of one another or that they are normally distributed with zero mean, the estimates of rhythm parameters (mesor, amplitude and acrophase) are not ordinarily affected and are valid. However, the validity of the probability of rejecting the null hypothesis of zero amplitude must be questioned as must be the confidence regions for the rhythm parameters.

In summary, cosinor analysis is a versatile and, when used appropriately, powerful technique. In common with any other method, it must be used with due recognition of its limitations and the factors that can undermine the validity of its results. In practice, the experimenter will be advised to inspect his data visually before undertaking cosinor analysis to assure himself of its worth and the interpretation to be placed on the acrophase. These comments will apply also when interpretation of the changes to cosinor parameters is considered (below).

Assessing changes in rhythm parameters using cosinor analysis
When the cosinor analysis is used to assess the rhythm parameters of a single time series covering many cycles of a rhythm, it must be assumed that the data are

stationary, that is, there is no change in the rhythm parameters with time. Sometimes this assumption cannot be made. For example, in an individual following the start of night work or after a time-zone transition, the phase and/or amplitude of a rhythm will change [20]. In such a case the cosinor analysis can still be used as part of a serial section analysis [21]. In this, the times series is divided into small sections (for example, one day's data per section) and the cosinor analysis performed on each section. In this way changes in a rhythm's parameters may be followed. If the number of data points from any one section is small, data from several successive sections can be combined to get a greater likelihood of a statistically significant fit. The process can then be repeated by adding on one section's data at the end of the data span and taking off another section's at the beginning. For example, the first analysis could be performed on the data from days 1–3, the second on the data from days 2–4 and so on. It has the effect of averaging any day-to-day changes and this might enable a general trend to be assessed more easily. However, such averaging will also mean that there will be some difficulty in calculating the 'daily' rate of change of the rhythm if it is not constant, or the exact day when a particular amount of change has taken place.

As indicated above, the serial section analysis has frequently been used to assess the change in phase of circadian rhythms following a change in the sleep/wake schedule. However, a change in acrophase detected by this method may not be an accurate measure of the amount by which a rhythm's phase has shifted. The shift in acrophase will be an accurate measure of the shift in rhythms only if the shape of the data within each section is the same. Why should the rhythm change its shape? There are two common reasons.

The first is because the overt circadian rhythm is determined by the sum of exogenous and endogenous components (see Chapter 1) and the internal clock is slow to adjust to any change (Chapter 11). Therefore, after a shift or change of exogenous factors, there might be a temporary loss of the normal phase relationship between the two components. The other reason is very similar insofar as two components adjusting at different rates are involved, but it postulates that the two components are both due to internal clocks.

Another result that might arise with the serial section analysis is that there appears to be a gradual loss of rhythmicity with successive sections, perhaps shown by a decrease in the 'percentage rhythm' or even the null hypothesis of zero amplitude cannot be rejected. There is an interpretative problem for there might be several explanations for such a result. For example, following administration of a drug, a variable may be elevated (or decreased) to some maximum (minimum) value so that rhythmic changes can no longer be seen. Alternatively, a normal rhythm may be produced by variation about some tonic mean value and a drug may inhibit such variation.

Another situation where a decrease in rhythmicity may be erroneously concluded is that when data pooled from many individuals are used. For example, if the individuals become desynchronized from one another, perhaps because some experimental manipulation prevents the internal clock from being synchronized by zeitgebers, then the combined rhythm from all individuals will decrease in amplitude and may become statistically insignificant. In such a case, analysis of rhythms from each individual would show a rhythm of unchanged amplitude but the change in phase will be different between individuals.

The serial section analysis has also been used by some to detect the period of a rhythm. The method assumes that provided the true period of the rhythm is not too different from the period assumed in the cosinor analysis, then over a limited

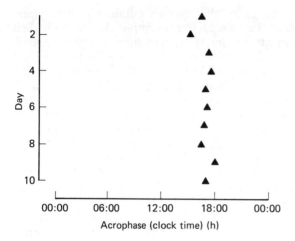

Figure 14.4 Serial section analysis. Cosinor analysis was performed on each successive day of the data of Figure 14.1. The figure shows the computed acrophase for successive days plotted from above, down

span of data (a cycle or so) the rhythm parameters calculated will not be too inaccurate. Thus, for example, to detect a near 24-h rhythm, a cosine curve with period of 24 h could be fitted to successive days' data. If the true period is not exactly 24 h then the calculated daily acrophase will become progressive later day-by-day (if the period is longer than 24 h) or earlier (if it is less than 24 h). A regression line through the daily acrophases will give the average shift per day and the deviation in the true period from an exact 24 h. Figure 14.4 shows the acrophase derived from fitting a 24 h cosine curve to successive days of the data shown in Figure 14.1. The consistency of the acrophase day-by-day confirms the 24-h period of the rhythm.

Some alternatives to the single cosinor

A major assumption of the cosinor analysis is that the data are approximately sinusoidal. Since the data may not conform to this shape there have been attempts to describe the data by other mathematical models.

One method that has been used by some, especially in assessing hormonal and body temperature rhythms, is to add various harmonics to the fundamental period given in Equation 14.1. Thus in the case of a description of circadian variation, Equation 14.1 has been expanded to contain not only the fundamental period of 24 h but also cosine terms with various harmonics of this, for example 12 h, 8 h and 6 h. However, such a procedure raises a general point with regard to the use of mathematical models in biological systems.

The question arises of how many harmonics should be added? Fourier's theorem (see under 'Spectral analysis') states that any waveform can be reproduced by an appropriate combination of cosine and sine terms. Thus, although the adding of harmonics will undoubtedly lead to a better description of the data, there is the difficulty of interpreting these in physiological, biochemical, etc. terms. In addition, a mathematical model that fits the data perfectly has also included the 'noise' term and so is not modelling the biological processes alone.

An alternative approach is to model the data mathematically by considering those biological factors likely to affect the variable under consideration. For example, in a recent paper [22] we have tried to model the mental performance of individuals leading irregular sleep/wake schedules in terms of: a trend throughout the experiment (T), the time of day (TOD) and the time since waking (TSW). Thus, performance, P, might be expressed by the equation:

$$P = C + f_1(T) + f_2(TOD) + f_3(TSW) + \text{error} \tag{14.6}$$

where C is a constant and f_1, f_2 and f_3 are mathematical functions. In general, the functions may have a linear, exponential or sinusoidal form. Biological theory might indicate the type of relationship to be expected. The solution of the equation is usually obtained by some iterative non-linear least squares technique (that is, the error term in Equation 14.6 is minimized by using different values of the functions). The advantage of this technique is that the time series has been modelled in terms of factors that are thought to affect it. However, there is the problem that other models, based on different premises, might fit the data equally well. In addition, it might not always be possible to assess that one particular set of parameters is, statistically, significantly better than another.

It has already been described how the cosinor method may be used to assess changes in a rhythm's phase. However, again the basic assumption of a sinusoidal rhythm must be made. As an alternative, the data before and after some experimental procedure may be cross-correlated after introducing various time lags into the premanipulation data until they match the postmanipulation data most closely. The time lag that yields the highest correlation is then used as the estimate of the phase shift produced [23]. The advantage of this technique is that it makes no assumption about the absolute shape of the data. Furthermore, if there is reason to believe that the data are influenced by two factors and that these responded differently to the experimental manipulation, the technique can be modified to describe the postmanipulation data in terms of two components phase-shifted independently [24,25]. Although the method was originally intended for data that had been equidistantly sampled [24], more recently we have used it for irregularly sampled data also [25].

Assessing the period of a rhythm when it is unknown

The methods described thus far have assumed that the period of the rhythm is known or can be assumed *a priori*. However, if individuals are denied exposure to zeitgebers (e.g. patients in intensive care units), have a weakened perception of zeitgebers (the blind), or are living on irregular sleep/wake schedules, no such assumption can be made. Furthermore, it is now recognized that there are certain diseases that seem to result in an abnormal circadian timing mechanism (e.g. periodic psychoses). In these circumstances, the period of the rhythm must be sought. (Having gained such knowledge, the other rhythm parameters – mesor, amplitude and phase – may be sought by the methods described in the previous section.)

The search for unknown periodicity involves more complex techniques than those described thus far. Furthermore, the requirements of the data format (frequency, regularity and duration of collection) are more rigorous. In the following sections we will outline the major methods that are used. It is to be noted from the outset that all these methods require data that are equidistantly sampled and, in general, they are of use only if several (at least four) cycles of the periodicity being sought are available.

Autocorrelation

This method estimates the correlation between observations made at different intervals. In practice, this involves the correlation of the time series with a duplicate of itself after the introduction of various time lags. Thus, if a time series is periodic then a high autocorrelation will be obtained as the lag approaches the period of the rhythm. A plot of the correlation coefficient against the lag is called the correlogram. A correlogram derived from the data shown in Figure 14.1 is shown in Figure 14.5.

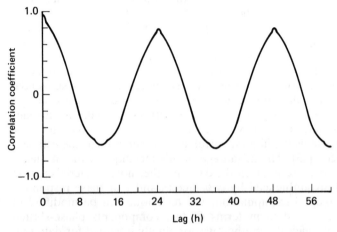

Figure 14.5 Correlogram of the data shown in Figure 14.1. The autocorrelation coefficient is plotted against lag; lags were incremented by 12 min (corresponding to interval between successive data points)

To calculate the autocorrelation coefficients consider a time series in which a variable x is measured at hourly intervals over N hours. Thus we have a time series $x_1, \ldots x_N$ with measurements being taken at times $t_1, \ldots t_N$. For a lag of $1\,h$ the coefficient of correlation (r_1) is calculated between the $N-1$ pairs, (x_1, x_2), (x_2, x_3), $\ldots (x_{N-1}, x_N)$ using normal equations for calculation of the Pearson product–moment correlation coefficient, that is:

$$r_1 = \frac{\sum_{t=1}^{N-1} (x_t - \bar{x}_{(1)})(x_{t+1} - \bar{x}_{(2)})}{\left(\sum_{t=1}^{N-1} (x_t - \bar{x}_{(1)})^2 \sum_{t=1}^{N-1} (x_{t+1} - \bar{x}_{(2)})^2 \right)^{1/2}}$$

where $\bar{x}_{(1)} = \sum_{t=1}^{N-1} x_t/(N-1)$

and $\bar{x}_{(2)} = \sum_{t=2}^{N} x_t/(N-1)$

The calculation can then be repeated introducing lags in hourly increments. In general terms then for a lag of k hours:

$$r_k = \frac{\sum_{t=1}^{N-k} (x_t - \bar{x}_{(1)}) (x_{t+k} - \bar{x}_{(2)})}{\left(\sum_{t=1}^{N-k} (x_t - \bar{x}_{(1)})^2 \sum_{t=1}^{N-k} (x_{t+k} - \bar{x}_{(2)})^2 \right)^{1/2}} \qquad (14.7)$$

Since $\bar{x}_{(1)} \simeq \bar{x}_{(2)} \simeq \bar{x}$, if N is large, then Equation 14.7 can be simplified to:

$$r_k = \frac{\sum_{t=1}^{N-k} (x_t - \bar{x})(x_{t+k} - \bar{x})}{\sum_{t=1}^{N} (x_t - \bar{x})^2}$$

It is to be noted that this method requires equidistantly sampled data. Furthermore, the method will detect multiples of the fundamental period. Thus if a period of, say, 25 h is present in the data, a high correlation will be obtained not only at a lag of 25 h but also at 50 h, 75 h etc. This can be seen in Figure 14.5 where not only is a peak seen at the expected period of 24 h, but also at 48 h. Further limitations of the method are that the data should be stationary; for example, there should be no trend in the data (other than the periodicity being sought), that is, the amplitude, mesor and period must remain constant throughout the time series, and at least four cycles of the period being sought should be available (thus lags greater than $N/4$ should not be attempted).

Spectral analysis

Spectral analysis is essentially a modification of Fourier analysis and is based upon approximating a function by a sum of sine and cosine terms, called the Fourier series representation. In fact any waveform can be represented by a Fourier series. For a full description of the methods readers are referred to Priestley [4].

In spectral analysis, sometimes also called harmonic analysis, a time series is represented by cosine and sine terms which have a period equal to the length of the time series plus all harmonics of this.

For example, with 240 hourly data points the periods that may be investigated are:

$$\frac{240}{1}, \frac{240}{2}, \frac{240}{3}, \frac{240}{4}, \frac{240}{5}, \ldots \frac{240}{120} \text{ h}$$

In general, then, for N data points sampled at intervals of k hours, the periods that can be assessed are:

$$\frac{Nk}{1}, \frac{Nk}{2}, \frac{Nk}{3}, \frac{Nk}{4}, \frac{Nk}{5}, \ldots \frac{Nk}{N/2} \text{ h}$$

The last term is equal to $2k$. This indicates that the longer the period to be detected the longer the duration of time measurements must be taken, whereas the smaller the period to be detected, the more frequently must observations be made.

A measurement x_t at time, t, ($t = 1k, 2k, 3k, \ldots Nk$) is then represented as the sum of these harmonic components. Namely

$$x_t = M + \sum_{p=1}^{N/2} [a_p\cos (\omega_p t) + b_p\sin (\omega_p t)] \tag{14.8}$$

where $M = \bar{x}$, $\omega_p = 2\pi p/N$, $a_p = 2/N [\Sigma x_t\cos (\omega_p t)]$ and $b_p = 2/N [\Sigma x_t\sin (\omega_p t)]$ (where $p = 1, 2 \ldots N/2$).

(Strictly this equation is correct only if N is even. If N is odd, a modified equation must be used; alternatively the first or last data point can be dropped from the time series.) It will be noted that the coefficients a_p and b_p are similar to β and γ (Equation 14.2) for the cosinor analysis (indeed it will be noticed that the calculation of β and γ for the special case of equidistant data is identical to above).

The overall effect of harmonic analysis of the data is to partition the variability of the time series into components at periods Nk, $Nk/2$, $Nk/3$, $\ldots$ $2k$. The contribution of the p harmonic component is then represented by its amplitude (A_p) where:

$$A_p = (a_p^2 + b_p^2)^{1/2}$$

A graphical presentation of amplitude versus the period of each harmonic component is termed the periodogram [26] or power spectrum. (In fact, most authors represent the ordinate as the amplitude squared or some variant of this.) Peaks in this plot are taken to represent the periodic components present in the data. The statistical significance of any period can be assessed by using the data in a cosinor analysis with this period and then performing the zero amplitude test (page 280, Equation 14.5). Figure 14.6 shows the periodogram for the data of Figure 14.1; a peak at a period of 24 h is evident.

The major limitation of this method is that only periods that are integral divisors of the series length can be resolved. Thus, in the above example where 240 hourly data points are available, the nearest the periods approaching circadian values are:

$$\frac{240}{8} = 30 \text{ h}; \frac{240}{9} = 26.67 \text{ h}; \frac{240}{10} = 24 \text{ h}; \frac{240}{11} = 21.82 \text{ h and} \frac{240}{12} = 20 \text{ h}$$

To be able to include more periodic components in the circadian range would require a much longer time series. For example, to be able to include components with periods of 24 and 25 h would require 25 days of hourly data. In general, a distinction between periods of length X and Y requires hourly data covering a span $(XY)/(X - Y)$ h. Because of this limitation, Van Cauter [27,28] has suggested varying the length of the time series by omitting data points from the beginning or end of the series. In this way, a range of circadian periods can be obtained. However, the exact effect of using different amounts of data for the analyses is not known.

Finally it should be noted that this analysis gives information about the periodic components present in the data, not necessarily the apparent period of the overt rhythm. For example, consider data containing periodic components with periods of 6 and 8 h with identical phases (say zero). The 6-h component will give peaks

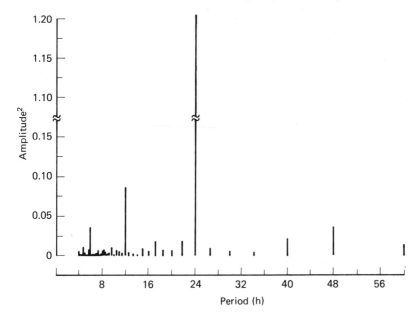

Figure 14.6 Spectral analysis of the data shown in Figure 14.1. The 'power' of each spectral component is shown as the amplitude squared

in the data at 0, 6, 12, 18, 24, etc. and the 8-h component yields peaks at 0, 8, 16, 24, 32 etc. h. Note that both produce peaks at 0 and 24 h so that when they are present simultaneously a period of 24 h will be evident in the data, even though this will not be detected by spectral analysis (which will detect the 6- and 8-h periodic components only).

Modern periodogram analysis

As described above, a periodogram is a plot of period against some measure of the intensity or power of the periodic component. In the previous section, the power was estimated from the amplitudes of the Fourier series. Modern periodogram analyses use a different method of estimating the power of each period component. Most are based upon the method first described by Whittaker and Robinson [29] which is summarized in the following.

Consider a time series which is made up solely of a periodic component with period, P (that is there is a pure rhythm with no residual errors). Then if this time series is divided into sections having length P, all sections will be identical to each other and to the average of all the sections. However, if a section length not equal to P is chosen, the sections will differ from one another and from their average. Thus, differences between sections and their average can be used to indicate whether the section length represents a true period in the entire time series.

The method involves drawing the data up in the form of a Buys-Ballot table (Table 14.1) and deriving the form estimate, as previously described, for different trial periods, P. The mean and standard deviation of each column in the table is then calculated. As the trial period approaches the true period of any periodic component in the data, the sections become more synchronous and so the standard deviation of the column means will increase. It will be a maximum when the trial and true periods are identical. In the method of Whittaker and Robinson [29], the power of each periodic component is derived by expressing the standard deviation of the column means as a proportion of the standard deviation of the entire series. Others [30,31] have used slightly different methods to estimate the power of each period. The method most frequently used is that of Dorrescheidt and Beck [32] in which the power of each period, $q(p)$, is estimated as:

$$q(p) = \frac{n \times \text{between-column sum of squares}}{\text{total sum of squares}}$$

where n is the number of rows in the Buys-Ballot table. Thus, considering a time series x_t, consisting of N data points taken at hourly intervals, for a trial period of p hours, the data can be drawn up into a Buys-Ballot table consisting of p columns and n rows where n is the integer part of N/p. The power, $q(p)$, of this period is then estimated as:

$$q(p) = \frac{n \sum_{i=1}^{p} (C_i - \bar{x})^2}{\sum_{j=1}^{np} (x_j - \bar{x})^2}$$

where C_i is the mean of the ith column (Table 14.1) and $\bar{x}$ is the mean of all data points.

Figure 14.7 shows this value for several trial periods using the data shown in Figure 14.1. Again, a clear peak is seen at a period of 24 h (though, as with the correlogram, a peak at the integer multiple of this – 48 h – is seen also).

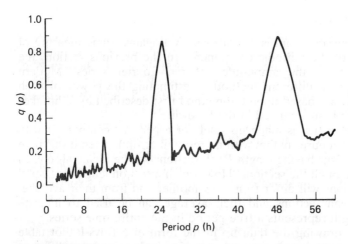

Figure 14.7 Whittaker periodogram analysis of the data shown in Figure 14.1. Since the data were measured at 12 min intervals, periods incremented by 12 min are shown. $q(p)$ is the 'power' of each period

The advantage of the method of Dorrescheidt and Beck is that the statistical significance of any period can then be assessed. For this a variance ratio, F, is calculated in which:

$$F = \frac{\text{variance between columns}}{\text{within-column variance}}$$

This variance ratio is then compared with F tables for $p-1$ and $np-p$ degrees of freedom. Note this method is the same as that described by Dorrescheidt and Beck [32], though the degrees of freedom have been corrected as suggested by Harris and Morgan [33].

Note also with this technique that the length of the data series must be adjusted to be a multiple of the period being sought by omitting data from the end of the time series, if necessary. The effects of using different amounts of the entire time series upon the assessment of the best fitting period is not known. However, for this reason, at least four cycles of the period being sought should be available.

Like the autocorrelation and spectral analyses, this analysis requires equidistant data and cannot be used with irregularly sampled or time-averaged (e.g. urinary) data. However, it is able to give better resolution of the period than spectral analysis. Periods can be assessed with a resolution equal to the frequency of measurement. For example, with data measured at hourly intervals, the modern periodogram analysis will allow the presence of periods incremented by 1-h steps to be assessed.

Concluding remarks

It is obvious from the above that the detection of an unknown period imposes many more constraints on the data span. Thus, in general, the determination of period frequently requires equidistantly sampled data over many cycles. By contrast, if the period is known or can be assumed, the detection of a rhythm (by ANOVA) is simple. Characterization of the rhythm (its phase, amplitude, etc.) is often more difficult. If the data approximate to a sine curve, then the cosinor analysis can be used but otherwise an alternative model must be used. The problem is to decide which model and even when a model is chosen, how can one be sure that it is the correct model? It is to be noted that estimates of the period of a rhythm, its time of peak and amplitude that are based upon data that have not been collected in accord with the principles discussed above appear all too frequently in the scientific literature. In such cases, the results seldom justify the confidence placed in them by those who have performed the study, and they can even be misleading. It is for these reasons that a description of the raw data will remain an important part of rhythm analysis. Thus, for example, even though it may not be possible to quantify (model) the rhythm mathematically, it may be sufficient to show that the form of the rhythm is reproducible in many individuals or may be changed in a reproducible way with some (fixed) experimental manipulation.

References

1. Anderson, T.W. *The Statistical Analysis of Time Series*, Wiley, New York (1971)

2. Box, G.E.P. and Jenkins, G.M. *Time Series Analysis, Forecasting and Control*, Holden-Day, San Francisco (1976)
3. Chatfield, C. *The Analysis of Time Series: An Introduction*, 3rd edn, Chapman and Hall, London (1984)
4. Priestley, M.B. *Spectral Analysis and Time Series*, Academic Press, London (1981)
5. De Prins, J., Cornelissen, G. and Malbecq, W. Statistical procedures in chronobiology and chronopharmacology. *Annu. Rev. Chronopharmacol.*, **2**, 27–142 (1986)
6. Minors, D.S. and Waterhouse, J.M. Mathematical and statistical analysis of circadian rhythms. *Psychoneuroendocrinology*, **13**, 443–464 (1988)
7. Krieger, D.T. Rhythms in CRF, ACTH and corticosteroids. In *Endocrine Rhythms* (ed. D.T. Krieger), Raven Press, New York, pp. 123–124 (1979)
8. Veldhuis, J.D. and Johnson, M.L. Cluster analysis: a simple, versatile and robust algorithm for endocrine pulse detection. *Amer. J. Physiol.*, **250**, E486–493 (1986)
9. Monk, T.H. Parameters of the circadian temperature rhythm using sparse and irregular sampling. *Psychophysiology*, **24**, 236–240 (1987)
10. Monk, T.H. and Fookson, J.E. Circadian temperature rhythm power spectra: is equal sampling necessary? *Psychophysiology*, **23**, 472–479 (1986)
11. Motohashi, Y., Reinberg, A., Nougier, J., Bourdeleau, P., Benoit, O., Foret, J. and Levi, F. A circadian marker rhythm for shift workers: the axillary temperature. Method for data gathering and analysis. *Ergonomics*, **30**, 1235–1247 (1987)
12. Halberg, F., Johnson, E.A., Nelson, W., Runge, W. and Sothern, R.B. Autorhythmometry – Procedures for physiologic self-measurements and their analysis. *Physiol. Teacher*, **1**, 1–11 (1972)
13. Nelson, W., Tong, Y.L., Lee, J-K. and Halberg, F. Methods for cosinor-rhythmometry. *Chronobiologia*, **6**, 305–323 (1979)
14. Fort, A. and Mills, J.N. Fitting sine curves to 24 h urinary data. *Nature (London)*, **226**, 657–658 (1970)
15. Monk, T.M. and Fort, A. 'Cosina': A cosine curve fitting program suitable for small computers. *Int. J. Chronobiol.*, **8**, 193–224 (1983)
16. Vocak, M. A comprehensive system of cosinor treatment programs written for the Apple II microcomputer. *Chronobiol. Int.*, **1**, 87–92 (1984)
17. Hsi, B.P. Rhythmometry analysis on personal computers for applications to chronopharmacology studies. *Annu. Rev. Chronopharmacol.*, **1**, 181–182 (1984)
18. Marquardt, D.W. An algorithm for least square estimation of nonlinear parameters. *J. Soc. Indust. Appl. Math.*, **11**, 431–441 (1965)
19. Greenhouse, J.B., Kass, R.E. and Tsay, R.S. Fitting nonlinear models with ARMA errors to biological rhythm data. *Stat. Med.*, **6**, 167–183 (1987)
20. Minors, D.S. and Waterhouse, J.M. *Circadian Rhythms and the Human*, Wright, Bristol (1981)
21. Arbogast, B., Lubanovic, W., Halberg, F., Cornelissen, G. and Bingham, C. Chronobiologic serial sections of several orders. *Chronobiologia*, **10**, 59–68 (1983)
22. Minors, D.S., Nicholson, A.N., Spencer, M.B., Stone, B.M. and Waterhouse, J.M. Irregularity of rest and activity: studies on circadian rhythmicity in man. *J. Physiol.*, **381**, 279–295 (1986)
23. Mills, J.N., Minors, D.S. and Waterhouse, J.M. Adaptation to abrupt time shifts of the oscillator(s) controlling human circadian rhythms. *J. Physiol.*, **285**, 455–470 (1978)
24. Minors, D.S. and Waterhouse, J.M. The use of constant routines in unmasking the endogenous components of human circadian rhythms. *Chronobiol. Int.*, **1**, 205–216 (1984)
25. Minors, D.S. and Waterhouse, J.M. Effects upon circadian rhythmicity of an alteration to the sleep–wake cycle: problems of assessment resulting from measurement in the presence of sleep and analysis in terms of a single shifted component. *J. Biol. Rhythms*, **3**, 23–40 (1988)
26. Schuster, A. On the investigation of hidden periodicities with application to a supposed 26-day period of meteorological phenomena. *Terr. Magn. Atmos. Elect.*, **3**, 3–41 (1898)
27. Van Cauter, E. Methods for the analysis of multifrequential biological time series. *J. Interdiscipl. Cycle Res.*, **5**, 131–148 (1974)
28. Van Cauter, E. and Huyberechts, S. Problems in the statistical analysis of biologic time series: the cosinor test and the periodogram. *J. Interdiscipl. Cycle Res.*, **4**, 41–57 (1973)
29. Whittaker, E.T. and Robinson, G. *The Calculus of Observations*, Blackie, London (1964)

30. Enright, J.T. The search for rhythmicity in biological time series. *J. Theor. Biol.*, **8**, 426–468 (1965)
31. Williams, J.A. and Naylor, E. A procedure for the assessment of significance of rhythmicity in time series data. *Int. J. Chronobiol.*, **5**, 435–444 (1978)
32. Dorrescheidt, G.T. and Beck, L. Advanced methods for evaluating characteristic parameters (α, ρ,τ) of circadian rhythms. *J. Math. Biol.*, **12**, 107–121 (1975)
33. Harris, G.J. and Morgan, E. Estimates of significance in periodogram analysis of damped oscillations in biological time series. *Behav. Anal. Lett.*, **3**, 221–230 (1983)

Index